NURSING PHOTOBOOK™

Ensuring Intensive Care

NURSING84 BOOKS™
SPRINGHOUSE CORPORATION
SPRINGHOUSE, PENNSYLVANIA

NURSING84 BOOKS™

NURSING PHOTOBOOK™ SERIES
Providing Respiratory Care
Managing I.V. Therapy
Dealing with Emergencies
Giving Medications
Assessing Your Patients
Using Monitors
Providing Early Mobility
Giving Cardiac Care
Performing GI Procedures
Implementing Urologic Procedures
Controlling Infection
Ensuring Intensive Care
Coping with Neurologic Disorders
Caring for Surgical Patients
Working with Orthopedic Patients
Nursing Pediatric Patients
Helping Geriatric Patients
Attending Ob/Gyn Patients
Aiding Ambulatory Patients
Carrying Out Special Procedures

NEW NURSING SKILLBOOK™ SERIES
Giving Emergency Care Competently
Monitoring Fluid and Electrolytes Precisely
Assessing Vital Functions Accurately
Coping with Neurologic Problems Proficiently
Reading EKGs Correctly
Combatting Cardiovascular Diseases Skillfully

NURSE'S REFERENCE LIBRARY®
Diseases
Diagnostics
Drugs
Assessment
Procedures
Definitions
Practices

NURSING NOW™
Shock
Hypertension

NURSE'S CLINICAL LIBRARY™
Cardiovascular Disorders
Respiratory Disorders

Nursing84 **DRUG HANDBOOK™**

NURSING PHOTOBOOK™ Series

PUBLISHER
Eugene W. Jackson

EDITORIAL DIRECTOR
Jean Robinson

CLINICAL DIRECTOR
Barbara McVan, RN

ART DIRECTOR
Lisa A. Gilde

**Springhouse Corporation
Book Division**

DIRECTOR
Timothy B. King

DIRECTOR, RESEARCH
Elizabeth O'Brien

VICE-PRESIDENT, PRODUCTION AND
PURCHASING
Bacil Guiley

Staff for this volume

BOOK EDITOR
Katherine W. Carey

CLINICAL EDITOR
Kathleen Soneki Waring, RN

ASSOCIATE EDITOR
Patricia K. Lawson

PHOTOGRAPHER
Paul A. Cohen

ASSOCIATE DESIGNERS
Linda Jovinelly Franklin
Scott M. Stephens
Carol Stickles

DESIGN ASSISTANT
Darcy Moore Feralio

ASSISTANT PHOTOGRAPHER
Thomas Staudenmayer

EDITORIAL/GRAPHIC COORDINATOR
Doreen K. Stowers

CLINICAL/GRAPHIC COORDINATOR
Evelyn M. James

COPY EDITOR
Sharyl D. Wolf

EDITORIAL STAFF ASSISTANT
Cynthia A. O'Connell

PHOTOGRAPHY ASSISTANT
Frank Margeson

ART PRODUCTION MANAGER
Robert Perry

ARTISTS
Diane Fox   Joan Walsh
Robert H. Renn   Robert Walsh
Sandra Simms   Ron Yablon
Louise Stamper

TYPOGRAPHY MANAGER
David C. Kosten

TYPOGRAPHY ASSISTANTS
Janice Auch Haber
Nancy Boesch
Ethel Halle
Diane Paluba

PRODUCTION MANAGERS
Wilbur D. Davidson
Robert L. Dean, Jr.

PRODUCTION ASSISTANT
Donald G. Knauss

ILLUSTRATORS
Larry Cetlin   Polly Krumbhaar Lewis
Jack Freas   Pat Macht
Jean Gardner   John Murphy
Tom Herbert   Ron Yablon
Bob Jackson   Bud Yingling

SERIES GRAPHIC DESIGNER
John C. Isely

COVER PHOTO
Seymour Mednick

**Clinical consultants
for this volume**

Cathy Gozensky, RN
Director of Education
L.W. Blake Memorial Hospital
Bradenton, Fla.

Joanne M. Seasholtz RN, MSN, CCRN
Cardiovascular Clinical Nurse Specialist
North Hills Passavant Hospital
Pittsburgh

Amended reprint, 1984
© 1981 by Springhouse Corporation,
1111 Bethlehem Pike, Springhouse, PA 19477
All rights reserved. Reproduction in
whole or part by any means
whatsoever without written permission
of the publisher is prohibited by law.
Printed in the United States of America.

PB-031283

Library of Congress Cataloging in Publication Data

Main entry under title:

Ensuring intensive care.

  (Nursing Photobook)
  "Nursing81 books"
  Bibliography: p.
  Includes index.
  1. Intensive care nursing. I. Springhouse
Corporation II. Series.
RT120.I5E57   610.73'61   81-6995
ISBN 0-916730-37-9   AACR2

Contents

Introduction

Understanding intensive care

CONTRIBUTORS TO
THIS SECTION INCLUDE:
June L. Stark, RN
Valerie Hunt, RN, MS

8 Total patient care

Caring for the respiratory patient

CONTRIBUTORS TO
THIS SECTION INCLUDE:
Virginia Barrett, RN

18 Respiratory basics
28 Airway management
43 Respiratory support

Caring for the cardiovascular patient

CONTRIBUTORS TO
THIS SECTION INCLUDE:
Cathy Gozensky, RN
Sue Mead, RN
Julia Ann Purcell, RN, MN

60 Cardiovascular basics
72 Cardiac monitoring
84 Hemodynamic monitoring
100 Cardiovascular emergencies

Caring for the gastrointestinal patient

CONTRIBUTORS TO
THIS SECTION INCLUDE:
Majorie L. Beck, RN

108 Gastrointestinal basics
114 Tube care
124 Total parenteral nutrition

Caring for the neurologic patient

CONTRIBUTORS TO
THIS SECTION INCLUDE:
Linda Dexter, RN, BSN
Karen March, RN

128 Neurologic basics
137 Special procedures

Managing special ICU challenges

CONTRIBUTORS TO
THIS SECTION INCLUDE:
June L. Stark, RN
Valerie Hunt, RN, MS

142 Fluids and electrolytes
149 Common problems
154 Stress management

155 Acknowledgements
156 Selected references
158 Index

Contributors

At the time of original publication, these contributors held the following positions.

Virginia Barrett is an inservice team leader at Abington (Pa.) Memorial Hospital. A graduate of Hahnemann Hospital School of Nursing in Philadelphia, she is working toward a BSN degree at LaSalle College, Philadelphia. Ms. Barrett is a member of the American Association of Critical-Care Nurses.

Marjorie L. Beck is a charge nurse on Abington (Pa.) Memorial Hospital's gastrointestinal procedure unit. A member of the American Nurses' Association and the Society of Gastrointestinal Assistants, Ms. Beck graduated from Abington (Pa.) Memorial Hospital School of Nursing.

Linda Dexter is a head nurse on the neurological unit at the Hospital of the University of Pennsylvania in Philadelphia. She has associate and BSN degrees from Gwynedd-Mercy College in Gwynedd Valley, Pennsylvania.

Cathy Gozensky, an advisor for this PHOTOBOOK, is director of education at L.W. Blake Memorial Hospital in Bradenton, Florida. She is a graduate of St. Joseph Hospital School of Nursing, Reading, Pennsylvania and a member of the American Association of Critical-Care Nurses and the American Heart Association. She is an editor for *Critical Care Nurse* and president of Health Education Associates, St. Petersburg, Florida. Trained in coronary care studies by H.J.L. Marriott, she has lectured on critical care throughout the United States.

Valerie Hunt is assistant director of staff education at Brigham and Women's Hospital in Boston. She graduated from Boston College School of Nursing with a BS degree and earned an MS degree in psychiatric nursing at the Medical College of Virginia, in Richmond.

Karen March is a staff nurse on the surgical intensive care unit at the Hospital of the University of Pennsylvania in Philadelphia. She earned her nursing diploma at the Hospital of the University of Pennsylvania and is a member of the American Association of Neurosurgical Nurses and the American Association of Critical-Care Nurses.

Sue Mead is a supervisor of the Cardiovascular Data Bank and a coronary care unit staff nurse at Atlanta's Emory University Hospital. She earned her associate degree in nursing at Alfred (N.Y.) State College and is enrolled in a Bachelor of Independent Studies degree program at the University of South Florida in Tampa.

Julia Ann Purcell is a cardiology clinical nurse specialist at Emory University Hospital in Atlanta. She earned her BSN degree at the University of South Carolina in Columbia and her MN degree at Emory University. Ms. Purcell is a member of the American Heart Association and Sigma Theta Tau.

Joanne M. Seasholtz, an advisor for this PHOTOBOOK, is a cardiovascular clinical nurse specialist at North Hills Passavant Hospital in Pittsburgh. She has a BSN degree from Widener College in Chester, Pennsylvania and an MSN degree from Philadelphia's University of Pennsylvania. Ms. Seasholtz is a member of the American Association of Critical-Care Nurses and Sigma Theta Tau.

June L. Stark is a critical care instructor and renal nurse consultant at Boston's Tufts-New England Medical Center Hospital. She has a nursing diploma from Jackson Memorial Hospital School of Nursing in Miami and a BSN degree from Salem (Mass.) State College. She is a member of the American Association of Critical-Care Nurses.

Introduction

If you had to pick one word to describe intensive care nursing, which would you choose: demanding, exhilarating, frustrating, rewarding? Chances are, you'd have a hard time deciding on just one. Instead, you might respond like this: *"All of those words describe my job. Intensive care nursing just can't be characterized so easily."*

And no wonder. In the intensive care unit (ICU), you care for patients with a wide variety of physical problems. Each is critically ill—yet each may require distinctly different care.

This PHOTOBOOK will help you meet this challenge. First, we'll tell you how to minimize the inevitable emotional stress for your patient and his family. Then, we'll focus on nursing care according to body systems: respiratory, cardiovascular, gastrointestinal (GI), and neurologic. For each system, we'll show you how to do a thorough assessment, which provides an indispensable baseline for ongoing care. Next, we'll explain the procedures and equipment you'll rely on to manage each patient's particular problem.

For example, when you care for a respiratory patient, you'll need to know about airway management. We've provided information on all types of artificial airways. For the patient who needs improved oxygenation and ventilation, we'll show you how to use oxygen delivery systems, how to administer positive end-expiratory pressure, and how to cope with ventilator problems. You'll also learn how to care for a chest tube drainage system.

Suppose your patient has a cardiovascular problem. Can you initiate continuous monitoring? Run a 12-lead EKG? Manage invasive and noninvasive hemodynamic monitoring systems? Respond confidently to a code for cardiac arrest? Use the cardiovascular section to sharpen your skills.

For the GI patient, you need to know how to manage nasogastric and gastric intubation, and what to do if your patient begins to hemorrhage from his GI tract. In addition, we'll spell out the basics of total parenteral nutrition, a potential lifesaver for a patient with impaired GI function.

Does your patient suffer from a lesion, injury, or disease affecting his brain? Learn how to routinely assess his condition with a thorough neurocheck. We'll also give you pointers on caring for a patient with increased intracranial pressure, and show you how to use a hypothermia blanket.

Of course, some ICU problems are common to all the patients you treat. That's why, in the last section, we discuss maintaining fluid and electrolyte balances, preventing infection, avoiding safety hazards, and minimizing the ill effects of long-term immobility.

Now, how about you? Could you use some help dealing with the pace and intensity of ICU nursing? If so, consider the suggestions we've provided for avoiding emotional burnout, another ever-present hazard for ICU nurses.

Yes, intensive care nursing can be demanding and, at times, frustrating. But it can also be exhilarating and uniquely rewarding. You'll find this PHOTOBOOK to be an invaluable aid to complete, satisfying ICU nursing.

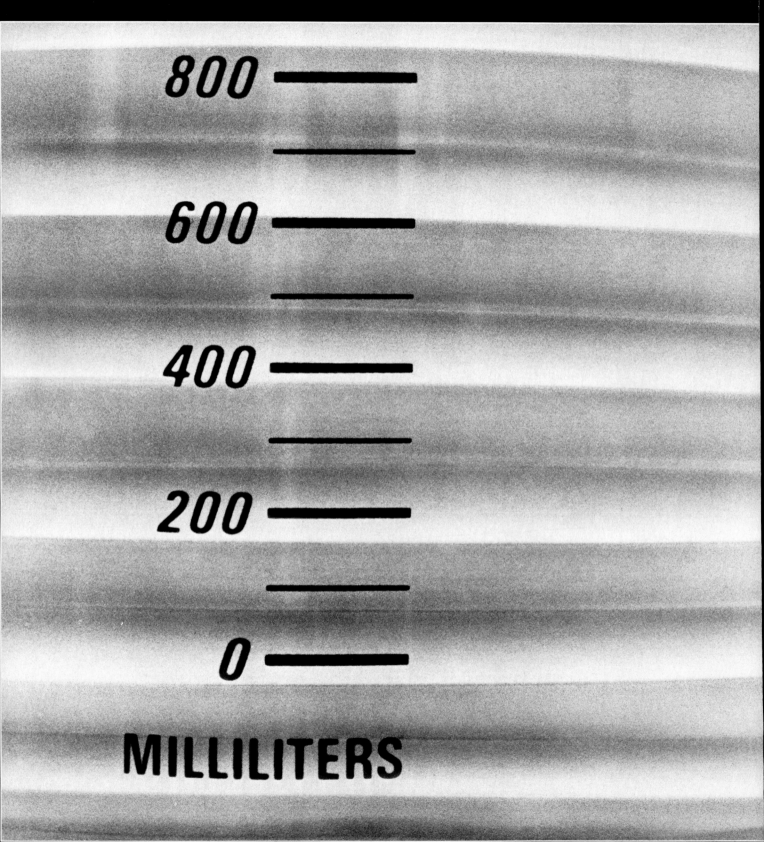

Understanding Intensive Care

Total patient care

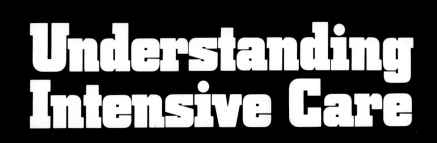

Total patient care

Total patient care. As an intensive care nurse, what does this nursing concept mean to you?

Of course, it means providing the best nursing care possible. But total patient care goes beyond that.

Consider your patient's emotional needs. Can you help him cope with his loss of control and changed body image? Have you thought about protecting him from the constant bombardment of noise, lights, and health-care procedures?

Then stop and consider the patient's family. They need your help, too. They're suffering from the stress and emotional turmoil caused by their loved one's serious condition. *Remember:* The family's emotional state will affect your patient. So, by helping the family, you're helping your patient, too.

Providing total patient care is a challenge. In the following pages, you'll see how to meet it.

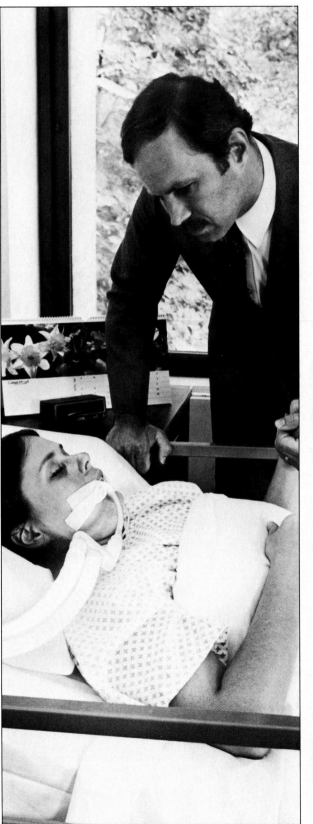

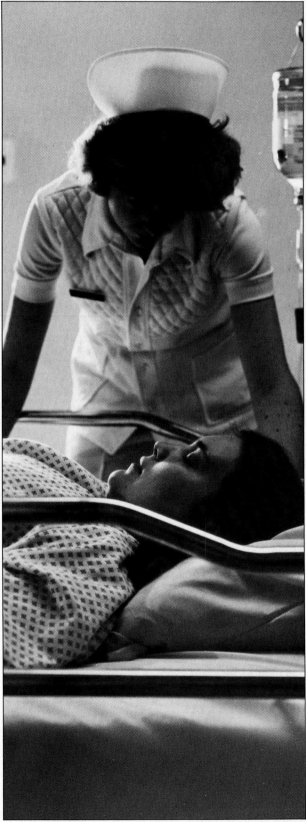

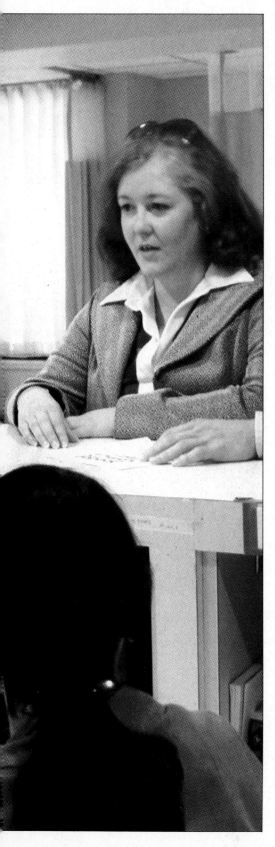

Intensive care:
A special nursing challenge

What makes intensive care so special? Stop and think about it. Is it the highly sophisticated and complex equipment? Perhaps knowing that a patient's life depends on your quick and accurate judgment makes intensive care unique. But, one thing's for sure. Before you can begin to learn about intensive care nursing, you have to understand the special challenges and problems it presents.

In intensive care, your patient's condition is too serious to be managed in a conventional hospital setting. He needs close observation and constant monitoring with special medical equipment. You must have special training to care for him.

Consider vital signs and hemodynamics, for example. In intensive care, every detail matters. You have to note the quality, duration, and pattern of those signs. Then ask yourself how these signs relate to one another. After you've gathered this information, your nursing knowledge and experience will help you decide what your patient needs. In intensive care, these decisions often must be made during a crisis, when every second counts.

Now let's look at your patient. The intensive care unit poses some special problems for him. He may be on a ventilator and unable to talk. His senses are overloaded by all the activity and frightening equipment. He may be worried about how he'll pay his medical expenses. Or, maybe he's worried about how his family is managing at home while he's hospitalized. And what if he dies? How will his family adjust?

Nowhere is the nurse-patient relationship more intimate than in the intensive care unit. Here, your patient depends totally on you. You're the one who maintains his life-support equipment. You administer his medications. You participate in critical decisions regarding his life. When his sensory patterns are altered, he depends on you to help him cope with his environment.

Then, consider the patient's family. Intensive care nursing extends to them, too. Engulfed by the flurry of medical procedures, they feel helpless. In some ways, the family is more emotionally strained than the patient. Occasionally, they may feel guilty or responsible for contributing to their loved one's hospitalization. In the face of all their concerns, they can only wait endlessly for a few minutes every hour to visit him.

While you're giving your all to your patient and his family, do you stop to consider yourself? You too, have special needs in the stressful atmosphere of an intensive care unit. You're more susceptible to professional burnout than you would be in a less hectic unit. Much of your energy may go into finding ways of coping with the tension. And remember, your co-workers are undergoing the same stresses that you are. (We'll tell you how to combat burnout in Section 6.)

In short, you need boundless energy and unfailing dedication to be an intensive care nurse. That's why being an intensive care nurse is so special.

Explaining the intensive care unit to your patient

Your patient's critically ill. He's anxious and afraid. To complicate matters, he may not be able to talk, so he can't ask questions about his condition or what's happening to him. In short, your patient's experiencing severe stress. What can you do to help put him more at ease?

To begin, explain your patient's immediate environment. Tell him about each piece of equipment and how it's helping him. But avoid using medical terminology. This will only confuse and frighten him. Instead, use simple, understandable terms. For example, show him the electrodes on his chest and explain that these monitor his heart rhythm. Also, explain any other equipment in use, such as a ventilator, oxygen mask, or arterial line.

Prepare him for any alarms he may hear. Explain that the alarm sounds as a warning, indicating a change in his condition or that the equipment needs to be checked. It does not necessarily mean he's in danger.

Then, tell him about some of the restrictions in the intensive care unit. Explain your hospital's policy on visiting hours. For example, if your patient understands his family may visit again in another hour, he won't be so upset when they must leave. However, before you make promises, determine if the family is planning to stay.

Be sure to include these guidelines, too, if they apply to your hospital:
• Tell your patient that he must remain in bed. If he's not permitted to use the bathroom or bathe himself, explain why.
• Explain that televisions, radios, and electric hair dryers and razors are not permitted because they may interfere with the unit's electrical equipment.
• Check your hospital's policy regarding gifts of flowers, food, or candy, and inform your patient. He may receive greeting cards. (Remember to open and read them to him if he can't.)
• Provide a list of personal items your patient may keep by his bedside.

Total patient care

Understanding your patient's emotional stress

You've probably seen it a hundred times. A patient is admitted on Monday. He's understandably anxious and upset because he knows he's seriously ill. But he's alert and doesn't fight your attempts to treat him. By Wednesday morning, he's sullen and withdrawn. He doesn't want to talk and responds belligerently when you question him. You recognize his behavior, but do you know what to do about it?

No doubt a serious illness will affect your patient psychologically. But you don't need to stand by passively. Before you can begin to help, you need to understand how your patient's being stressed. To do so, review these psychological concepts:

Self-image: How has your patient's self-image been changed? Does he feel inadequate and helpless? Perhaps he feels he's not quite the same person he was before his illness because he can't perform the same activities. He probably fears his illness means giving up most of the things he enjoys. He may dread having to change his life-style, or maybe he believes everyone expects him to be irritable. Exactly how your patient responds depends on his personality, social and economic status, education, age, and prior experiences, and what he's been told about his condition. Also, his relationship with his family and his confidence in the medical personnel caring for him will influence how he perceives himself during the illness and how much stress he experiences.

Body image: How has your patient's body image been altered? Has he been disfigured or scarred? Has his body been invaded with tubes, monitors, and intravenous lines? With his physical appearance altered, he may become anxious and defensive. Because of his illness, he's suddenly confronted with his own mortality. Sometimes a patient may react by denying his illness or speaking of it in a joking, carefree manner. He may also react with tremulousness, excessive perspiration, restlessness, and rapid speech.

Loss: Has your patient experienced a loss of identity, individuality, and independence? No doubt he's lost the ability to function as he would like. He's isolated from most of his family and friends. He's unable to care for his own body. To resolve this loss, he must have time to grieve.

Control: Does your patient feel he's lost control over his life? You need only look at him for the answer. He's tied to monitors and tubes. He can't wear his own clothes. His diet is selected for him, if he's permitted to eat at all. At any moment, a doctor or nurse may appear to perform another uncomfortable procedure. This lack of control over his own life diminishes his self-esteem.

When you recognize your patient's stress, you can help minimize some of it. But, you'll need his confidence and cooperation. Try to establish a trustful, caring relationship. Encourage him to relax as much as possible. Then, follow these guidelines to help lessen your patient's emotional stress:
• Be optimistic without being unrealistic. Emphasize your patient's progress, no matter how small.
• Restore some feeling of control to your patient. Whenever possible, let him make a decision. Avoid restraining him, if possible.
• Explain what's going on. Never assume your patient's not interested. Keeping him informed is one way of showing your respect for him. As a result, his self-image will improve.
• Take care to address your patient by name. Doing so will help him feel more like an individual and restore his identity.
• Personalize your patient's surroundings as much as possible. Display some of his personal possessions, such as family photographs, where he can easily see them. (For more information on adapting the intensive care environment, see the following page.)
• Provide adequate rest periods for your patient. If he's well rested, he'll be better equipped to cope with stress.
• If appropriate, remind your patient that he'll eventually be able to resume his normal life-style.

Combating sensory imbalance

Imagine what happens to your patient's senses when he's admitted to the intensive care unit. On one hand, his senses are overloaded with strange and frightening sounds and sights. On the other hand, he's deprived of his normal routine and habitat. He's isolated and immobile. He may not be able to talk. He has few diversions. Consequently, he can only reflect on himself and his condition.

Before you can help him cope, review these phenomena that contribute to his sensory imbalance:

Sensory overload: Your patient's subjected to many high-intensity stimuli that he doesn't understand and can't control or change. For example, he's constantly prodded, turned, and checked. He hears strange sounds from the cardiac monitor, ventilator, and oxygen valves. His sense of touch is restricted.

Sensory distortion: Your patient's sense of the sequence and timing of sights, sounds, and sensations is altered.

Sensory deprivation: Your patient becomes disoriented when he loses contact with the outside world. For example, he may lose track of the day or time from the continuous activity and lights in the unit. His eyeglasses or hearing aid may be taken from him, adding to his confusion about what's going on around him.

When you know that your patient's suffering from sensory imbalance, what can you do to help? Your most important task is to restore a balance between too much sensory stimulation and not enough. Here are some guidelines:
• Orient your patient to reality. Frequently tell your patient where he is, why he's there, and what day it is. To help, place a clock and calendar where he can see them. Speak calmly and reassuringly. Touch him gently to let him know you're there. But avoid startling him.
• Before you perform any nursing procedures, explain to your patient what you're about to do. By doing so, you'll avoid frightening him.
• Avoid conversations just outside his room or cubicle. Even if you're not talking about him, he may think you are and become confused or suspicious.
• If your hospital's policy permits, be flexible about visiting hours. Your patient's contact with his family has been severely limited. A few extra minutes may help him immensely.
• Adapt his environment. Place a few familiar objects where he can see them. Dim the lights. Draw the curtains, if appropriate, so he can sleep. (For more information on helping the patient adapt to his environment, see the following page.)
• Allow your patient to follow his normal routine as much as possible. For example, bathe him in the evening, if that's the time he prefers.
• Make him as comfortable as possible. Do what you can to reduce any painful or annoying stimuli. Adjust his pillow. Change his gown. Retape a bothersome indwelling (Foley) catheter.

Adapting your patient's environment

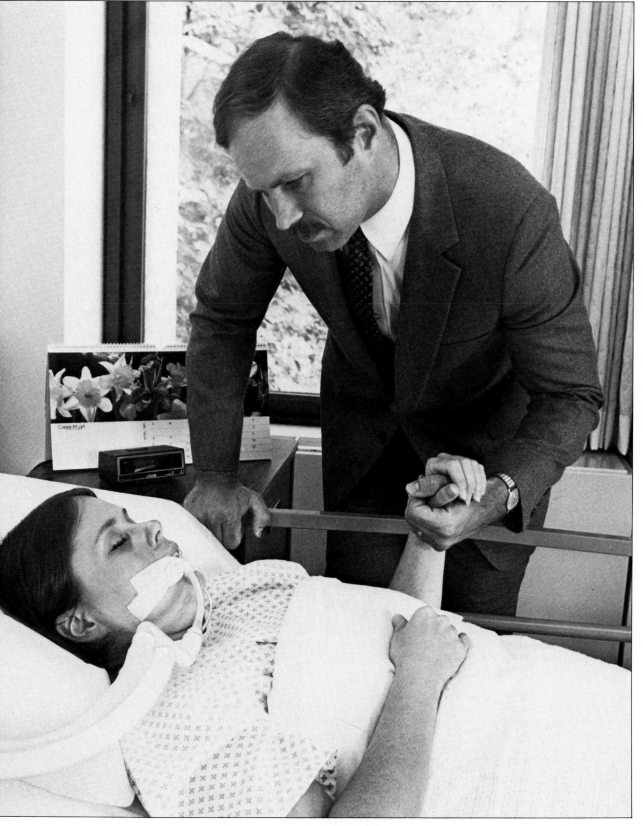

You're already familiar with the problems that may affect your patient in the intensive care unit and know what to do about many of them. But what can you do to help make his immediate environment less stressful and still maintain the unit's efficient functioning? Follow these guidelines.
• Respect the patient's privacy whenever possible.
• Provide the patient's eyeglasses and hearing aid, if appropriate.
• Ask the family to bring a few of the patient's small personal items.
• Ask the family to visit and talk to the patient frequently, even if he's unconscious or unable to talk.
• Display a clock and calendar where the patient can see them.
• Minimize the noise level throughout the unit at all times.
• Keep noisy equipment away from the patient's head. Explain any equipment sounds your patient may hear.
• If possible, position the patient's bed so he can look out the window.

Total patient care

Sleep in the ICU: The impossible dream

Sleep. Most of us take it for granted. But to the patient in the intensive care unit, deep, restful sleep may seem an unattainable feat. At times, he may wonder if the unit's staff hasn't conspired to keep him from getting the rest he desperately needs. What can you do to help him? To begin, let's review the basics of normal sleep.

A normal sleep cycle, which lasts 90 to 120 minutes, has two states: rapid eye movement (REM) sleep and non-REM (NREM) sleep. When a person falls asleep, he progresses through four stages of NREM sleep, each deeper than the last (see graph below). These four stages are characterized by muscle relaxation and drops in vital signs and metabolic activity. After reaching the fourth and deepest stage, the sleeper reverses the process and returns to stage two.

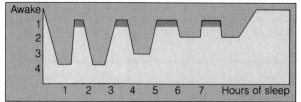

Next, the sleeper begins REM sleep, sometimes called paradoxical sleep because of the sudden increase in physiologic activity. (On the graph, REM sleep periods are shaded black.) In addition to the rapid eye movements that give it its name, REM sleep is characterized by rises in cardiac output, oxygen consumption, body temperature, and blood pressure. Respiratory rate fluctuates, and blood flow to the brain may double. Muscles become tense and immobile, except for intermittent twitching.

REM sleep is also distinguished by its dream activity. Although dreams may occur during any stage of sleep, they're most vivid--and frequently bizarre--during REM sleep.

After the REM stage, the sleeper returns to stage two and begins the cycle again. During an uninterrupted night's sleep, he experiences five or six sleep cycles. Toward morning, he spends more time in the REM stage of each cycle.

Research suggests that the deep sleep of stage four and the vivid dreaming of REM sleep are essential for mental stability. Consider what this means for your patient. In the ICU, his sleep cycle may be repeatedly disrupted by nursing measures, bright lights, and excessive background noise. Once awakened, he can't pick up the sleep cycle where he left it. Instead, he must begin the cycle again, from stage one. As a result, he may never get the sleep he needs.

Prolonged sleep deprivation depletes the patient's vital healing energy and jeopardizes his recovery. Eventually, the patient may exhibit some signs of ICU syndrome (see page 13). The longer the patient remains in intensive care, the more serious the outcome of sleep deprivation.

What can you do to help your patient? Review the following information to learn the signs and symptoms of sleep deprivation and some nursing interventions that may help prevent or correct it.

Sleep deprivation

Possible causes
- sensory disturbances including sensory deprivation, distortion, and overload
- continued sleep interruption
- excessive anxiety
- depression
- pain.

Signs and symptoms
- combativeness and noncompliance with treatment
- slurred, disordered speech, mumbling
- delusions, paranoia, excessive fear or anxiety, mood changes, depression, hallucinations, or nightmares
- loss of accurate time awareness, disorientation to persons or location, alteration in thought processes, diplopia
- mild to moderate motor impairment
- restlessness or hyperactivity.

Nursing interventions
- Schedule nursing care to permit uninterrupted periods of sleep. Try to have these sleep periods coincide with the patient's normal sleep pattern.
- Minimize background noise. Move equipment away from patient's head. Eliminate unnecessary conversation while patient's sleeping.
- Dim lights during specified sleep periods to reestablish diurnal rhythms.
- Provide reassurance and support. Encourage contact with family.
- Provide physical relaxation with backrubs, if possible, and medication, if ordered.
- Provide tactile stimulation by gently touching the patient's hand or shoulder.

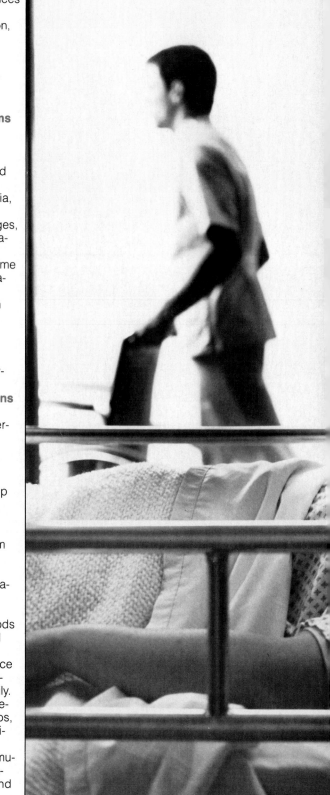

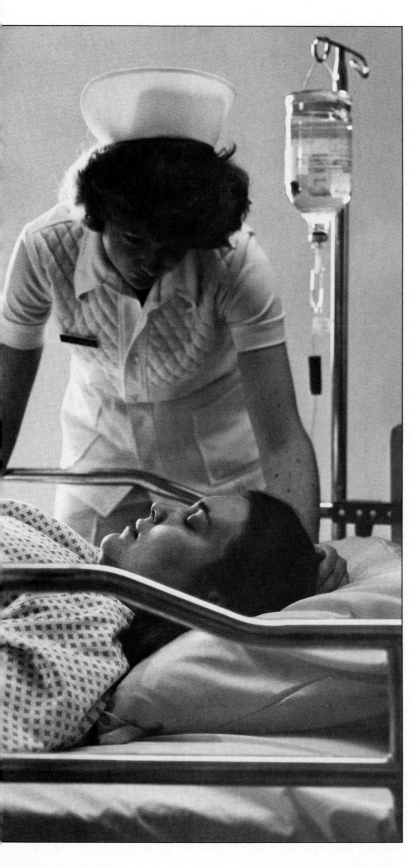

Coping with ICU syndrome

George Taper, a 57-year-old accountant, was admitted to the intensive care unit (ICU) after suffering a myocardial infarction (MI). During his first day in the unit, he was lucid. He knew where he was. He was aware of the day and time. But now, after almost a week, he begins to show signs of confusion. He's lost track of time and is beginning to resist your efforts to treat him. Do you know why he's behaving this way?

When a patient has been in intensive care for more than a few days, he may begin to exhibit signs of ICU syndrome. ICU syndrome results from sensory disturbances, prolonged sleep deprivation, immobilization, and lack of communication and meaningful interpersonal relationships. Also, the patient's age, severity of illness, medications, abnormal lab values (such as electrolyte imbalance), and pain may contribute to changes in his behavior.

Recognizing ICU syndrome

One distinguishing feature of ICU syndrome is that your patient will be lucid for 2 to 5 days before exhibiting behavior changes. The longer he remains in intensive care, the more likely he'll be to show some signs of ICU syndrome.

ICU syndrome usually develops in two stages. During the first stage, the patient may exhibit some or all of these signs and symptoms: subtle changes in mental status; changes in affect; sleeplessness; hyperactivity and restlessness; disorientation to place, time, and persons; inappropriate behavior; recent memory loss; mild perceptual distortion; and spatial distortion, such as floating sensations. During the second stage, he may experience delusions, visual and tactile hallucinations, and severe disorientation. In addition, he may become combative or paranoid, and refuse to comply with treatment.

When you notice any of these danger signs, alert the doctor. If untreated, ICU syndrome can pose a serious threat to your patient. As mental functioning deteriorates, your patient may lose his ability to cope. His healing resources may become depleted. In severe cases, your patient may develop hypertension, cardiac arrhythmia (for example, tachycardia), and hyperventilation.

Important: Avoid confusing ICU syndrome with organic brain syndrome. Although some signs of ICU syndrome and organic brain syndrome are similar, organic brain syndrome is caused by a physiologic abnormality, such as neurologic impairment or cerebrovascular damage. The patient with organic brain syndrome is severely disoriented. Signs of organic brain syndrome include drowsiness, reduced awareness, deteriorating mental function without hallucinations, and poor response to all mental function tests. Adapting the patient's environment will not prevent or improve organic brain syndrome.

How you can help

To help your patient suffering from ICU syndrome, follow these guidelines:
• Determine whether your patient's experiencing ICU syndrome or organic brain syndrome.
• Adapt your patient's environment to remove sources of sensory overload and supply sufficient sensory stimulation. (For tips on how to do this, review page 11.)
• Promote specified periods of restful sleep to avoid sleep deprivation.
• Ask the patient to report any feelings of confusion, misperception of time, floating sensations, or fatigue. Also, ask the family to tell you if they notice changes in the patient's behavior.
• Provide preoperative teaching, if appropriate, to prepare the patient and minimize the emotional trauma of intensive care.

Total patient care

Helping the patient's family

As an intensive care nurse, you give your patient the most professional nursing care available in a crisis. You deal with highly sophisticated equipment and health-care procedures. But how well do you deal with the patient's family?

As you know, giving total patient care means including the patient's family, especially in an intensive care situation. Why? Because the family is severely stressed. Their loved one is seriously ill, and they may not know whether he will live or die. In addition, they may have other worries, such as paying costly medical bills.

What can you do to help the family cope? First, recognize their state of crisis. Sound obvious? It is. But the family may be too anxious to know what they need. That's up to you.

Fortunately, a family in crisis is usually receptive to a sympathetic attempt to help. Show your concern for them as well as for the patient. The family may feel a need to talk about the circumstances that brought the patient to intensive care. Give them an opportunity to relive the events. This will give you insights into their feelings about the patient's illness, too.

Be sure the family knows what to expect when they see the patient. Is the patient on a ventilator? Explain any equipment being used, such as monitors or arterial lines, and why the patient needs them. Also, alert the family to changes in the patient's level of consciousness.

Suggest that the family be encouraging and supportive of the patient. Encourage them to touch him and reassure him. But warn them to avoid discussing any topics that may upset or worry him.

Note: If the patient is in a coma, remind the family he may be able to hear them. They should still be encouraged to talk to him. But warn them not to say anything in front of him they may not want him to hear.

Orient the family to the ICU and its immediate area. Show them the nearest waiting room or lounge, a public telephone, the rest room, and the snack bar. Make sure they understand ICU rules and policies, and explain why candy, food, and electrical appliances aren't allowed in the ICU. And don't forget to instruct them *not* to bring the patient money or valuables. (If the patient was admitted with money or valuables, ask the family to take them home.) If your hospital publishes an ICU brochure, give the family a copy.

Try to identify the family's concerns. For example, are they guilt-ridden because they believe they may have done something to cause the patient's illness? Are they undergoing another unrelated crisis that may place additional stress on them, such as a divorce? If indicated, refer the family for counseling or call their clergyman.

Help family members focus on their feelings and define their own roles. Let them participate in setting up a plan of action. Perhaps one family member can be appointed to make important phone calls, while another gets coffee. By being actively involved, if only in doing simple errands, the family will feel less helpless and more in control.

Finally, keep communication with the family ongoing. Make sure they know when visiting hours are, and encourage them to visit the patient. Then, seek them out during their visits and report any changes in the patient's condition. If hospital policy permits, allow them to call the nurses' station for information on the patient's condition. Tell them when you'll be free to talk with them. Or take a few minutes during the day and give them a call, especially if they're unable to visit. In short, do all you can to keep the family informed.

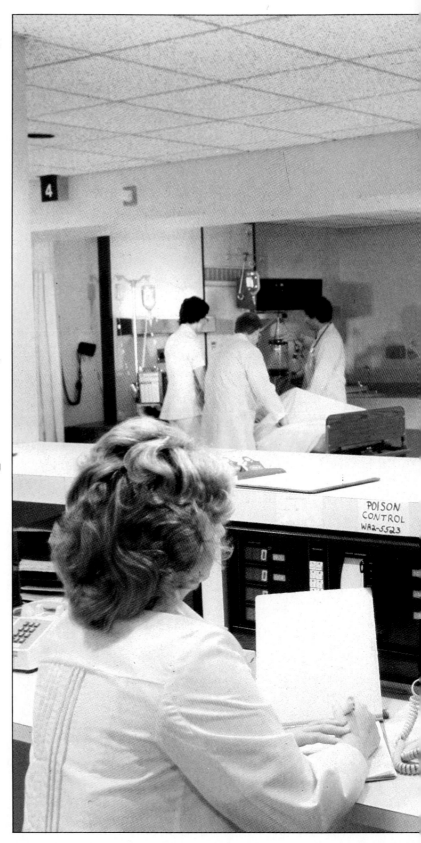

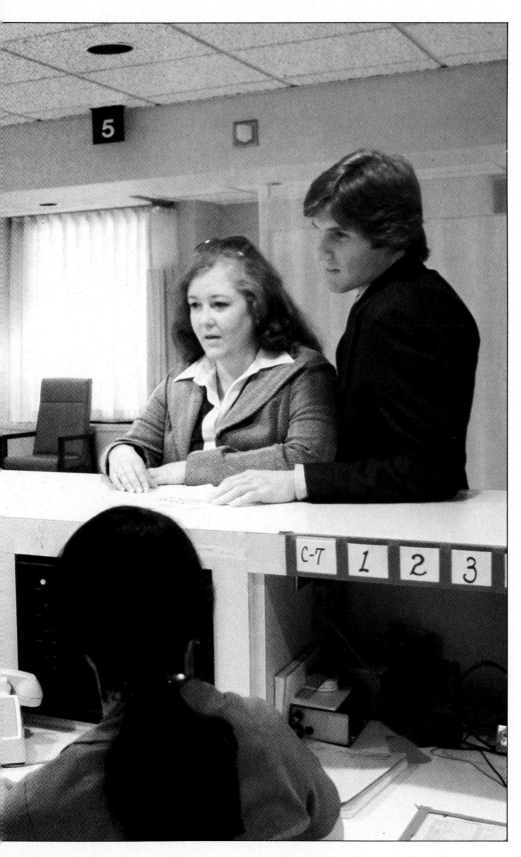

Helping the family confront death

Despite your best nursing efforts, some of your patients will die. This is especially true in the intensive care unit. You may not be able to change this fact, but you can help the patient's family prepare for and accept their loved one's eventual death. To do so, follow these guidelines:
• Listen to the family's concerns and fears. Answer their questions sympathetically, but avoid raising false hopes.
• Reassure the family that the patient's receiving the best health care available and tell them that everything's being done to make him as comfortable as possible. Try to establish a rapport with the family by showing genuine concern for them and their loved one. This will also help reassure the family that their loved one is receiving conscientious and sympathetic nursing care.
• Encourage the family to help with simple tasks to lessen their feeling of helplessness. For example, they can help bathe the patient or comb his hair. Also, encourage the family to touch the patient frequently and continue talking to him even if he's in a coma.
• Avoid doing or saying anything the family may misconstrue as indifference for the dying patient. Remember, the family's under great emotional stress. They will be especially sensitive to your words and actions.
   Follow these guidelines to help ease the family's grief if the patient dies:
• Realize that each person reacts to death in his own way. Allow the family to express their grief as they choose, as long as it doesn't endanger anyone or disrupt the unit's functioning. To help console them, offer to call a family friend or clergyman.
• Express your own grief, if appropriate. But remain in control, or you won't be able to help the family or continue with your duties.
• Remind the family of ways they helped make their loved one more comfortable before he died. Also, reassure them that the patient had the best health care available. These measures will help ease the common guilt associated with a loved one's death. *Remember:* Emotional stress may precipitate a medical crisis, such as myocardial infarction. Stay alert for danger signs. If a family member begins to experience pain in his arm or chest, shortness of breath, or dizziness, ask him to lie down. Then, see that he's taken to the emergency department for immediate assessment.
• Avoid letting a family member go home alone. If possible, call another relative or friend to meet him. Or, call the hospital clergy, if appropriate.

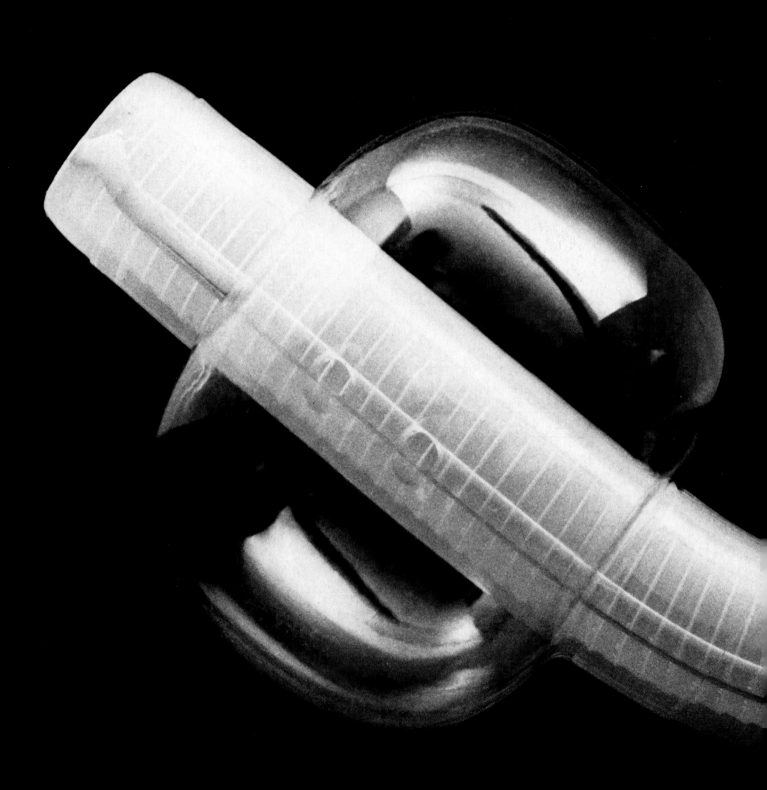

Caring for the Respiratory Patient

Respiratory basics
Airway management
Respiratory support

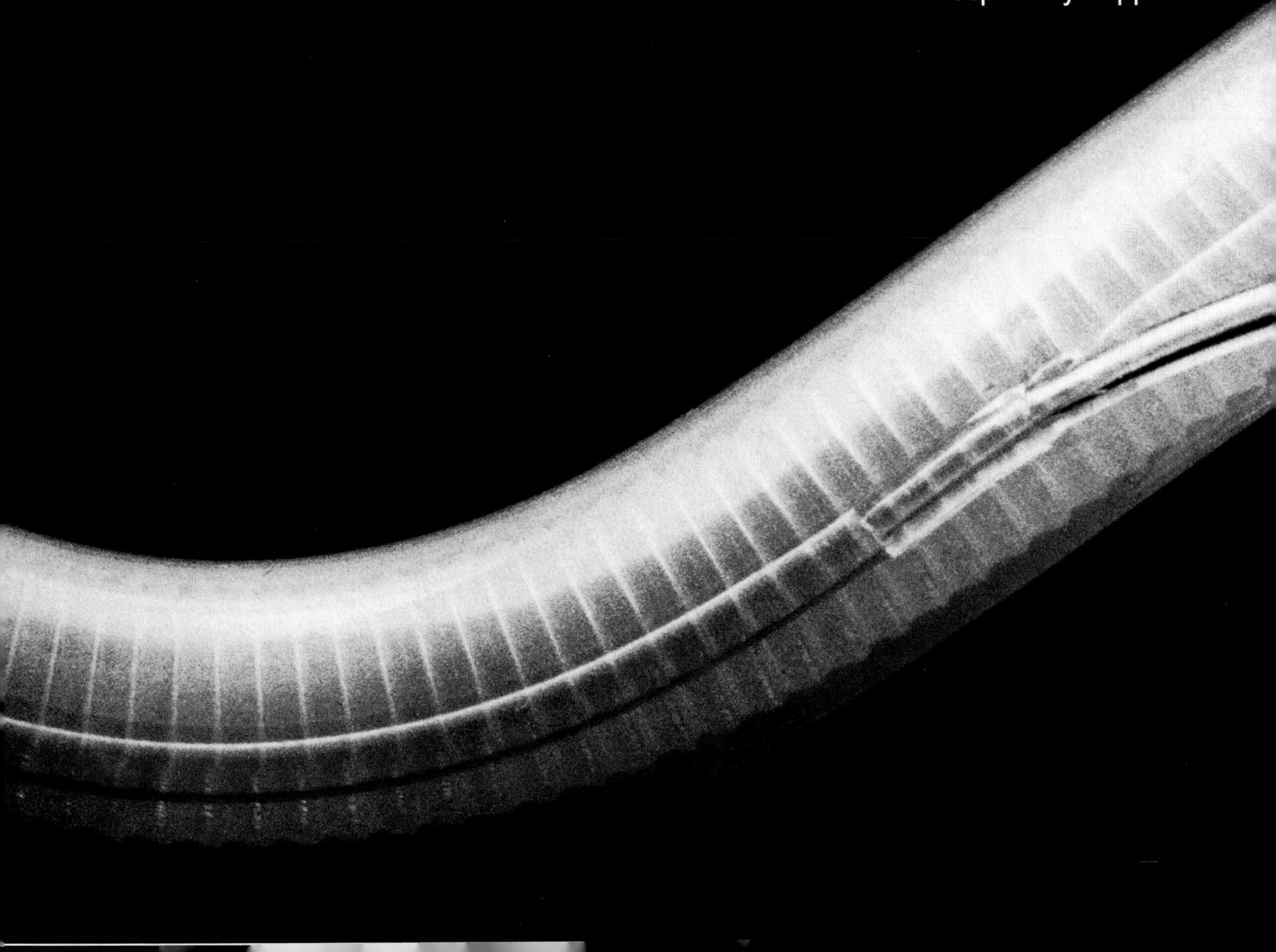

Respiratory basics

You're working in the intensive care unit, caring for severely ill patients. Your responsibilities are heavy and the pressure rarely lets up. Without question, you need to have instant recall of basic nursing knowledge. For that reason, we've included in the following pages a review of respiratory anatomy, physiology, and assessment.

We start by providing you with an anatomical illustration to help you visualize the respiratory tract. With a firm grasp of anatomy, you can better understand respiratory physiology. In discussing physiology, we briefly review respiratory mechanics, and then zero in on the fine points of gas exchange and pulmonary circulation.

Do you need to brush up on chest assessment procedures? You'll find explanations of the basic procedures, accompanied by charts that help you identify and interpret chest sounds. You'll also find charts that will clarify your understanding of arterial blood gas measurements.

Studying the text, charts, and illustrations on the next few pages will help you acquire (or regain) the foundation you need to provide good respiratory intensive care.

Understanding respiratory physiology

As you know, the lungs are a medium for the exchange of gases. During respiration, the lungs transport oxygen from the atmosphere to a person's tissue cells, and carbon dioxide from his tissue cells to the atmosphere.

Each respiratory cycle consists of an inspiratory and an expiratory phase. During inspiration, a person's diaphragm contracts and flattens to enlarge his thoracic cavity. This increase in lung volume creates negative pressure within the alveoli, which draws air into the lungs. The negative pressure also assists venous blood return to the heart. During expiration, the diaphragm relaxes and resumes its resting shape. The lungs compress, which creates positive pressure within the alveoli and forces air out of the lungs.

At the end of expiration, some air remains in the alveoli. This happens because a lipoprotein mixture called surfactant, secreted continuously by alveolar lining cells, reduces the surface tension of pulmonary fluids. Otherwise, the surface tension would cause the alveoli to collapse, forcing out all air. Sighing, which most people do 8 to 10 times every hour, stimulates production of surfactant.

A crucial characteristic of the lungs is their elasticity, called *compliance*. Conditions that reduce the lungs' efficiency by diminishing compliance include pneumothorax, pleural effusion, and adult respiratory distress syndrome (ARDS).

Respiration requires energy to power the respiratory muscles and to overcome pulmonary resistance. Airway resistance, a measure of the difficulty with which air moves through the bronchial passages, makes up about 80% of pulmonary resistance. Emphysema or airway obstruction can increase this resistance, hampering breathing.

Non-elastic tissue resistance, a measure of the difficulty with which viscous tissue cells slide past each other, is a lesser component of pulmonary resistance. Edema increases this resistance, making breathing more difficult.

Understanding gas exchange

Now that you've reviewed the mechanics of respiration, you'll want to take a closer look at the alveoli, the site of gas exchange. To do so, first study the top left illustration on the following page.

Follow the pulmonary artery with

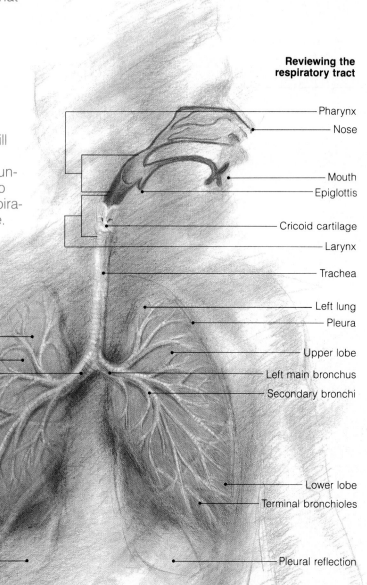

Reviewing the respiratory tract

Pharynx
Nose
Mouth
Epiglottis
Cricoid cartilage
Larynx
Trachea
Left lung
Pleura
Upper lobe
Left main bronchus
Secondary bronchi
Lower lobe
Terminal bronchioles
Pleural reflection

Right lung
Upper lobe
Right main bronchus
Middle lobe
Lower lobe
Pleural reflection

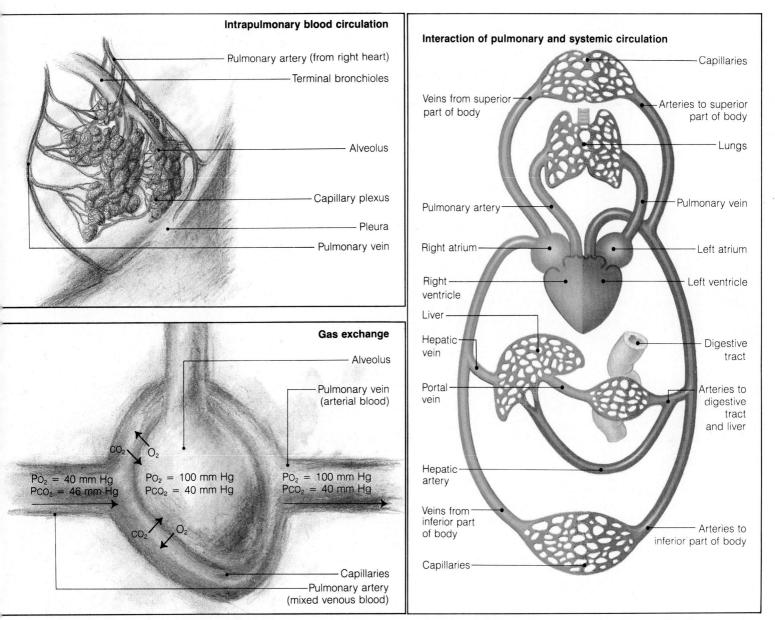

Intrapulmonary blood circulation

- Pulmonary artery (from right heart)
- Terminal bronchioles
- Alveolus
- Capillary plexus
- Pleura
- Pulmonary vein

Interaction of pulmonary and systemic circulation

- Capillaries
- Veins from superior part of body
- Arteries to superior part of body
- Lungs
- Pulmonary artery
- Pulmonary vein
- Right atrium
- Left atrium
- Right ventricle
- Left ventricle
- Liver
- Hepatic vein
- Digestive tract
- Portal vein
- Arteries to digestive tract and liver
- Hepatic artery
- Veins from inferior part of body
- Arteries to inferior part of body
- Capillaries

Gas exchange

- Alveolus
- Pulmonary vein (arterial blood)

CO_2 O_2

$PO_2 = 40$ mm Hg
$PCO_2 = 46$ mm Hg

$PO_2 = 100$ mm Hg
$PCO_2 = 40$ mm Hg

$PO_2 = 100$ mm Hg
$PCO_2 = 40$ mm Hg

CO_2 O_2

- Capillaries
- Pulmonary artery (mixed venous blood)

its supply of blood. When the artery reaches the lungs, its terminal branches enter the alveolar capillary network shown in the middle of the illustration. Gas exchange takes place here.

During the gas exchange process, oxygen and carbon dioxide diffuse across the very thin pulmonary membrane. This membrane makes up the alveolar sac and all other surfaces in the respiratory cavity that permit gas exchange.

To understand gas exchange, keep in mind that gases move from areas of higher pressure to areas of lower pressure. Study the relationships of the pressures shown in the gas exchange diagram above. Then you'll understand how carbon dioxide diffuses from the venous end of the capillary to the alveolus, while oxygen diffuses from the alveolus into the arterial end of the capillary. The blood itself diffuses from the venous capillary to the arterial capillary. Newly oxygenated, the blood then flows into a pulmonary vein branch. From there, it's carried back to the heart, which pumps it through-

out the body, delivering oxygen to the tissue cells. (See the illustration directly above.)

Most oxygen in the blood binds with hemoglobin. Hemoglobin ultimately releases the oxygen to the tissues. A very small fraction of the oxygen simply dissolves in the blood.

Most carbon dioxide in the blood takes the form of bicarbonate ion. But small amounts of carbon dioxide combine with hemoglobin or dissolve in the blood.

During rest, most people require 16 to 18 breaths per minute to replenish oxygen and eliminate carbon dioxide. The brain stem's respiratory centers (in the medulla and the pons) maintain a basic, unvarying respiratory rhythm. But, respiratory rate and depth change frequently, in response to four variables. Listed in order of importance, these variables are: carbon dioxide concentration, hydrogen ion concentration, oxygen concentration, and exercise or activity level.

Respiratory basics

Review of basic respiratory terms

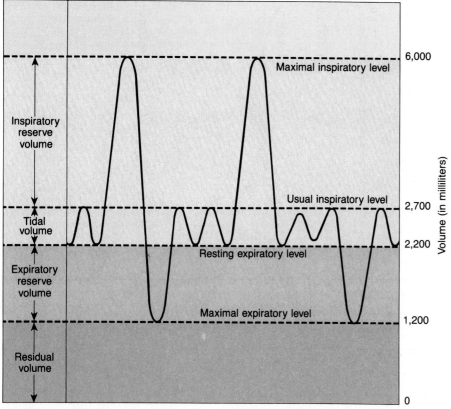

Nurses' guide to respiratory patterns

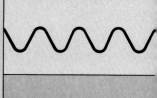

Is your patient breathing fast or slow? Is he gasping for breath, or not breathing at all for as long as a minute? To learn to identify respiratory patterns, study this chart.

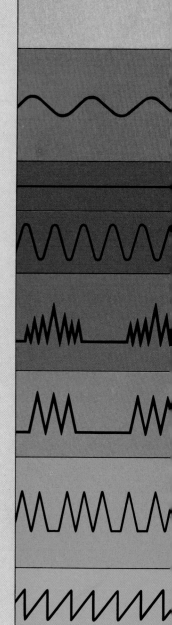

The terms below refer to measurements of respiratory function. You'll need to know these terms when you care for respiratory patients, particularly those on mechanical ventilation. The lung volumes listed here are illustrated in the graph above.

Tidal volume: Volume of air moved in and out of the lungs with each normal respiration. Equals about 500 ml in a normal adult (male or female).

Inspiratory reserve volume: Volume inhaled during forced inspiration (above tidal volume). Equals about 3,300 ml in a normal male, and 1,900 ml in a normal female.

Expiratory reserve volume: Volume of forced expiration (above tidal volume). Equals about 1,000 ml in a normal male, and 700 ml in a normal female.

Residual volume: Volume of air remaining in lungs after forced expiration. Can only be measured by indirect spirometry. Equals about 1,200 ml in a normal male, and 1,100 ml in a normal female.

Functional residual capacity: Expiratory reserve volume plus residual volume. The amount of air remaining in the lungs after a normal expiration. Equals about 2,300 ml in a normal male, and 1,800 ml in a normal female.

Vital capacity: Sum of inspiratory reserve volume, tidal volume, and expiratory reserve volume. Equals about 4,900 ml in a normal male, and 3,100 ml in a normal female.

Total lung capacity: Sum of inspiratory reserve volume, tidal volume, expiratory reserve volume, and residual volume. Volume of lung expansion possible with the greatest inspiratory effort. Equals about 6,000 ml in a normal male, and 4,200 in a normal female.

Resting minute ventilation: Respiratory rate multiplied by tidal volume. Should be less than 10 liters per minute, but should double with a maximal voluntary ventilation.

Negative inspiratory pressure: Amount of negative pressure the patient generates to initiate a breath. Should be greater than 20 cm H_2O pressure.

Alveolar-arterial oxygen gradient (A-aDO_2): Measure of the difficulty with which oxygen moves from the alveolus, across the alveolar-capillary membrane, and into the arterial blood. Indicates a ventilation/perfusion imbalance. Normal value is less than 15 mm Hg in room air. Value for mechanically ventilated patients should be under 350 mm Hg.

Graph modified from J.H. Comroe, et al, THE LUNG: CLINICAL PHYSIOLOGY AND PULMONARY FUNCTION TESTS, 2nd ed. Copyright © 1962, Year Book Medical Publishers, Inc., Chicago. Used by permission.

Eupnea
Normal respiratory rate and depth, regular rhythm. Expiration lasts twice as long as inspiration. Adult rate equals 16 to 18 breaths per minute.

Tachypnea
Increased respiratory rate (usually over 30 breaths per minute); shallow depth; regular or irregular rhythm. Often accompanies fever, as the body tries to rid itself of excess heat. Respirations increase about four breaths per minute for every degree Fahrenheit above normal. Respiration rate also increases with pain, anxiety, pneumonia, compensatory respiratory alkalosis, respiratory insufficiency, lesions in the brain's respiratory centers, and aspirin poisoning.

Bradypnea
Decreased respiratory rate (usually less than 12 breaths per minute); variable depth; and irregular rhythm. Normal during sleep. Abnormal when the brain's respiratory control center is affected by opiate drugs, tumor, alcohol, metabolic disorder, or respiratory decompensation.

Apnea
Absence of breathing; may be periodic.

Hyperpnea
Increased respiratory rate; increased depth; regular rhythm.

Cheyne-Stokes
Gradually increasing, then decreasing rate and depth, in a cycle lasting 30 to 170 seconds. Alternates with 20 to 60 second periods of apnea. Occurs with increased intracranial pressure, severe congestive heart failure, renal failure, meningitis, and drug overdose.

Biot's
Increased respiratory rate and depth, with irregular periods of apnea between respirations. Each breath has the same depth. Usually seen with central nervous system (CNS) disorders.

Kussmaul's
Increased respiratory rate (usually over 20 breaths per minute); increased depth; irregular rhythm. Patient's breathing usually sounds labored; breaths resemble sighs. Also called air hunger or paroxysmal dyspnea. Occurs in renal failure or metabolic acidosis, particularly diabetic ketoacidosis.

Apneusis
Prolonged, gasping, cramplike inspiration, followed by extremely short, insufficient expiration. Caused by lesions in the brain's respiratory centers.

Learning about chest assessment
When a patient is first admitted to the intensive care unit, you'll perform a chest assessment to determine his status and identify any problems. Repeat this assessment periodically to determine the effects of therapy.

For a complete chest assessment, you must obtain a detailed respiratory history from your patient (see box below). Then you'll perform the following four procedures: inspection, palpation, percussion, and auscultation. The doctor will also order arterial blood gas (ABG) measurements, pulmonary function tests, X-rays, and any indicated lab tests, such as a complete blood cell count (CBC). In the next few pages, we'll show you how to perform inspection, palpation, percussion, and auscultation. For more details on performing chest assessment, refer to the NURSING PHOTOBOOK PROVIDING RESPIRATORY CARE.

DOCUMENTING

Obtaining a respiratory history

Before you inspect your patient's lungs, you must find out all you can about his past and present respiratory conditions. However, ask him about his present problem first; a severely ill patient's condition requires prompt assessment, so treatment can be quickly initiated. If your ICU patient can't talk, question a family member.

In your questions, cover the date the problem started, and the patient's signs and symptoms (including their severity and duration). Find out if anything alleviates or worsens his symptoms. If you see a pattern developing, ask your patient about other symptoms he might be expected to have. Also, obtain a summary of any previous therapy for the condition. Finally, ask your patient to describe how he felt immediately before the condition's onset.

Use the following questions as guidelines:
• Do you have trouble breathing? Do you have shortness of breath? When does it occur? Does anything relieve it?
• Do you feel unusually fatigued? If so, describe your feeling.
• Are you experiencing chest pain? If so, describe the pain.
• Do you have a cough? If so, when did it start? Do you cough anything up? If so, how much, and what color is it? Is it bloody?
• Do you have allergies? What kind?
• Do your ankles ever swell? Have you noticed a recent weight gain?
• Do you—or did you ever—smoke cigarettes, a pipe, or cigars? If you smoke now, how much do you smoke each day? How long have you been smoking? If you no longer smoke, how long has it been since you quit?
• Do you work around chemicals, fumes, asbestos, dust, or coal? If so, describe your work environment.
• Have you traveled recently? If so, where? Did you feel ill while you were there or upon returning? Describe the symptoms.
• Do you have any other lung problems?

After you've established the patient's present problem, review his health before the problem's onset. Cover his early growth and development, childhood diseases, adult diseases, immunizations, previous hospitalizations (if any), and current medications. Use the questions we've just listed, but apply them to his past. Also ask him:
• Have you ever been treated for a lung problem? If so, when and what type of problem?
• Have you ever had a blood clot in your lungs? When?
• Have you ever been exposed to tuberculosis? If so, when was your last tuberculin test? Have you ever had tuberculosis? If so, when? Were you treated for it? What medication did you take?
• When was your last chest X-ray taken? Was it normal?

Respiratory basics

Performing inspection

Begin your assessment by inspecting your patient. To do so, seat your patient upright and remove his clothing above the waist.

However, if your ICU patient can't sit upright, position him on his side. If he can't maintain that position by himself, get help to support him.

In inspecting your patient, use the following guidelines:
• First, observe the patient for neurologic signs of hypoxia, such as decreased level of consciousness, lethargy, restlessness, drowsiness, confusion, or irritability.
• Next, observe your patient's unassisted respirations to determine their rate, depth, and rhythm. When observing his respirations, remember to count them for at least one minute. Otherwise, your assessment may be off by as much as four per minute. Be sure to check for apnea. To review the basic respiratory patterns, study the chart on pages 20 and 21.
• Observe your patient's chest wall movement. Asymmetric

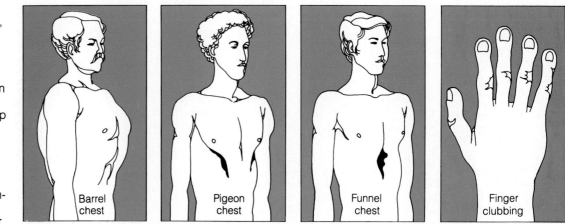

Barrel chest

Pigeon chest

Funnel chest

Finger clubbing

expansion may indicate pneumothorax, an endotracheal tube inadvertently lodged in the right mainstem bronchus, or other obstruction of a major bronchus.
• Determine the anterior-posterior diameter of his chest. The transverse diameter—axilla-to-axilla width—should be twice the anterior-posterior width. Abnormal configurations include a barrel chest, indicating chronic obstructive pulmonary disease (COPD); a pigeon

chest, indicating rickets or emphysema; or a funnel chest, indicating rickets.
• Note whether the patient uses his accessory muscles to breathe; for example, the intercostal muscles, the sternocleidomastoid, or the abdominal wall muscles. Using accessory muscles to breathe indicates poor compliance.
• Check the patient for signs of cyanosis, but distinguish between peripheral and central cyanosis. Poor circulation or

vasoconstriction cause peripheral cyanosis, which involves the fingertips, earlobes, and toes. Severe hypoxia causes central cyanosis, which involves the mucous membranes, chest, and trunk, as well as the remainder of the body. In a respiratory assessment, central cyanosis is of greater concern than peripheral cyanosis.
• Check patient's fingers for clubbing from chronic hypoxia.
• Document your findings in your nurses' notes.

Performing percussion

Percussing your patient's chest reveals changes in the tones normally emitted by the thoracic cavity. To perform percussion, place the tip of one middle finger on the patient's chest between two ribs. Apply only light pressure, to avoid distorting the percussion note. Don't touch his chest with your other fingers. Moving your wrist, tap your middle finger's first joint with the middle fingertip of your

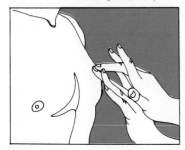

opposite hand (see illustration at lower left).

Percuss your patient's chest anteriorly and posteriorly, following the sequences shown in the diagrams at right. As you move from his upper to lower chest, compare the sounds on each side of his chest. Expect to hear the following:
• resonance (a hollow sound) over normal, air-filled lungs
• dullness (a thudding sound) over fluid-filled organs such as the heart and the liver, or in pleural effusion
• flatness (an extremely dull sound) over the sternum, muscle, or an atelectatic lung
• tympany (a drum-like sound) over the air-filled stomach. When heard over the lungs, this signifies increased air volume.
• hyperresonance (a booming

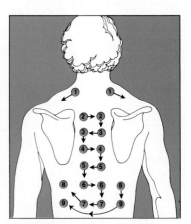

sound) over hyperinflated airways, as in emphysema or pneumothorax.

Make sure your patient's diaphragmatic excursion measures between 3 and 5 cm. It should be equal bilaterally.

Finally, have your patient rest

his forearm on his head, if possible, while you percuss his lateral chest at 2″ intervals. *Remember:* For best results, always percuss between his ribs, not directly over them.

Document all findings in your nurses' notes.

Performing palpation

Palpation entails checking the patient's anterior and posterior chest for symmetric expansion and tactile fremitus. Tactile fremitus is the vibration you feel when the patient speaks.

To check for symmetric expansion of your patient's upper chest, place your palms on either side of his upper chest. Rest your fingers on his shoulders and extend your thumbs until they meet. Have your patient inhale and exhale deeply. Observe the movement of your thumbs on his chest for unilateral lag, which may indicate thickening pleura, atelectasis, obstruction of a major bronchus, pneumothorax, or a misplaced endotracheal tube.

Then, examine his midchest by placing your hands on the sides of his chest. Rest your thumbs on the sixth rib level and extend them so they meet. Again, have the patient inhale and exhale deeply. As he inhales, your thumbs will separate (see illustration). Repeat the examination on his lower chest.

To assess tactile fremitus, position your hands on either side of your patient's upper chest. Place your palms flat against his chest, but don't touch him with your fingers. Move your palms from his upper to lower chest, both anteriorly

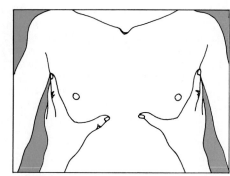

and posteriorly, as he repeats the words "ninety-nine." In doing so, follow the sequence indicated in the percussion diagram (see page 22). Expect to feel fremitus in the upper chest, close to the bronchi. However, you should feel little or no fremitus in the lower chest.

In his upper chest, you should feel vibrations of equal intensity on either side. Greater intensity on one side may signify tissue consolidation. Lesser intensity on one side may signify emphysema, pneumothorax, or pleural effusion.

Document all findings.

For details on how to perform these basic palpation techniques, see the NURSING PHOTOBOOK ASSESSING YOUR PATIENTS.

Performing auscultation

Auscultate your patient's lungs to detect abnormal breath sounds. To do so, listen with a stethoscope over all lung fields, anteriorly, posteriorly, and laterally. Apply the stethoscope diaphragm firmly against the patient's skin. (If necessary, wet his chest hairs to reduce rubbing sounds.) As you do this, have your patient breathe in and out slowly and deeply through his mouth (if possible). Follow the same sequence you used to percuss your patient.

As you descend from the patient's upper chest to his lower chest, compare the sounds on each side of his chest. Concentrate on distinguishing between normal and abnormal sounds. For help, see Nurses' guide to breath sounds (below) and Nurses' guide to adventitious sounds (on page 24).

If your intensive care patient is lying on his side, his uppermost lung will be better ventilated. Keep this in mind when you compare breath sounds.

Nursing tip: Suppose your patient has difficulty breathing and you hear rhonchi. Ask him to cough. Some breath sounds become evident only after the patient has cleared his airway of secretions.

Document any abnormal breath sounds in your nurses' notes. Be sure to record which lobe or lobes are affected.

Nurses' guide to breath sounds

Breath sounds	Description	Position in respiratory cycle	Typical respiratory cycle	Normal findings	Abnormal findings
Vesicular	• High-pitched and loud on inspiration; low-pitched and soft on expiration	• More prominent during inspiration than during expiration	• Inspiration is longer than expiration, with no pause between them.	• Over peripheral lung fields, you'll hear sounds that have a soft, swishy quality.	• Decreased sounds over peripheral lung fields; may indicate emphysema or early pneumonia
Bronchial or tracheal	• High-pitched, loud, harsh, hollow	• Less prominent during inspiration than during expiration	• Inspiration is shorter than expiration, with a pause between them.	• Over the trachea or the mainstem bronchus, you'll hear a sound like air blown through a hollow tube.	• Bronchial sounds over peripheral lung fields; may indicate atelectasis or consolidation
Bronchovesicular	• Medium-to-high-pitched, muffled	• Equally prominent during inspiration and expiration	• Inspiration and expiration are equal, with no pause between them.	• Over large airways, either side of the sternum, the Angle of Louis, and between the scapulae, you'll hear a blowing sound.	• Bronchovesicular sounds over peripheral lung fields; may indicate consolidation

Respiratory basics

Understanding abnormal breath sounds

Abnormal breath sounds include mislocated bronchial/broncho-vesicular sounds (explained under abnormal findings on the chart on page 23), and adventitious sounds. Also included in this category are absent breath sounds.

Absent breath sounds indicate a loss of functional ventilating power, and may signify:
• obstruction of larynx, trachea, or bronchus.
• laryngeal bronchospasm.

• pneumonectomy or phrenic nerve palsy.
• endotracheal tube malpositioning.
• pleural abnormalities.

During auscultation, you may hear adventitious sounds superimposed over your patient's normal breath sounds. To perform an accurate assessment, you must learn to recognize these sounds. Study the following chart to understand each sound's significance. Also refer to the chart on lung conditions on the opposite page.

Nurses' guide to adventitious sounds

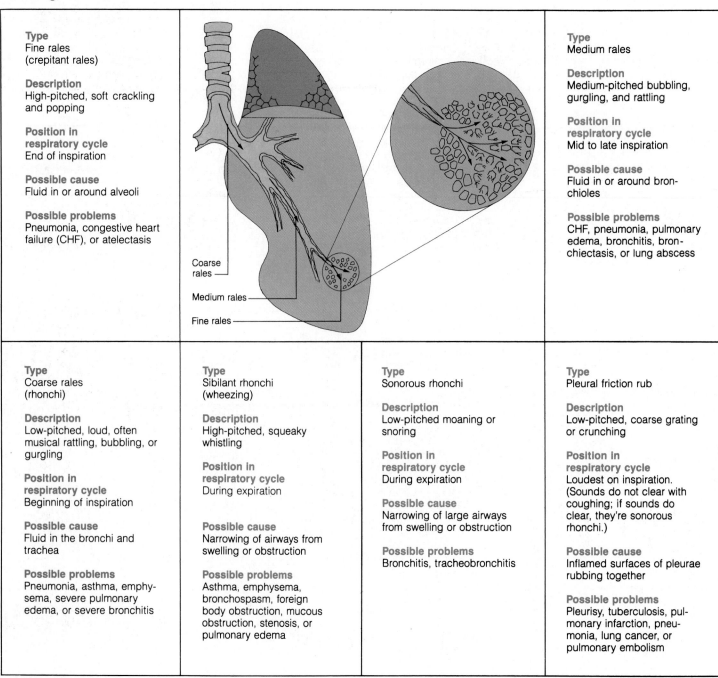

Type
Fine rales
(crepitant rales)

Description
High-pitched, soft crackling and popping

Position in respiratory cycle
End of inspiration

Possible cause
Fluid in or around alveoli

Possible problems
Pneumonia, congestive heart failure (CHF), or atelectasis

Coarse rales
Medium rales
Fine rales

Type
Medium rales

Description
Medium-pitched bubbling, gurgling, and rattling

Position in respiratory cycle
Mid to late inspiration

Possible cause
Fluid in or around bron-chioles

Possible problems
CHF, pneumonia, pulmonary edema, bronchitis, bron-chiectasis, or lung abscess

Type
Coarse rales
(rhonchi)

Description
Low-pitched, loud, often musical rattling, bubbling, or gurgling

Position in respiratory cycle
Beginning of inspiration

Possible cause
Fluid in the bronchi and trachea

Possible problems
Pneumonia, asthma, emphysema, severe pulmonary edema, or severe bronchitis

Type
Sibilant rhonchi
(wheezing)

Description
High-pitched, squeaky whistling

Position in respiratory cycle
During expiration

Possible cause
Narrowing of airways from swelling or obstruction

Possible problems
Asthma, emphysema, bronchospasm, foreign body obstruction, mucous obstruction, stenosis, or pulmonary edema

Type
Sonorous rhonchi

Description
Low-pitched moaning or snoring

Position in respiratory cycle
During expiration

Possible cause
Narrowing of large airways from swelling or obstruction

Possible problems
Bronchitis, tracheobronchitis

Type
Pleural friction rub

Description
Low-pitched, coarse grating or crunching

Position in respiratory cycle
Loudest on inspiration. (Sounds do not clear with coughing; if sounds do clear, they're sonorous rhonchi.)

Possible cause
Inflamed surfaces of pleurae rubbing together

Possible problems
Pleurisy, tuberculosis, pulmonary infarction, pneumonia, lung cancer, or pulmonary embolism

Common lung conditions: Signs and symptoms

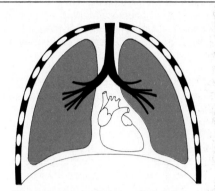

Suppose you've just performed a chest assessment. The results indicate that your patient has a respiratory problem, but you're not sure which one. Compare his signs and symptoms with those listed in this chart. He may have one of the following common lung conditions.

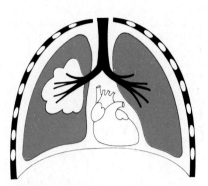

PNEUMOTHORAX

Inspection
Dyspnea; less motion on affected side. Trachea deviates away from affected side.

Palpation
Decreased fremitus

Percussion
Hyperresonance

Auscultation
Decreased or absent breath sounds over affected side

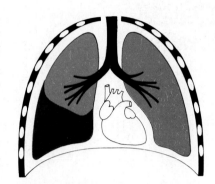

CONSOLIDATION

Inspection
Less motion on affected side

Palpation
Increased fremitus

Percussion
Dullness to flatness

Auscultation
Medium to coarse rales; transient friction rub

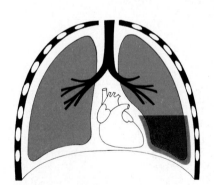

PLEURAL EFFUSION

Inspection
Dyspnea; less defined intercostal spaces on affected side

Palpation
Decreased fremitus

Percussion
Flatness; decreased diaphragmatic excursion

Auscultation
Decreased or absent breath sounds over involved area

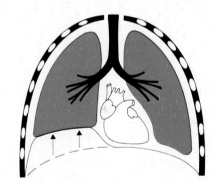

ATELECTASIS

Inspection
Less motion and lowered volume of thorax on affected side. Trachea deviates toward affected side.

Palpation
Varied fremitus

Percussion
Dullness

Auscultation
Transient fine rales

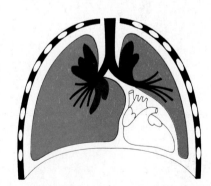

CONGESTIVE HEART FAILURE (CHF) WITHOUT EFFUSION

Inspection
Mostly normal

Palpation
Normal

Percussion
Normal

Auscultation
Fine to medium rales, louder on right than left side

Respiratory basics

Common lung conditions:
Signs and symptoms continued

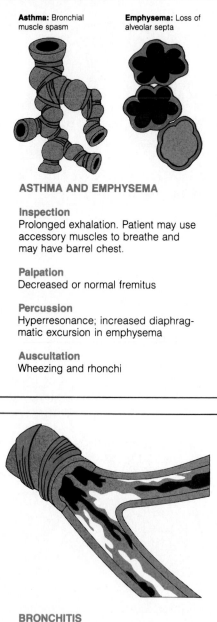

Asthma: Bronchial muscle spasm

Emphysema: Loss of alveolar septa

ASTHMA AND EMPHYSEMA

Inspection
Prolonged exhalation. Patient may use accessory muscles to breathe and may have barrel chest.

Palpation
Decreased or normal fremitus

Percussion
Hyperresonance; increased diaphragmatic excursion in emphysema

Auscultation
Wheezing and rhonchi

BRONCHITIS

Inspection
Variable, depending on amount of secretions and airway edema

Palpation
Variable

Percussion
Variable

Auscultation
Localized rales, rhonchi, and wheezing

Interpreting arterial blood gas measurements

To monitor your intensive care patient's respiratory status, you must frequently draw blood to obtain arterial blood gas (ABG) measurements. For detailed instructions on drawing blood for these measurements, see the NURSING PHOTO-BOOK PROVIDING RESPIRATORY CARE.

After you obtain the blood gas measurements, can you interpret them? First, study the chart on the opposite page—it shows the blood gas factors measured. Note among these the patient's acid-base status (pH), how much oxygen his lungs deliver to the blood (PaO_2), and how well his lungs eliminate carbon dioxide ($PaCO_2$). You'll measure these three factors directly. You'll calculate the others shown in the chart from these first three—except for oxygen saturation (SaO_2), which may be measured by a special device.

In interpreting your patient's values, you must answer the following important questions. To help find the answers, refer to the chart.

• *Does the patient's pH level show acidosis, alkalosis, or a normal acid-base balance?* Look at his pH value and compare it with the normal and abnormal pH values in the chart.

• *If his pH level shows acidosis, does he have respiratory or metabolic acidosis?* Look for $PaCO_2$ greater than 45 mm Hg. Retention of carbon dioxide by the lungs, which leads to increased carbonic acid in the blood, causes respiratory acidosis.

Or look for decreased HCO_3^-. Renal excretion of large amounts of a base may reduce bicarbonate levels, causing metabolic acidosis.

• *If his pH level shows alkalosis, does he have respiratory or metabolic alkalosis?* Look for $PaCO_2$ less than 35 mm Hg. Excessive loss of carbon dioxide and water from the lungs leads to reduced carbonic acid levels, causing respiratory alkalosis.

Or look for increased HCO_3^-. Renal retention of excessive alkali leads to increased bicarbonate levels, causing metabolic alkalosis.

• *If your patient has an acid-base imbalance, has his body's buffer system begun to compensate for it? Or, if his pH is within normal limits, but just barely, are his compensatory mechanisms masking an acid-base imbalance?* Use the diagram on evaluating acid-base compensation to help answer these questions. Compensation means that one organ of the body's lung-kidney buffer system tries to make up for the malfunction of the other. For example, if the patient has respiratory acidosis, the kidneys will raise the bicarbonate

(base) level in the blood. On the other hand, if the patient has metabolic acidosis, the lungs compensate by blowing off more CO_2 and H_2O, reducing the carbonic acid level in the blood.

• *Is his PaO_2 normal, considering his age and the level of oxygen he's receiving?* Look at his PaO_2 level and compare it with the chart. Remember, if the patient's breathing room air (which has 21% oxygen), he may have lower PaO_2 than a patient breathing 40% oxygen through a venturi mask. Also, the normal range for infants and elderly adults is lower than the typical adult normal range.

• *Does the relationship between SaO_2 and PaO_2 confirm well-oxygenated blood, or hypoxia?* The curve depicted below shows the relationship between the level of oxygen dissolved in the blood and the amount of hemoglobin carrying oxygen. This curve is called the oxygen dissociation curve. As you can see, oxygen has a very strong affinity for hemoglobin. Only after PaO_2 decreases below 50 mm Hg, will SaO_2 begin to drop significantly.

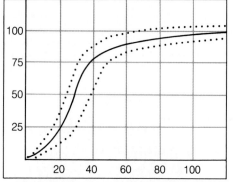

The oxygen dissociation curve can shift to either the right or left, as the dotted lines indicate. Higher pH, decreased temperature, and reduced carbon dioxide levels cause a shift to the left. With this shift, relatively more oxygen combines with hemoglobin, leaving less available for release to the tissues. Lower pH, increased temperature, and increased carbon dioxide levels cause a shift to the right. With this shift, hemoglobin readily releases oxygen to the tissues.

Note: In interpreting blood gas measurements, keep your patient's history in mind. Remember, a chronic obstructive pulmonary disease (COPD) patient may have chronically abnormal blood gas levels. But these levels are typical for him in his disease's non-acute phases. Always compare a COPD patient's ABG measurements with his typical blood gas levels, to see if his condition has worsened.

Nurses' guide to arterial blood gas measurements

Pao_2 Oxygen tension. Partial pressure exerted by the small amount of oxygen dissolved in arterial blood. **Normal values** 80 to 100 mm Hg **Abnormal values** Value less than 50 mm Hg signifies hypoxia. Pao_2 between 50 and 80 mm Hg may or may not signify hypoxia, depending on age of patient and oxygen concentration he's receiving. A newborn infant has a Pao_2 between 40 and 60 mm Hg. After age 60, the adult may show a Pao_2 below 80 mm Hg, without being hypoxic.	**$Paco_2$** Carbon dioxide tension. Partial pressure exerted by carbon dioxide dissolved in arterial blood. Primarily influenced by lung disorders and respiratory pattern. **Normal values** 35 to 45 mm Hg **Abnormal values** Value above 45 mm Hg signifies hypoventilation (hypercarbia). Value below 35 mm Hg signifies hyperventilation (hypocarbia). $Paco_2$ level may also indicate respiratory (lung-regulated) acid-base imbalance. If patient's pH shows an imbalance, $Paco_2$ above 45 mm Hg indicates respiratory acidosis; $Paco_2$ below 35 mm Hg indicates respiratory alkalosis.	**H_2CO_3** Carbonic acid, formed by carbon dioxide and water. Source of acid hydrogen ions and basic bicarbonate ions. Always 3% of $Paco_2$. **Normal value** 1.05 to 1.35 mEq/L 1:20 ratio with bicarbonate ions **Abnormal value** The important value here is the ratio of carbonic acid to bicarbonate. More carbonic acid, as in a 1:16 ratio, indicates acidosis. More bicarbonate, as in a 1:23 ratio, indicates alkalosis. But very close ratios such as 1:19 or 1:21 may indicate compensation for acidosis or alkalosis.
HCO_3^- Amount of bicarbonate dissolved in blood. Primarily influenced by metabolic changes. Determined by calculation involving pH and $Paco_2$. **Normal value** 22 to 26 mEq/L **Abnormal value** Value greater than 26 mEq/L indicates metabolic (kidney-regulated) alkalosis. Value less than 22 mEq/L indicates metabolic acidosis.	**pH** Expression of hydrogen ion concentration. Clinical measure of blood acidity. **Normal value** 7.35 to 7.45 **Abnormal value** Value greater than 7.45 signifies alkalosis. Value less than 7.35 signifies acidosis. If the patient has either imbalance, check his $Paco_2$ and HCO_3^- measurements to see if it's respiratory or metabolic. Then, to see if his system has begun to compensate, look at the chart below. Also check for compensation if his value is borderline (for example, 7.37).	**Sao_2** Oxygen saturation (percentage of hemoglobin carrying oxygen). Hemoglobin carries most of the oxygen in the blood. **Normal value** 95% to 100% **Abnormal value** If Pao_2 is between 60 and 95 mm Hg, Sao_2 should remain above 85%. Sharply decreased values usually indicate drop in Pao_2 below 50 mm Hg.

Evaluating acid-base compensation

Has your patient's system compensated for an acid-base imbalance? Use this diagram to find out. If your patient's primary imbalance is from an abnormal $Paco_2$ level (indicating a respiratory

ACID-BASE IMBALANCE

imbalance), first check his HCO_3^- level. Or, if his primary imbalance is from an abnormal HCO_3^- level (indicating a metabolic imbalance), check his $Paco_2$ level. Then, consult this diagram.

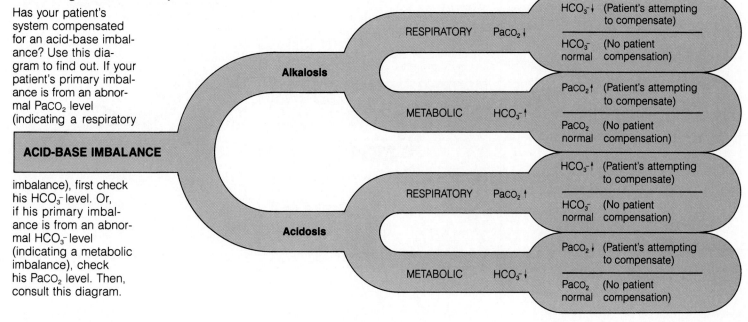

Airway management

What's the first nursing measure to consider when caring for a respiratory patient—or any patient for that matter? Maintaining a patent airway, of course. Sometimes your patient needs only an oropharyngeal airway inserted. But, if his arterial blood gases can't be maintained at a normal level, or his condition fails to improve or deteriorates, the doctor will order an endotracheal tube inserted. If long-term intubation with an artificial airway is needed, the doctor may perform a tracheotomy.

Read the following pages for the information you need to care for a patient with any type of artificial airway. For example, the chart below shows you how artificial airways differ. In this section, you'll also find out how to insert an oropharyngeal airway, how to care for a patient with an endotracheal tube, and how to care for a tracheostomy patient. Finally, we'll tell you how to cope with such common intubation problems as a ruptured cuff or a tracheoesophageal fistula.

Nurses' guide to artificial airways

Oropharyngeal

Indications
- Airway obstruction, when nasopharyngeal airway is contraindicated because of nasal obstruction or predisposition to epistaxis
- Short-term intubation

Contraindications
- Trauma to lower face
- Before, during, or after oral surgery

Advantages
- Inserted easily
- Holds tongue away from pharynx
- Tolerated well by patients

Disadvantages
- Dislodged easily
- May stimulate gag reflex
- May cause obstruction if airway size is incorrect

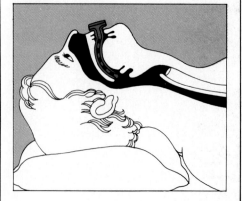

Nasopharyngeal

Indications
- Airway obstruction, when oropharyngeal airway is contraindicated because of trauma to lower face or oral surgery
- Surgery, to maintain patent airway until patient recovers from anesthesia

Contraindications
- Nasal obstruction
- Predisposition to epistaxis

Advantages
- Inserted easily
- Tolerated better than oropharyngeal airway by conscious patients
- Allows for suctioning without displacing the patient's nasal turbinates

Disadvantages
- May cause severe epistaxis if inserted too forcefully
- Kinks and clogs easily, obstructing airway
- May cause pressure necrosis of nasal mucosa
- May cause air passage obstruction, if artificial airway is too large

Oral esophageal

Indications
- Airway obstruction, when all other efforts to maintain an open airway have failed. (Used primarily in emergency departments or by trained paramedics.)

Contraindications
- Trauma to lower face
- Before, during, or after oral surgery

Advantages
- Inserted quickly and easily
- Prevents aspiration of stomach contents while tube is in place

Disadvantages
- May cause pharyngeal trauma during insertion
- May be accidentally inserted into trachea
- May cause gastric distention and impair ventilation if cuff is improperly inflated
- Allows possible aspiration of stomach contents during tube removal

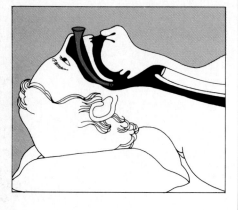

Oral endotracheal

Indications
• Cardiopulmonary resuscitation or other airway obstruction, when all other efforts to maintain an airway have failed, and when patient has nasal obstruction or predisposition to epistaxis
• Mechanical ventilation, when patient has nasal obstruction or predisposition to epistaxis
• Short-term intubation

Contraindications
• Trauma to lower face
• Before, during, or after oral surgery
• Long-term intubation

Advantages
• Inserted quickly and easily
• Causes less intubation trauma than nasal endotracheal airway
• Permits use of a larger diameter tube
• Eliminates danger of introducing infection or blood from nasal fossae into trachea
• Involves less tissue destruction than with trach tube
• Prevents aspiration of stomach contents, if cuff is inflated

Disadvantages
• May damage teeth or lacerate lips, mouth, pharyngeal mucosa, or larynx during insertion
• May cause aspiration of blood or vomitus during insertion
• Activates gag reflex in conscious patients
• Kinks and clogs easily, obstructing airway
• Interferes with cough reflex
• Prevents patient from talking, if cuff is inflated
• May be bitten or chewed
• May cause pressure necrosis
• May stimulate retching, which can lead to gastric distention
• May cause laryngeal edema, apnea secondary to reflexive breath holding, bronchospasms, or infection
• May cause tracheal damage

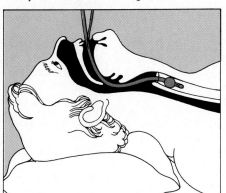

Nasal endotracheal

Indications
• Airway obstruction, when all other efforts to maintain an open airway have failed, and when patient has facial trauma
• Mechanical ventilation
• Long-term intubation

Contraindications
• Nasal obstruction
• Fractured nose
• Sinusitis
• Predisposition to epistaxis

Advantages
• Feels more comfortable than oral endotracheal tube, making it preferable for long-term therapy
• Permits good oral hygiene
• Can't be bitten or chewed
• Provides a channel for suctioning
• May be adapted easily if patient requires continuous ventilation
• Can be anchored in place easily
• Causes less tissue destruction than trach tube
• Prevents aspiration of stomach contents, if cuff is inflated

Disadvantages
• May be more traumatic to insert than oral endotracheal tube for conscious patient
• May lacerate pharyngeal mucosa or layrnx during insertion
• Kinks and clogs easily, obstructing airway
• Interferes with cough reflex
• Prevents patient from talking, if cuff is inflated
• Increases airway resistance because of small lumen size needed to fit nasal passages
• May cause pressure necrosis of nasal mucosa
• May cause laryngeal edema
• May cause tracheal damage

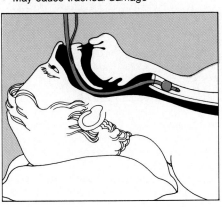

Tracheostomy

Indications
• Complete upper airway obstruction, when endotracheal intubation is impossible
• Long-term intubation

Contraindications
• Intubation of infants
• Whenever patient's highly susceptible to infection; for example, when he's receiving an immunosuppressant drug
• Short-term intubation

Advantages
• Suctioned more easily than endotracheal tube
• Decreases dead air space in respiratory system more than other airways do
• Permits patient to swallow and eat
• Feels more comfortable than other tubes
• Prevents aspiration of stomach contents, if cuff is inflated

Disadvantages
• Requires surgery to insert
• Can't be used for infants
• May cause laceration or pressure necrosis of trachea, especially in children
• May cause tracheoesophageal fistula
• Increases risk of tracheal and stomal inflammation
• Entails major risk of infection
• Increases risk of mucous plugs
• Prevents patient from talking, if cuff is inflated

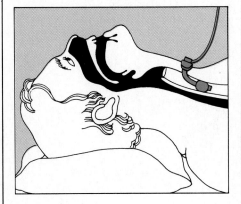

Airway management

Inserting an oropharyngeal airway

1 *Jenna Crisler, your 25-year-old ICU patient, was admitted for severe injuries incurred in an automobile accident. Suddenly, she loses consciousness. You must immediately insert an oropharyngeal airway, to prevent her tongue from resting against her posterior pharyngeal wall. Doing this will keep her airway open until her condition stabilizes. Here's how to insert an oral airway:*

If your patient's mouth is closed, immediately open it with the crossed-finger technique, as shown here. Or, use a tongue depressor.

Note: For a patient with neck injuries, use a modified jaw thrust. But be gentle to avoid injuring teeth or gums.

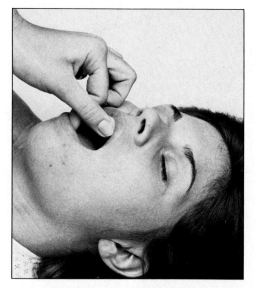

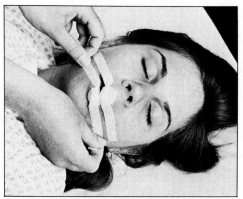

3 If the artificial airway is positioned incorrectly, your patient may vomit. As a precaution, turn her head to the side immediately after you've inserted the airway. This position will decrease the possibility of aspiration if she does vomit. Reposition the airway, as necessary.

Now, tape the airway in place. To do so, wind two 4″ wide, 3″ long nonallergenic tape strips around the tabs on the top and bottom of the airway. Then, secure the tape to the patient's cheeks. *Important:* Make sure you've allowed enough room to insert a suction tube past the airway.

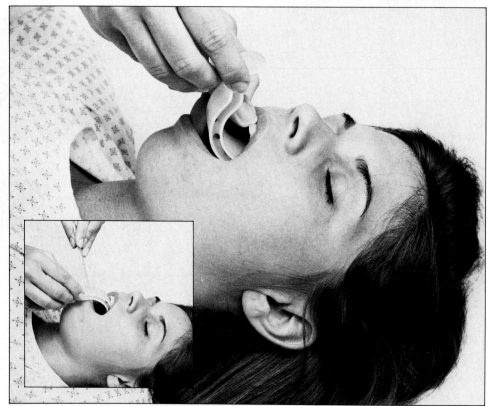

2 Now you're ready to insert the oropharyngeal airway. To make this easier, wet the airway with water to lubricate it. However, never use water-soluble lubricating jelly. It contributes to mucous build-up on the airway, and it may be aspirated.

For quick insertion, point the tip of the artificial airway toward the roof of your patient's mouth. When the tip of the airway has passed her uvula, rotate the airway 180° as you gently advance it into position.

If your patient gags, hold the airway in place for a few seconds until she relaxes. However, if she begins to vomit, turn her on her side immediately.

[Inset] Here's another insertion method, which works particularly well with infants: Hold your patient's tongue down with a tongue depressor, and guide the artificial airway over the back of it, as shown here.

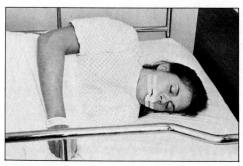

4 Turn the patient fully on her side for continued protection against aspiration.

Remove your patient's artificial airway when she's fully conscious and can swallow on her own. *Note:* If your patient tries to pull the airway out, she probably no longer needs it.

Or, if her condition hasn't stabilized, the doctor may order the oropharyngeal airway replaced with an endotracheal tube, for long-term intubation and mechanical ventilation.

To remove the airway, gently pull it out and down, following the mouth's natural curvature. *Important:* After removal, check your patient's gag and cough reflexes. If neither is present (and you're not going to insert an endotracheal tube), you've probably removed the airway prematurely. Reinsert it immediately.

Suctioning your patient's mouth and trachea

1 *To prevent accumulated secretions from obstructing your patient's air passages, suction first her mouth, then her trachea. Here's how:*
To begin the procedure, obtain two sterile suction kits, each of which includes a suction catheter, disposable basin, 4 oz. packet of sterile water, and a sterile glove. Also, obtain a sterile tongue depressor, two lengths of suction tubing, suction canister and regulator (not shown), and a hand-held resuscitator (not shown). If your catheter has no control valve, also obtain a sterile Y connector.
Ask another nurse to assist you. Wash your hands before proceeding.

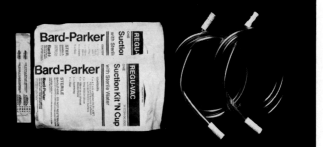

2 Explain the procedure to your patient. Position her in semi-Fowler's position, if possible. Or, if her condition requires it, keep her flat on her back.

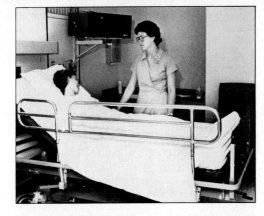

4 Now, open one suction kit. Slip a glove on the hand you'll be working with. Be sure to maintain strict aseptic technique throughout the procedure.

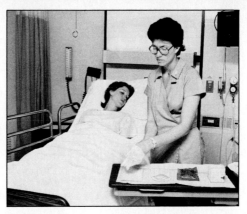

3 Next, attach one end of the suction tubing to the suction regulator.
[Inset] Attach the other end of the suction tubing to the suction canister you've mounted on the wall.

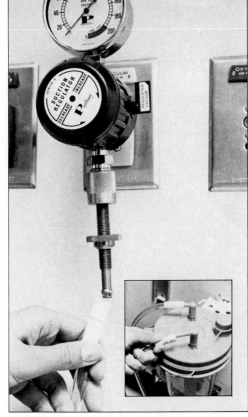

5 Then, open the sterile water and pour it into the basin.

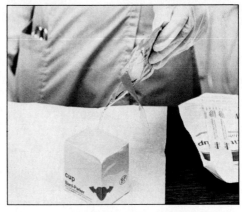

6 Next, use your gloved hand to pull the catheter from its wrapper.

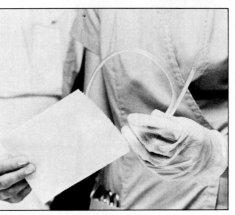

Airway management

Suctioning your patient's mouth and trachea

7 Now, you're ready to connect the catheter to the suction tubing. Continue to hold the catheter in your gloved hand as you do so.

[Inset] If the catheter lacks a control valve, first place a sterile Y connector on its distal end. Then, attach the Y connector to the suction tubing.

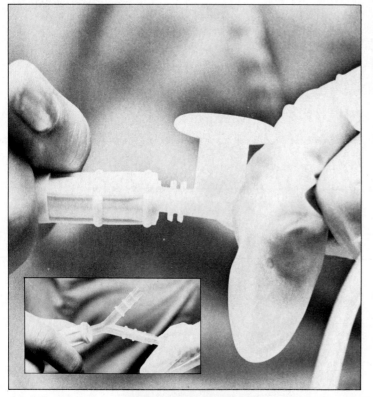

8 Prepare for suctioning by setting the suction regulator dial to 120 mm Hg. Turn on the suction regulator. Then, dip the catheter tip in sterile water to lubricate it.

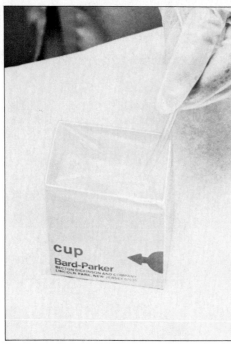

9 Now, have your assistant firmly depress your patient's tongue, so you can see better. This will also prevent the patient from biting the catheter. Begin suctioning, controlling it by intermittently covering the valve with your thumb.

[Inset] If you're using a Y connector, intermittently cover the open end with your thumb.

Nursing tip: You can also control suctioning by bending and pinching the catheter between your fingers.

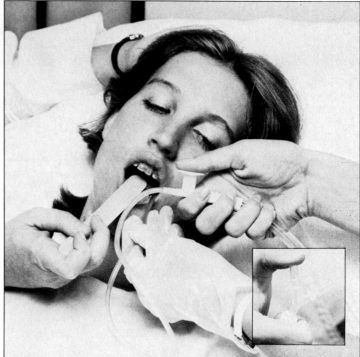

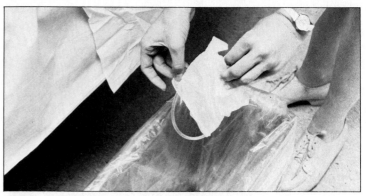

10 After you've suctioned your patient's mouth, dispose of the contaminated catheter and glove this way: Use your ungloved hand to pull the glove inside out and down over the catheter. Avoid touching your ungloved hand to either the outside of the glove or the catheter. Drop both into a wastebasket, as shown here.

Important: Never use the same catheter to suction both the mouth and trachea. Doing so may introduce oral bacteria into the patient's respiratory tract. Keep in mind that her defense mechanisms are already compromised.

Now you're ready to suction her trachea, using the second sterile suction kit.

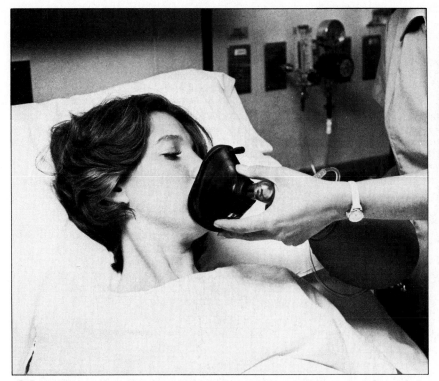

11 Before you begin, hyperventilate your patient with 100% oxygen, using a hand-held resuscitator with a reservoir (see the NURSING PHOTOBOOK PROVIDING RESPIRATORY CARE).

Now, open the second sterile kit, and put on the sterile glove. Open the sterile water packet and pour the sterile water into the basin. Connect the suction catheter to the suction tubing, as described in step 7. Lubricate the catheter by dipping the tip into the sterile water.

12 Now, you're ready to insert the catheter into your patient's trachea. Ask your assistant to hold down the patient's tongue with a tongue depressor. Gently insert the catheter through your patient's mouth into the trachea. If possible, have your patient take slow, deep breaths through her mouth as you advance the catheter as far as it will go (about 12" to 18"). Don't start suctioning yet. Instead, withdraw the catheter slightly (about 1 to 2 cm).

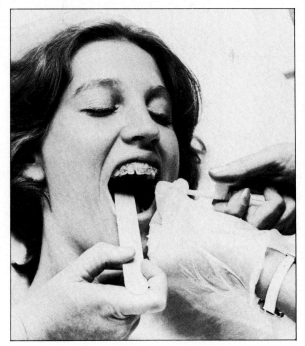

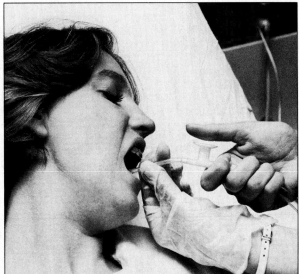

13 Now, turn your patient's head to one side, to facilitate suctioning of the main bronchus on the opposite side. To do this, you may need to remove the pillow from under your patient's head.

Begin suctioning the patient. To do so, completely withdraw the catheter with a twirling movement while you apply intermittent suction. Rinse the catheter with sterile water each time you reinsert it.

Note: Never plunge the catheter up and down rapidly, or you may traumatize the patient's tracheal mucosa.

Caution: To prevent hypoxia or possible cardiac arrest, never suction longer than 10 or 12 seconds at a time. If your patient is hypoxic, hyperventilate her with oxygen between suctioning.

Date/ Time	Vital signs	Notes
6/25/81	99-86-26	*Procedure explained to patient. Small amount of*
10:00 AM	130/74	*clear secretion suctioned from patient's*
		mouth. Moderate amount of thin yellow
		secretion suctioned tracheally. No foul odor
		or blood present in oral or tracheal
		secretions. Patient tolerated procedure
		well, with no cyanosis. Vital signs stable.
		—Kathleen S. Waring, RN

14 To ensure removal of all secretions, turn your patient's head to the opposite side and suction her. Finally, position her with her face forward and suction her.

When you've completed the procedure, instruct the patient to breathe deeply. Hyperventilate her with oxygen. Dispose of the catheter and glove as in step 10.

Finally, document the suctioning procedure in your nurses' notes. Record the amount, consistency, and color of the secretions; presence of blood in the secretions; and how the patient tolerated the procedure.

Airway management

How to tape an oral endotracheal tube

1 *Suppose the doctor decides to insert an oral endotracheal tube in your patient. To find out how to assist him, see the* NURSING PHOTOBOOK PROVIDING RESPIRATORY CARE. *Immediately after the tube's in place, tape it securely. We'll show you two taping methods here. For either, you may have another nurse assist you by holding the tube steady. (Change the tape at least every 24 hours or as needed.)*

First, wipe your patient's cheeks with a Skin-Prep® swab. Then, for the first taping method, cut two 6″ pieces of 1″ wide nonallergenic tape. Take one piece and wrap it around the tube, chevron style, leaving at least 2″ of tape at each end. Extend the tape ends upward, and press them to the patient's cheeks.

Using the same technique, wrap the tube with the second piece of tape. This time, extend the tape ends downward. When you're finished, the tape will make an X-shape across the patient's cheeks, as shown in the photo.

This method of taping holds the tube very securely, because it exerts equal stabilizing pressure from above and below.

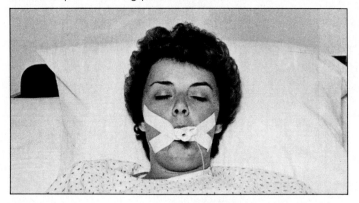

2 Here's the alternative taping method: After preparing your patient's skin, cut two 2″x2″ squares of nonallergenic tape. Press them in place on each of your patient's cheeks. Then, cut a 6″ long piece of 1″ wide nonallergenic tape. Leaving 2″ of tape at each end, wrap it once around the tube's end, chevron style.

This method of taping allows you to remove the tape around the endotracheal tube (when repositioning, for example), without irritating the patient's skin.

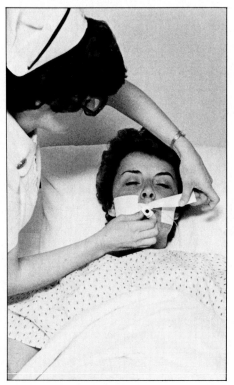

Suctioning your patient's endotracheal or trach tube

1 *If your patient has been intubated, she usually can't cough up her own secretions. And, if she's receiving oxygen or mechanical ventilation, the humidification will increase her secretions. Here's what to do to suction her:*

First, assemble the necessary equipment, listed on page 31. Explain the procedure to your patient and place her in semi-Fowler's position. Drape a towel across her chest. Prepare the suction device. Open your sterile suction kit.

Now, instill 5 ml of saline solution into the patient's endotracheal or trach tube. Doing this will thin and loosen the secretions, making suctioning easier.

Next, disconnect the wide-bore oxygen tubing attached to her endotracheal or trach tube, and lay the tubing on the towel. Hyperventilate her with a hand-held resuscitator. Then, reconnect the patient to the ventilator.

Note: If your patient's on a ventilator, check to see if her ventilator tubing has a flip-top port. If so, you can suction her without disconnecting the ventilator. If not, hyperventilate her before disconnecting it. Do this by increasing the oxygen concentration to 100% and depressing the manual sigh button on the ventilator. Next, reduce the oxygen level to its usual setting. Then, disconnect the ventilator tubing and lay it on the towel.

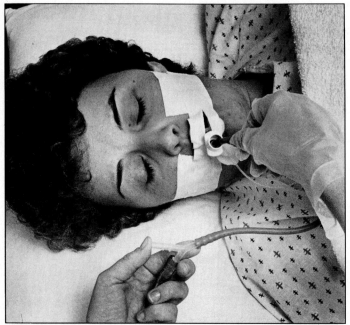

2 Next, put on the sterile glove. Then, fill the basin with the sterile water contained in the kit. Open the catheter and lubricate it as instructed on page 32. Disconnect the ventilator tubing, and lay it on the towel. Gently insert the suction catheter into the patient's endotracheal or trach tube. Proceed with suctioning. After each suction aspiration, hyperventilate the patient with a hand-held resuscitator. If necessary, suction her mouth and around the outside of the endotracheal tube. Don't forget to reconnect the wide-bore oxygen tubing or the ventilator to the endotracheal tube.

Important: After suctioning in or around the mouth, replace suction catheter with a new one if you need to suction through the endotracheal tube. Document the procedure in your nurses' notes.

Repositioning an oral endotracheal tube

1 *Does your patient have an oral endo-tracheal tube in place? You'll have to reposition it at least once every 4 hours to prevent mouth irritation.*

To do this, you may disconnect the ventilator or T tube. If you do so, rest the tubing on a towel on your patient's chest. Then, if your patient has an oropharyngeal airway in place as a bite block, untape the airway and temporarily remove it. Immerse the airway in a hydrogen peroxide solution. Next, insert a suction catheter into the patient's mouth, as shown in this photo. (For complete details on how to suction properly, using aseptic technique, see the preceding page and page 31.)

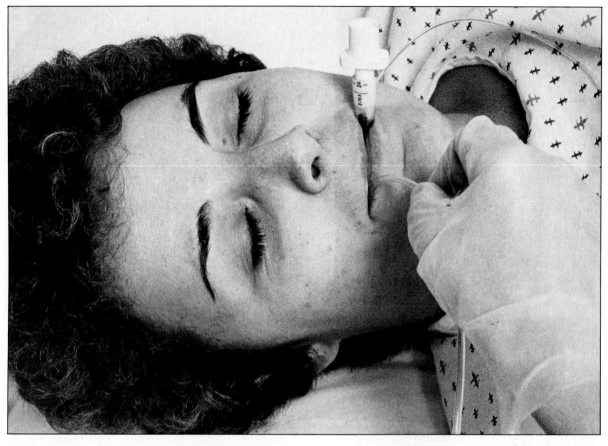

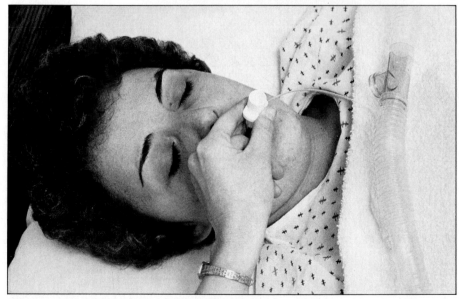

2 After you've suctioned one side of the patient's mouth, reposition the endotracheal tube, and suction the other side. But take care when you move the tube that you don't jostle the patient's trachea. You may also suction the patient's trachea at this time. When you've finished suctioning, perform mouth care (see the following page). *Note:* You may need to suction the patient once or twice each hour between regular repositioning times.

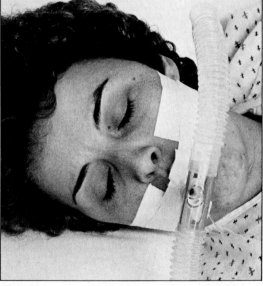

3 After performing mouth care, rinse the oro-pharyngeal airway with water and reinsert it. Retape the endotracheal tube and the airway. Then, reconnect the ventilator or T tube, if you've disconnected it. Document the care you've provided in your nurses' notes.

Airway management

Performing mouth care

Any patient with an artificial airway in place requires special mouth care. When you perform it, don't settle for simply applying mouthwash with a tongue depressor, or using lemon/glycerine swabs. Instead, brush the patient's teeth, using mouthwash or half-strength hydrogen peroxide solution. As you do so, suction any accumulating fluid.

After brushing his teeth, clean your patient's mouth and tongue by taping a gauze pad around a tongue depressor, dipping it in mouthwash, and wiping out the roof and sides of the patient's mouth. Also wipe his lips. Check his tongue and the roof of his mouth for the white patches that indicate monilia.

If the patient has monilial infection, the doctor will probably prescribe mycostatin suspension. To administer this medication, dip a cotton-tipped applicator into the suspension, and swab the patient's mouth and tongue.

However, use only a moderate amount of this solution, or you'll need to suction out the excess.

Now, swab his lips with glycerine swabs to lubricate them. Also, use acetone or nail polish remover to remove any tape marks from his face.

How to use an endotracheal tube holder

Instead of using an oropharyngeal airway as a bite block, you may substitute an endotracheal tube holder. As the illustration shows, the holder provides a protective sheath for the endotracheal tube. The holder's flange extends over the patient's lips.

Tape the tube holder and the tube together securely. Then attach the holder's cotton tie tapes to the flange covering the patient's lips, and tie the tapes behind the patient's head.

Important: Never use a holder if the patient has no teeth. The hard plastic may damage his gums.

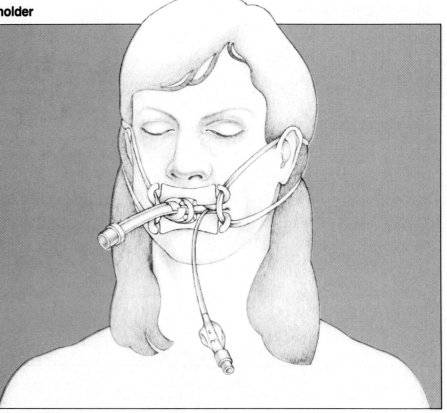

Removing an oral endotracheal tube

1 *Has the doctor ordered removal of your patient's oral endotracheal tube? If so, follow these steps:*

Place the patient in semi-Fowler's position. Then, wash your hands and explain the procedure to her. Next, suction inside the tube. To suction secretions that may have collected around the top of the tube's cuff, insert a catheter through the patient's nasopharynx and down into her trachea.

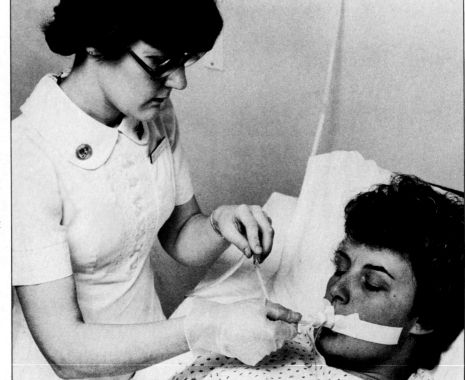

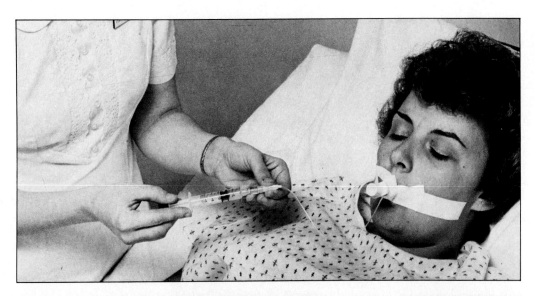

2 Now, you're ready to deflate the cuff. To do so, remove the needle from a syringe. Insert the tip of the syringe into the valve at the end of the cuff pillow. Draw back the plunger to remove all air from the cuff. Make sure the cuff pillow is flat. After you've deflated the cuff, suction the endotracheal tube again.

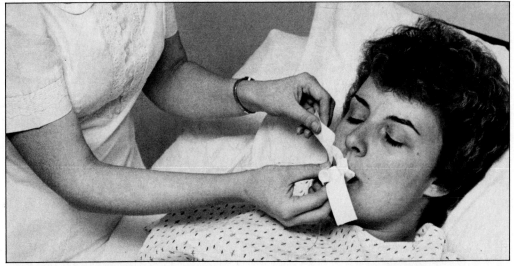

3 Then, with one hand, hold the end of the tube steady. With your other hand, remove the tape holding the tube in place.

Tell the patient that she should breathe deeply during the tube removal. Doing this will open her vocal cords and help prevent trauma.

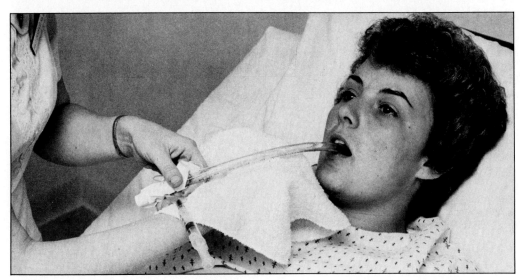

4 Now, you can remove the tube. To do so, hold a washcloth over the patient's chest, and pull the tube out in a smooth, slightly downward motion. Maneuver carefully, so you don't damage the patient's trachea. Give the patient an emesis basin if she needs it, because removing the tube may stimulate her gag reflex. Be prepared to suction her, if necessary.

Immediately after you remove the tube, give the patient humidified oxygen by face mask, at the prescribed flow rate. Help her to cough and deep-breathe. Let her expectorate. Then, perform mouth care, as instructed on the preceding page. Don't forget to remove the tape marks from her cheeks.

Document the procedure.

Airway management

Performing daily tracheostomy care

1 *Any patient who has a trach tube requires trach care at least once every 8 hours. By providing this care, you'll keep her artificial airway patent and help prevent infection. Remember, always use aseptic technique when performing trach care for an ICU patient. (In this story, the patient has a Shiley [double-cannula] trach tube.)*

First, assemble the equipment you'll need. Obtain a tracheostomy care kit, including two basins, trach bib, test tube brush, cotton-tipped applicators, pipe cleaners, forceps, sterile 4"x4" gauze pads, sterile gloves, and trach ties (not shown). In addition, you'll need a suction catheter and tubing, hydrogen peroxide solution, sterile water or normal saline solution, and a towel (not shown). If your patient's using a ventilator, also obtain an extra trach cannula. *Important:* Always keep a duplicate trach set handy for possible emergency trach tube reinsertion.

Wash your hands thoroughly. Explain the trach cleaning procedure to the patient.

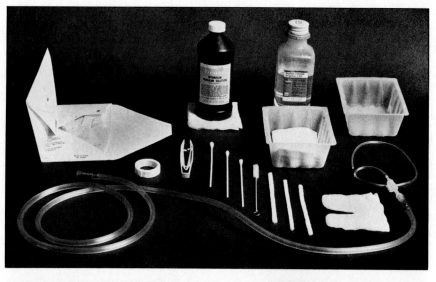

2 Open the kit, without contaminating the contents. Then, remove the caps from the solution bottles. To maintain sterility, upend the caps.

Slip on one glove, touching only its inside surface. With your gloved hand, separate the basins and place them side by side on the work surface. With your ungloved hand, pour hydrogen peroxide solution into the basin nearest the patient. Pour the water or saline solution into the other basin. Replace the bottle caps with your ungloved hand.

🔊 *Nursing tip:* To differentiate the water or saline solution from the hydrogen peroxide after you've poured it, you may place a sterile gauze pad in the water or saline solution basin (using your gloved hand).

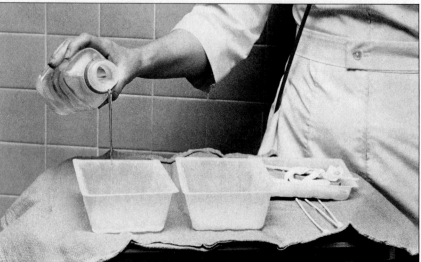

3 Now you're ready to suction the patient's trach tube to clear her airway of secretions. *Note:* Hyperventilate a mechanically ventilated patient with the machine's sigh mechanism. Then, disconnect the ventilator tubing, using your ungloved hand. Rest the tubing on a towel that you've placed on the patient's chest. (If your patient can't remain off the ventilator long enough for you to perform trach care, see the Special Considerations box on page 40.)

Suction the patient's trach tube, as instructed on page 34. Remember to hyperventilate her as necessary.

To clean the trach tube properly, you must remove its inner cannula. First, loosen the cannula with your ungloved hand. If your patient's trach tube locks in place, turn the inner cannula counterclockwise to unlock it. But don't pull it out yet. *Note:* If the patient's tracheostomy bib is soiled, remove it with your ungloved hand and discard it. If it's still clean, you may leave it in place to protect the patient's skin.

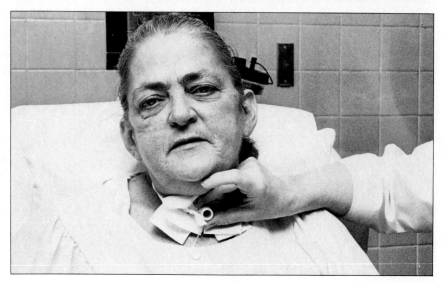

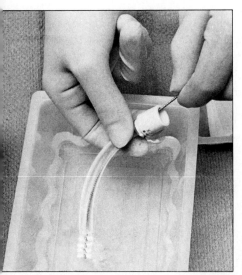

4 Now, slip on the second glove. Then, remove the loosened inner cannula by pulling it down and out.

Next, immerse the cannula in the hydrogen peroxide solution. You'll see foaming as the solution reacts to the secretions coating the cannula. Use the test tube brush to swab out the cannula. But don't force the brush. If you can't slide the brush in easily, use a pipe cleaner instead.

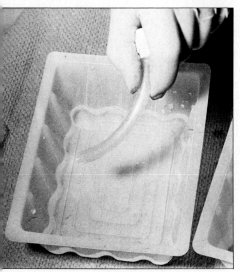

5 Now, drain the hydrogen peroxide from the clean cannula. Immerse the cannula in the sterile water or saline solution, and agitate it for about 10 seconds. Then, remove it from the basin and shake off the excess solution. Don't dry the cannula; the moisture helps ease reinsertion.

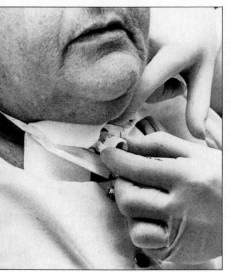

6 Now, you're ready to reinsert the cannula. As you insert it, keep the curved portion pointing down. With your free hand, hold the outer cannula steady to avoid jarring it. You don't want to irritate the patient's trachea and cause a coughing spasm. Then, lock the cannula securely in place by turning the hub clockwise.

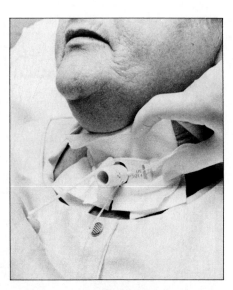

7 Now, clean the trach plate and outer cannula with a cotton-tipped swab dipped in hydrogen peroxide solution. *Caution:* Don't overload the swab with solution, or you might drip some down the patient's airway and trigger a coughing spasm.

When you've finished cleaning the trach plate and outer cannula, remove your gloves.

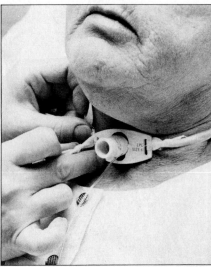

8 To replace the patient's trach ties, first remove the trach bib. Then, remove both ties from their wrapper.

An assistant may hold the trach plate steady as you slip the end of one tie through the trach plate. Using a square knot, tie it around the edge of the trach plate slot. Repeat the procedure with the other trach tie. Then, using another square knot, fasten both ties together on the side of the patient's neck (never in the back, or over the carotid artery).

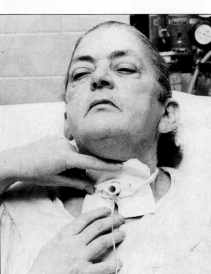

9 Finally, insert a new trach bib under the trach plate. *Note:* Always obtain a precut trach bib. Never simply cut a 4"x4" gauze dressing; the patient could aspirate lint from its frayed edges.

Use an adhesive strip to secure the bib to the plate's lower edge.

Nursing tip: If drainage is heavy, insert the bib from below to provide more absorption under the stoma.

Airway management

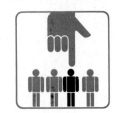

Trach care for the ventilator-dependent patient

What if your patient can't remain off the ventilator long enough for you to perform trach care? Follow this special procedure:

First, prepare the equipment as instructed in the preceding photostory. Then, hyperventilate the patient, using his ventilator's sigh mechanism. If his ventilator tubing has a flip-top port, you may suction him before disconnecting the tubing. Otherwise, disconnect the tubing and lay it on a towel on his chest. Then, suction the patient, hyperventilating him as necessary with a hand-held resuscitator. Working quickly, remove his inner cannula and replace it with a clean cannula from a trach set. Using 4"x4" sterile gauze pads to protect your gloves from contamination, immediately reconnect him to the ventilator. Proceed to clean the inner cannula, and store it in a sterile covered basin for future use. Then, clean the trach plate with hydrogen peroxide solution. Finally, remove your gloves and change the patient's trach ties and trach bib.

Reinserting a trach tube in an emergency

1 *Now you know how to perform daily trach care. But, do you know how to cope with a common trach tube emergency? Suppose your patient's trach ties are loose, and she coughs vigorously. She could completely dislodge her trach tube. For this reason, you should always keep a sterile replacement trach tube at the bedside. However, if you don't have one, reinsert the dislodged tube,* as we show here. Proceed as follows:

First, reassure the patient. Then, remove the inner cannula from the dislodged trach tube. Deflate the cuff. To do so, insert a syringe without a needle into the tube's pillow port. Withdraw all air.

[Inset] Take the obturator, which is usually taped to the head of the bed, and insert it into the trach tube's outer cannula.

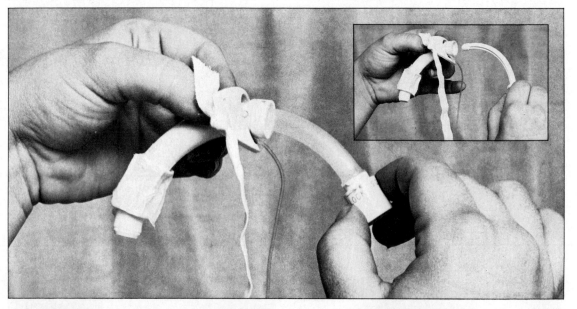

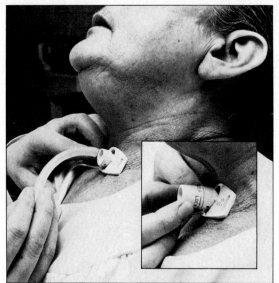

2 Then, reinsert the trach tube (with the obturator in place) into the patient's stoma. Hold the trach plate steady while you remove the obturator. Then, insert the inner cannula into the trach tube.

[Inset] Turn the inner cannula clockwise until it locks into place. Your patient will probably cough or gag while you're doing this, so hold onto the trach plate securely to prevent the tube from being dislodged again.

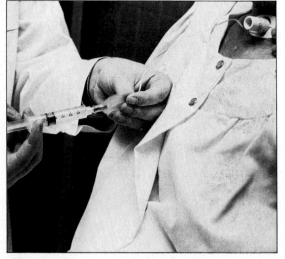

3 Now, using the same syringe without a needle, insert the tip of it into the tube's pillow port. Inflate the cuff.

Secure the trach ties and put a clean bib around the trach plate.

To complete the procedure, auscultate your patient's lungs to make sure she's getting air. Reassure her that she'll be able to breathe and tell her you've firmly secured her trach tube. When your patient's relaxed enough for you to leave, document the entire episode in your nurses' notes.

Coping with common endotracheal and trach tube problems

Your intubated patient may experience any of the following problems. Do you know how to solve them, and prevent their recurrence? The chart below will provide some helpful guidelines:

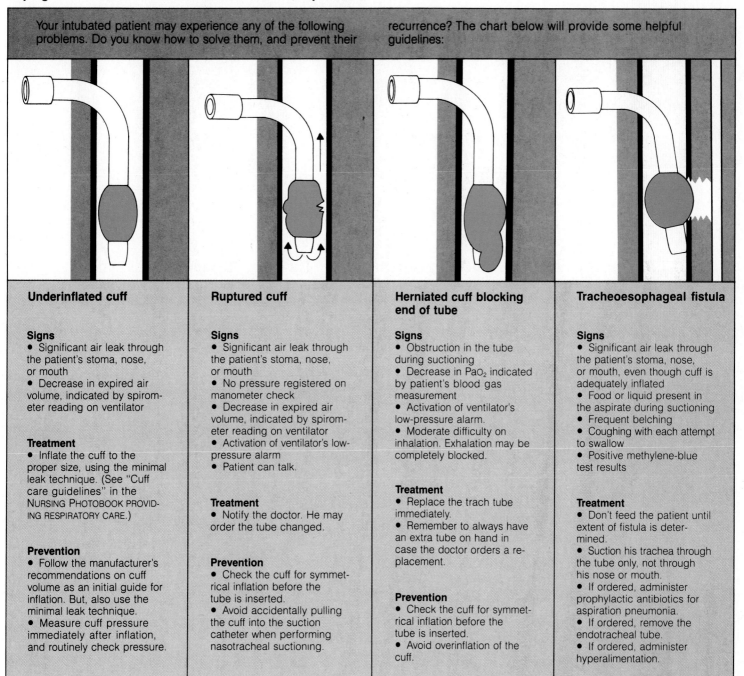

Underinflated cuff

Signs
• Significant air leak through the patient's stoma, nose, or mouth
• Decrease in expired air volume, indicated by spirometer reading on ventilator

Treatment
• Inflate the cuff to the proper size, using the minimal leak technique. (See "Cuff care guidelines" in the NURSING PHOTOBOOK PROVIDING RESPIRATORY CARE.)

Prevention
• Follow the manufacturer's recommendations on cuff volume as an initial guide for inflation. But, also use the minimal leak technique.
• Measure cuff pressure immediately after inflation, and routinely check pressure.

Ruptured cuff

Signs
• Significant air leak through the patient's stoma, nose, or mouth
• No pressure registered on manometer check
• Decrease in expired air volume, indicated by spirometer reading on ventilator
• Activation of ventilator's low-pressure alarm
• Patient can talk.

Treatment
• Notify the doctor. He may order the tube changed.

Prevention
• Check the cuff for symmetrical inflation before the tube is inserted.
• Avoid accidentally pulling the cuff into the suction catheter when performing nasotracheal suctioning.

Herniated cuff blocking end of tube

Signs
• Obstruction in the tube during suctioning
• Decrease in PaO_2 indicated by patient's blood gas measurement
• Activation of ventilator's low-pressure alarm.
• Moderate difficulty on inhalation. Exhalation may be completely blocked.

Treatment
• Replace the trach tube immediately.
• Remember to always have an extra tube on hand in case the doctor orders a replacement.

Prevention
• Check the cuff for symmetrical inflation before the tube is inserted.
• Avoid overinflation of the cuff.

Tracheoesophageal fistula

Signs
• Significant air leak through the patient's stoma, nose, or mouth, even though cuff is adequately inflated
• Food or liquid present in the aspirate during suctioning
• Frequent belching
• Coughing with each attempt to swallow
• Positive methylene-blue test results

Treatment
• Don't feed the patient until extent of fistula is determined.
• Suction his trachea through the tube only, not through his nose or mouth.
• If ordered, administer prophylactic antibiotics for aspiration pneumonia.
• If ordered, remove the endotracheal tube.
• If ordered, administer hyperalimentation.

Prevention
• Use a low-pressure cuff.
• Never overinflate the cuff; instead use the minimal leak technique.
• Exercise meticulous cuff care.
• Don't leave an oral endotracheal tube in place for extended periods of time.

Airway management

Coping with common endotracheal and trach tube problems continued

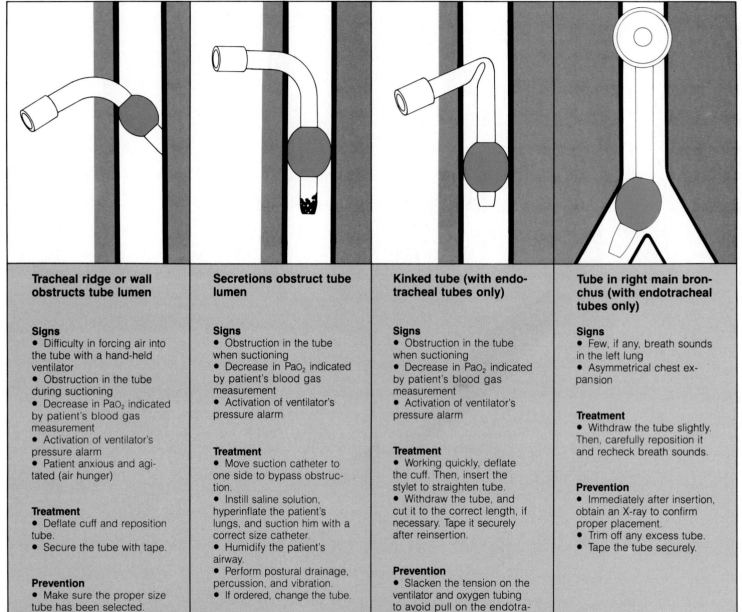

Tracheal ridge or wall obstructs tube lumen

Signs
- Difficulty in forcing air into the tube with a hand-held ventilator
- Obstruction in the tube during suctioning
- Decrease in PaO_2 indicated by patient's blood gas measurement
- Activation of ventilator's pressure alarm
- Patient anxious and agitated (air hunger)

Treatment
- Deflate cuff and reposition tube.
- Secure the tube with tape.

Prevention
- Make sure the proper size tube has been selected.
- Tape the tube securely.
- Tie the trach ties snugly.

Secretions obstruct tube lumen

Signs
- Obstruction in the tube when suctioning
- Decrease in PaO_2 indicated by patient's blood gas measurement
- Activation of ventilator's pressure alarm

Treatment
- Move suction catheter to one side to bypass obstruction.
- Instill saline solution, hyperinflate the patient's lungs, and suction him with a correct size catheter.
- Humidify the patient's airway.
- Perform postural drainage, percussion, and vibration.
- If ordered, change the tube.

Prevention
- As ordered, use humidified oxygen to keep secretions thin.
- If ordered, administer periodic cooled or heated aerosol treatments.
- Perform meticulous trach care.
- If ordered, administer forced fluids or I.V. therapy.

Kinked tube (with endotracheal tubes only)

Signs
- Obstruction in the tube when suctioning
- Decrease in PaO_2 indicated by patient's blood gas measurement
- Activation of ventilator's pressure alarm

Treatment
- Working quickly, deflate the cuff. Then, insert the stylet to straighten tube.
- Withdraw the tube, and cut it to the correct length, if necessary. Tape it securely after reinsertion.

Prevention
- Slacken the tension on the ventilator and oxygen tubing to avoid pull on the endotracheal tube.
- Make sure the proper size tube has been selected.

Tube in right main bronchus (with endotracheal tubes only)

Signs
- Few, if any, breath sounds in the left lung
- Asymmetrical chest expansion

Treatment
- Withdraw the tube slightly. Then, carefully reposition it and recheck breath sounds.

Prevention
- Immediately after insertion, obtain an X-ray to confirm proper placement.
- Trim off any excess tube.
- Tape the tube securely.

Respiratory support

As you know, proper oxygen delivery, mechanical ventilation, and thoracic drainage are three important elements of good respiratory support care. Do you understand the complex procedures and equipment involved in such care?

For example, do you feel confident about using a venturi mask? On the following pages, we'll explain how the mask works and how to use it to deliver exact oxygen concentrations.

Have you ever used a positive end-expiratory pressure (PEEP) attachment on your MA-1® ventilator? We'll tell you how and give you guidelines on caring for PEEP patients.

Does your patient need a chest tube? We'll show you how to connect it to a new type of underwater-seal drainage system.

You'll also find out how to deal with common ventilator complications and learn what the different ventilator alarms indicate. After reading these pages, you'll be better prepared to deal with your seriously ill respiratory patient.

Learning about the venturi mask

In a healthy person, or even a patient with an acute respiratory condition, hypercarbia triggers the breathing mechanism. But, in a patient with chronic obstructive pulmonary disease (COPD), hypoxia triggers the mechanism, because his body's accustomed to a low PaO_2 level.

So, if your COPD patient needs oxygen, you'll probably use a venturi mask to provide it (see photo below). Why? Because if your patient received excess oxygen, he might stop breathing altogether, since his brain's respiratory center responds only to low amounts of oxygen. But, a venturi mask can deliver an oxygen concentration as low as 24%, and accurate to within 1%. By using a low-oxygen concentration venturi mask, you can oxygenate your COPD patient safely.

How does the venturi mask work? It works through what's called the venturi effect, illustrated below. To explain, if a gas is flowing through a tube at a given flow rate, and the size of the tube decreases, the velocity of the gas increases to maintain the flow rate. As the velocity increases, the pressure exerted by the gas decreases.

To understand how this effect works in a venturi device, see the illustration below. As you can see, when oxygen flowing through a venturi apparatus enters a smaller tube (the jet adapter), the oxygen's speed increases. The faster it moves, the less pressure it exerts on the tube walls. This decreased pressure permits a certain amount of higher pressure room air to enter the apparatus through air entrainment ports. The room air dilutes the oxygen to the correct concentration. The larger the tube that the oxygen encounters, the less room air enters. Less room air means less oxygen dilution and a higher oxygen concentration.

The venturi mask delivers a fixed oxygen concentration as long as its total liter air flow exceeds the patient's peak inspiratory demand. This usually happens, because the mask takes in large enough amounts of room air to accommodate peak inspiratory demand. Also, since the entrainment ports are large, excess oxygen is vented, rather than increasing oxygen concentration above the desired level.

In spite of the accuracy of its oxygen delivery, the venturi mask has a few disadvantages:
• The entrainment ports may be occluded by bed linen, a gown, or the patient's body (depending on positioning).
• The mask precludes eating or talking.
• The mask prevents loss of body heat, causing facial sweating and skin irritation.
• High liter flow may dry out mucous membranes.

To find out how to use the Inspiron® venturi mask, including tips on avoiding or solving the problems listed, read the photostory on the next page.

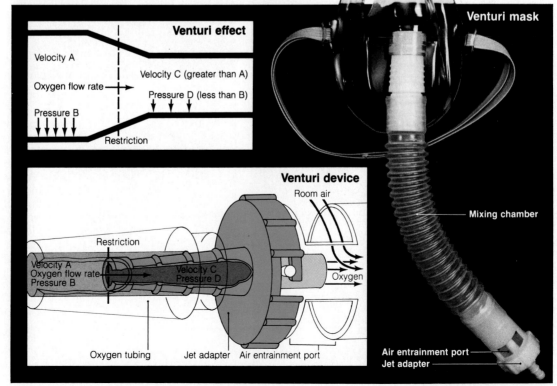

Venturi mask

Venturi effect

Velocity A

Oxygen flow rate →

Velocity C (greater than A)

Pressure D (less than B)

Pressure B

Restriction

Venturi device

Room air

Restriction

Velocity A
Oxygen flow rate
Pressure B

Velocity C
Pressure D

Oxygen

Oxygen tubing   Jet adapter   Air entrainment port

Mixing chamber

Air entrainment port
Jet adapter

Respiratory support

Using an Inspiron® venturi mask

1 *The Inspiron venturi mask is conveniently prepackaged, with wide-bore tubing, jet adapters, and an optional humidification adapter. The jet adapters are color-coded. Each color coincides with a specific liter flow of oxygen and an exact concentration of oxygen.*

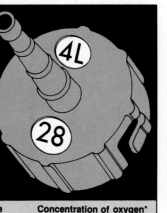

Color	Liters per minute	Concentration of oxygen*
Blue	4	24%
Yellow	4	28%
White	6	31%
Green	8	35%
Pink	8	40%

*Some companies supply venturi masks equipped with jet adapters that deliver oxygen concentrations up to 50%.

2 Now, here's how to use the venturi mask, which is illustrated in detail on the preceding page. First, attach the male adapter of the mask to the wide-bore tubing.

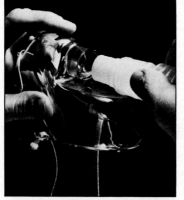

3 Select the prescribed jet adapter, and match the slots to the prongs on the entrainment collector. Push the jet adapter onto the entrainment collector, as shown here. Then, turn the jet adapter clockwise one half turn, locking it in place.

Nursing tip: Always keep the remaining jet adapters at the bedside. The doctor may prescribe a different oxygen concentration because of changes in the patient's blood gas measurements.

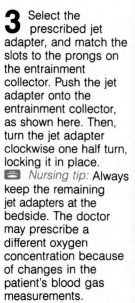

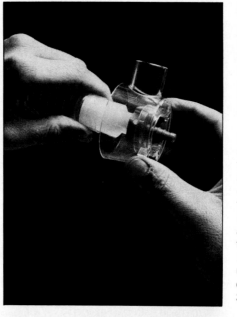

4 Some patients receive nonhumidified oxygen through the venturi mask. In such cases, attach one end of the oxygen tube to the jet adapter nipple, and twist it in place. Attach the other end of the oxygen tube to the nipple on the oxygen flowmeter.

For patients also requiring humidification, you'll need to attach a humidification adapter to the jet adapter before you attach the oxygen tube. To do this, grasp the wide-bore tubing and slip the humidification adapter over the jet adapter, as shown here. Keep the chimney straight up.

Remember: The doctor will usually order humidification if the oxygen concentration exceeds 30%.

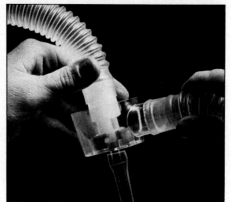

5 Connect one end of the wide-bore tube to the chimney of the humidification adapter, as the nurse is doing here. Connect the other end to the humidifier. Make sure the humidifier contains sterile or distilled water. Set the oxygen liter flow, referring to the code on the jet adapter. Flush the tubing with oxygen, and check it for air leaks. Be sure you see an adequate mist coming from the humidifier.

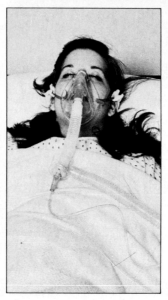

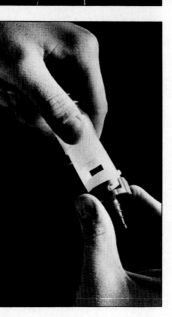

6 Place the venturi mask over the patient's nose and mouth. Slip the elastic strap around the back of her head, and position it above her ears. Prevent pressure sores by placing 4"x4" gauze pads under the strap where it touches her ears. Adjust the metal strip over her nose by pinching it into shape. The mask should fit snugly but not uncomfortably. Don't let the wide-bore tubing twist or kink. Also, don't let bed linen or the patient's body or gown cover the entrainment ports. Check the ports frequently to make sure they remain unobstructed.

Important: To prevent skin irritation, keep the patient's face dry and change her mask as needed.

Nursing tip: Keep a nasal cannula by the patient's bedside, for mealtime oxygen delivery. When you use it, set the cannula at a low flow rate and monitor the patient's blood gas measurements, if necessary.

Comparing pressure- and volume-cycled ventilators

Most ventilators are either pressure- or volume-cycled. This means that inspiration ends with delivery of a preset pressure or volume. A third ventilator type exists: the time-cycled ventilator, which ends inspiration after a preset time has elapsed. Use time-cycled ventilators primarily for infants.

The following chart compares pressure- and volume-cycled ventilators.

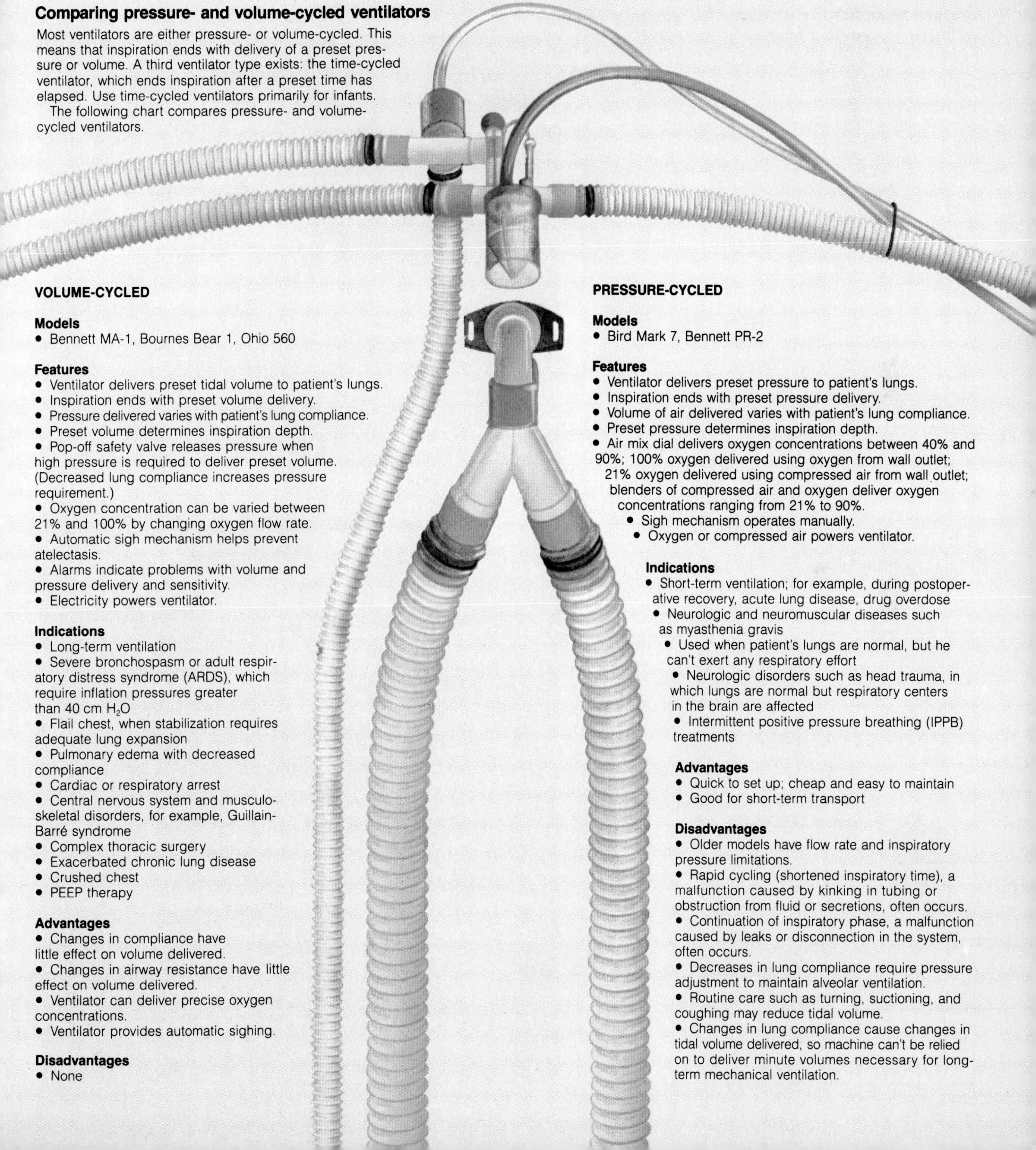

VOLUME-CYCLED

Models
- Bennett MA-1, Bournes Bear 1, Ohio 560

Features
- Ventilator delivers preset tidal volume to patient's lungs.
- Inspiration ends with preset volume delivery.
- Pressure delivered varies with patient's lung compliance.
- Preset volume determines inspiration depth.
- Pop-off safety valve releases pressure when high pressure is required to deliver preset volume. (Decreased lung compliance increases pressure requirement.)
- Oxygen concentration can be varied between 21% and 100% by changing oxygen flow rate.
- Automatic sigh mechanism helps prevent atelectasis.
- Alarms indicate problems with volume and pressure delivery and sensitivity.
- Electricity powers ventilator.

Indications
- Long-term ventilation
- Severe bronchospasm or adult respiratory distress syndrome (ARDS), which require inflation pressures greater than 40 cm H_2O
- Flail chest, when stabilization requires adequate lung expansion
- Pulmonary edema with decreased compliance
- Cardiac or respiratory arrest
- Central nervous system and musculo-skeletal disorders, for example, Guillain-Barré syndrome
- Complex thoracic surgery
- Exacerbated chronic lung disease
- Crushed chest
- PEEP therapy

Advantages
- Changes in compliance have little effect on volume delivered.
- Changes in airway resistance have little effect on volume delivered.
- Ventilator can deliver precise oxygen concentrations.
- Ventilator provides automatic sighing.

Disadvantages
- None

PRESSURE-CYCLED

Models
- Bird Mark 7, Bennett PR-2

Features
- Ventilator delivers preset pressure to patient's lungs.
- Inspiration ends with preset pressure delivery.
- Volume of air delivered varies with patient's lung compliance.
- Preset pressure determines inspiration depth.
- Air mix dial delivers oxygen concentrations between 40% and 90%; 100% oxygen delivered using oxygen from wall outlet; 21% oxygen delivered using compressed air from wall outlet; blenders of compressed air and oxygen deliver oxygen concentrations ranging from 21% to 90%.
- Sigh mechanism operates manually.
- Oxygen or compressed air powers ventilator.

Indications
- Short-term ventilation; for example, during postoperative recovery, acute lung disease, drug overdose
- Neurologic and neuromuscular diseases such as myasthenia gravis
- Used when patient's lungs are normal, but he can't exert any respiratory effort
- Neurologic disorders such as head trauma, in which lungs are normal but respiratory centers in the brain are affected
- Intermittent positive pressure breathing (IPPB) treatments

Advantages
- Quick to set up; cheap and easy to maintain
- Good for short-term transport

Disadvantages
- Older models have flow rate and inspiratory pressure limitations.
- Rapid cycling (shortened inspiratory time), a malfunction caused by kinking in tubing or obstruction from fluid or secretions, often occurs.
- Continuation of inspiratory phase, a malfunction caused by leaks or disconnection in the system, often occurs.
- Decreases in lung compliance require pressure adjustment to maintain alveolar ventilation.
- Routine care such as turning, suctioning, and coughing may reduce tidal volume.
- Changes in lung compliance cause changes in tidal volume delivered, so machine can't be relied on to deliver minute volumes necessary for long-term mechanical ventilation.

Respiratory support

Understanding positive end-expiratory pressure (PEEP)

As you know, a ventilator breathes for a patient who can no longer breathe for himself. But, did you know that the MA-1 ventilator has an attachment for improving a ventilated patient's gas exchange? It's called a positive end-expiratory pressure (PEEP) attachment, and it works by preventing air from being exhaled from the alveoli at the end of expiration. The alveoli then remain expanded longer, providing more surface area for oxygen diffusion into the blood.

You may wonder which patients benefit from this therapy. To find out, see the box below. As you read it, keep in mind that no matter which of these problems the patient has, the general indication for PEEP is the following: The patient can't maintain a PaO_2 above 50 mm Hg when he's receiving a 50% oxygen concentration. You'd avoid using a higher oxygen concentration to produce a higher PaO_2, because prolonged use of high oxygen concentrations can cause serious side effects. But with PEEP, you can keep the oxygen concentration low, yet still increase PaO_2, since you're keeping the alveoli open longer.

Before you initiate PEEP therapy, the doctor will probably order sedation for your patient. He'll do this because completely ventilator-controlled respiration best maintains the PEEP effect. The patient's own inspiratory effort could interfere with delivery of the preset PEEP pressure. To sedate the patient, the doctor will order a skeletal muscle relaxant, a tranquilizer, or both. However, in some cases, the doctor may choose to work with the assist or assist-control mode of ventilation, instead of sedating the patient.

The patient undergoing PEEP treatment must be carefully and continuously evaluated to determine whether the treatment's effective. If effective, the PEEP treatment will:
* increase the lung's functional residual capacity (FRC).
* increase lung compliance.
* reduce the imbalance between the amount of oxygen inspired and the amount perfused into the blood.
* improve arterial oxygenation. (However, PEEP will not reduce carbon dioxide levels in the blood.)

To find out how to use the PEEP attachment to deliver PEEP to your patient, read the photostory on the following page. *Note:* Some ventilators have a built-in PEEP mode.

For information on patient care during PEEP therapy, see the guidelines in the box on page 49.

INDICATIONS/CONTRAINDICATIONS

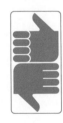

Who receives positive end-expiratory pressure (PEEP) therapy

You'll probably give PEEP therapy to the patient who has:
* adult respiratory distress syndrome (ARDS).
* reduced surfactant production from smoke inhalation, toxic lung damage, or hyaline membrane disease.

You'll rarely give PEEP therapy to a patient who has:
* bullous disorder of the lung.
* hypotension.
* pneumothorax.
* hypovolemia.
* chronic obstructive pulmonary disease (COPD).

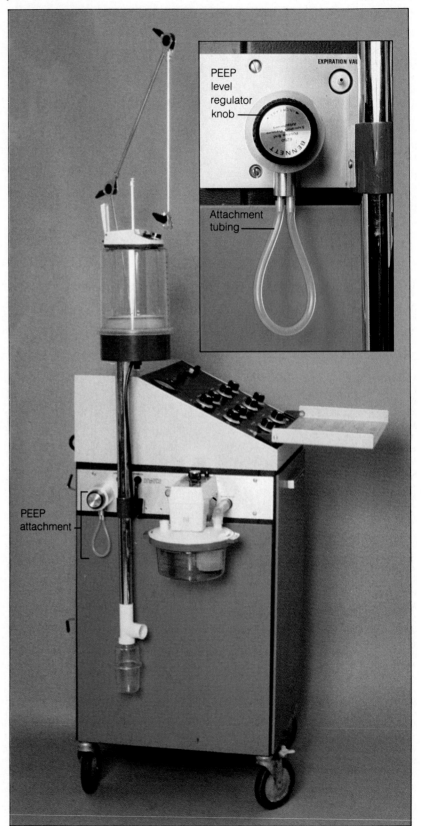

PEEP level regulator knob

EXPIRATION VAL

Attachment tubing

PEEP attachment

Using the MA-1 ventilator PEEP attachment

1 *How do you use the positive end-expiratory pressure (PEEP) attachment to administer PEEP to your patient?*

First, briefly explain to your patient how PEEP will affect his mechanical ventilation. Then, set up the ventilator for conventional ventilation. (For instructions, refer to the NURSING PHOTOBOOK PROVIDING RESPIRATORY CARE.)

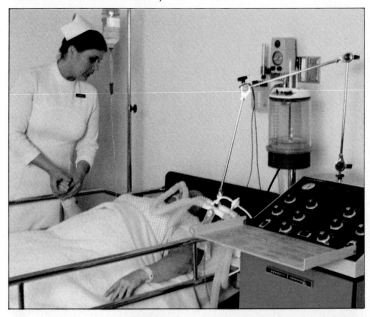

4 Then, remove the tubing from one of the outlet ports on the bottom of the PEEP attachment.

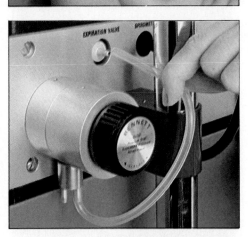

2 Attach the PEEP component to the side of the machine. To do this, first plug the attachment into the PEEP outlet.

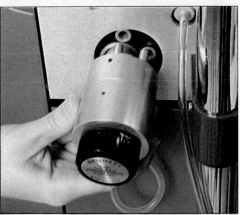

5 Take the end of this tubing and insert it into the expiration valve.

3 Next, remove the tubing from the expiration valve.

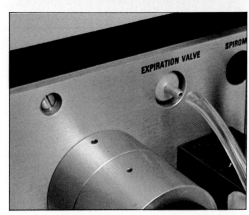

6 Attach the expiration valve tubing to the open outlet port on the bottom of the PEEP attachment.

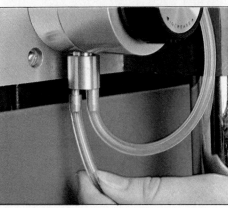

Respiratory support

Using the MA-1 ventilator PEEP attachment continued

7 Now, adjust the machine by setting the prescribed volume, rate, and pressure limit. Be sure to adjust the mode to assist-control ventilation, unless the doctor specifically orders otherwise.

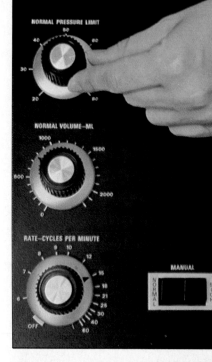

9 If the manometer ever reads zero after expiration, the patient's not receiving PEEP. If this happens when you're initiating PEEP, continue to gradually turn the dial counter-clockwise until the correct level registers on expiration. If it happens during PEEP treatment, check for leaks or a disconnection, like the one shown here.

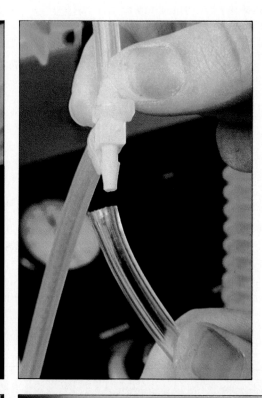

8 To set the required PEEP level, turn the uncalibrated knob on the PEEP attachment clockwise, while observing the pressure manometer on the left top corner of the machine's control panel (see inset). Usually, the doctor will order less than 15 cm H_2O pressure, the maximum deliverable by the attachment shown here. Adjust the dial in small increments until the manometer gives the correct reading after expiration. Be sure to turn the dial gradually.

Important: Never adjust the dial more than 2 cm H_2O at a time.

Note: Although the manometer will give a higher reading during inspiration, the reading after expiration should equal the PEEP level. Remember, PEEP keeps the alveoli open after expiration.

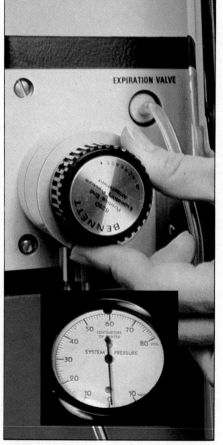

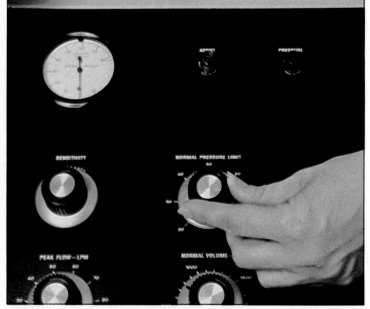

10 The pressure alarm may sound as you increase the PEEP level. If the alarm sounds, adjust the ventilator's pressure limit setting upward to accommodate the reading on the manometer. (Keep in mind that more pressure's required to maintain PEEP volume in the lungs than to deliver a tidal volume for non-PEEP ventilation.) Reset pressure limit to 10 cm H_2O above average pressure required to deliver ventilation with PEEP. If alarm rings again, don't simply reset the limit. Instead, follow steps indicated on the warning signals chart on page 50. This time, the problem may be with your patient. If so, he'll need immediate attention.

How to care for your patient receiving PEEP therapy

After connecting your patient to a positive end-expiratory pressure (PEEP) system, follow these guidelines:

• Take vital signs before and after you begin PEEP treatment; any time you change the PEEP level; and 15 and 30 minutes after a change. Be especially careful to watch for hypotension or tachycardia. Since PEEP impedes venous return to the heart, the resulting decrease in cardiac output may cause these complications.

• Monitor urinary output for a decrease, which may indicate hypovolemia, another result of reduced cardiac output.

Note: Hypovolemia must always be corrected before a patient begins PEEP therapy, because PEEP may aggravate his condition. At PEEP pressures higher than 10 to 15 cm H_2O, the doctor may order a pulmonary artery catheter inserted, for early detection of hypovolemia.

• Monitor your patient for signs of increasing intracranial pressure, a possible PEEP complication caused by decreased venous return. Signs include confusion or other changes in consciousness level, papilledema, decreased blood pressure, elevated temperature, and sensory and motor dysfunction.

• Monitor the patient for hypervolemia by checking for edema and increased blood pressure, pulse, and respiratory rate. An increase in antidiuretic hormone (ADH), which PEEP produces in some patients, may cause hypervolemia. If ordered, administer diuretics to counteract the effects of ADH.

• Auscultate the patient's lungs and immediately report to the doctor any change in breath sounds. Check carefully for the sounds that indicate pneumothorax, a common PEEP complication.

• Draw blood for arterial blood gas measurements, as ordered. Obtain a venous oxygen measurement periodically. This measurement indicates tissue oxygenation and cardiac output.

• Monitor the manometer gauge closely to be sure the patient's receiving the prescribed PEEP levels.

• Check the pressure alarm frequently to make sure it's set correctly and operating properly.

Learning about continuous positive airway pressure (CPAP)

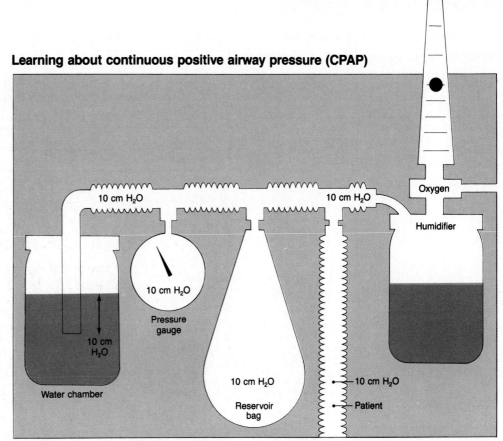

For a patient who can breathe on his own, but needs improved oxygen perfusion, a mode of ventilatory assistance similar to PEEP exists. It's called continuous positive airway pressure (CPAP). With this form of ventilatory assistance, the patient remains off a ventilator. Instead, he's connected to an oxygen delivery system that maintains continuous positive pressure in the alveoli, even after expiration.

CPAP therapy effectively treats the same conditions PEEP therapy treats. (See the Indications/contraindications box on page 46.) The general indication for CPAP is the same as for PEEP: The patient can't maintain a PaO_2 above 50 mm Hg on an oxygen concentration of 50%. Usually, the doctor will order CPAP therapy attempted before initiating PEEP therapy (providing the patient can breathe on his own.)

As the illustration shows, the CPAP system includes an oxygen/air source, a humidifier, a reservoir bag, a water chamber, and a pressure gauge, all of which are connected by flexible corrugated tubing. Oxygen and air flow from the wall unit to the patient. The reservoir bag retains extra oxygen for rebreathing, to guarantee the patient an adequate oxygen concentration. At the opposite end of the system, the tubing's immersed in water in the water chamber. The depth of the water around the tubing determines the level of pressure in the system. For example, if 10 cm H_2O pressure is required, the

water will be 10 cm deep. The system vents air and oxygen by bubbling it through the water. But a continuous replacement inflow helps preserve the positive pressure level. The pressure gauge monitors the system to ensure that the patient's actually receiving the desired level of CPAP.

Equipment set-ups vary, depending on specific use. Some may require a humidifier that can be heated. CPAP is usually delivered through an endotracheal tube.

When you administer CPAP treatment, gradually apply pressure increments of 2 to 5 cm H_2O by adding water to the water chamber, until the prescribed level's reached. At this level (usually 10 cm H_2O) the patient should be adequately oxygenated when he's receiving an oxygen concentration of 50% or less.

Successful CPAP therapy has the same effects as PEEP: arterial oxygenation improves, functional residual capacity (FRC) increases, and lung compliance increases. CPAP's advantage over PEEP is a reduced chance of barotrauma and other complications associated with mechanical ventilation (see the complications chart on page 51). But, if CPAP doesn't work effectively, or the patient develops breathing difficulties, the doctor will probably replace CPAP with PEEP therapy.

To wean your patient from CPAP, follow the same procedure you'd use for PEEP, as explained on page 53.

Respiratory support

TROUBLESHOOTING

Ventilator warning signals: How to respond

Signals	Problem	Cause	Nursing considerations
Pressure alarm sounds when delivery of preset volume requires higher pressures than pressure limit permits.	• Airway obstruction	• Secretions	• Suction the patient, instilling saline solution to loosen secretions.
		• Kink in tubes	• Straighten tubes and provide support for them.
		• Endotracheal or trach tube out of position	• Reposition tube.
	• High resistance	• Secretions	• Suction the secretions. • Provide chest physiotherapy.
		• Bronchospasm	• Administer bronchodilators, as ordered. • Decrease flow rate and tidal volume.
		• Water from humidifier in ventilator tubing	• Drain the water. • Check to see if water temperature's higher than 36° C.
	• Decrease in compliance	• Pulmonary edema	• Administer diuretics and restrict fluids, as ordered.
		• Adult respiratory distress syndrome (ARDS)	• Doctor will probably order continuous positive airway pressure (CPAP) or positive end-expiratory pressure (PEEP).
		• Pneumothorax	• Doctor will insert chest tubes.
		• Pneumonia	• Administer antibiotics, as ordered. • Give fluids, as ordered. • Provide chest physiotherapy.
	• Patient fighting ventilator	• Hypoxia	• Inspect patient for symptoms of hypoxia, such as confusion, dyspnea, cyanosis, and tachycardia. • Draw arterial blood to obtain arterial blood gas measurements. If ABG measurements indicate hypoxia, notify doctor so he can adjust the oxygen concentration order. • Suction patient and hyperinflate his lungs, as needed.
		• Fear, anxiety	• Ask patient if he feels he's getting enough air. • To make sure the patient's not actually hypoxic, inspect him for hypoxia symptoms. If inspection indicates hypoxia, draw arterial blood for blood gas measurements. • Try to calm patient. Give him writing materials so he can communicate. Give sedative or muscle relaxants, if ordered.
		• Improvement in patient's condition	• Begin weaning when ordered by doctor. • Adjust sensitivity setting, as needed.
Spirometer alarm sounds when tidal volume is less than preset volume.	• Leak or disconnection	• Loose connection in tubing, nebulizer, humidifier, endotracheal tube, or trach tube	• Carefully check each connection in system. • Reconnect tubing if it's loose. • Be sure humidifier or nebulizer lids fit tightly. • Check to see that the spirometer's rubber seal fits tightly.
		• Cuff insufficiently inflated	• Deflate cuff and inflate again. If cuff won't seal and patient's still not getting prescribed tidal volume, call the doctor. Use a hand-held resuscitator to ventilate patient's lungs until a new tube can be inserted.
	• Defect in spirometer action	• Water or dirt in spirometer	• Dry or clean the spirometer.
		• Spirometer incorrectly attached	• Check the manufacturer's instructions.
		• Defective spirometer	• Check position of diaphragm on the spirometer's base. • Check dump valve (black tube) fit on spirometer base. • Replace the spirometer, if necessary.
		• Tubing support arm leaning on dipstick, interfering with bellows movement	• Readjust arm so that it clears the dipstick.
	• Power interruption	• Faulty electrical connection	• Check circuit breaker. • Check whether plug's firmly in wall outlet.
Oxygen light activates because of incorrect oxygen concentration	• Oxygen not connected to ventilator	• Disconnection or failure to connect properly	• Connect ventilator tubing to oxygen outlet.
	• Dirty oxygen filter or dirty air intake filter	• Improper maintenance	• Remove filter, clean with warm, soapy water, and dry.

Coping with mechanical ventilation complications

Problem	Signs and symptoms	Treatment	Prevention
Barotrauma: Takes the form of pneumothorax, subcutaneous emphysema, or mediastinal emphysema. Usually caused when volume and pressure settings are too high or during administration of positive end-expiratory pressure (PEEP).	Sudden cyanosis; sudden drop in blood pressure; sudden decrease in lung compliance; increased anxiety. With pneumothorax, patient may have absent or diminished breath sounds over affected lung segment, acute pain on affected side, and trachea deviated away from pneumothorax. With subcutaneous emphysema, patient may have crepitus of face, abdomen, and extremities. With mediastinal emphysema, patient shows signs of reduced cardiac output and of crepitus over heart area.	• Call doctor immediately; he may insert chest tubes.	• Avoid high-pressure settings for high-risk patients; for example, those with chronic obstructive pulmonary disease (COPD), emphysematous blebs, or pulmonary scar tissue.
Atelectasis: Caused by insufficient deep breathing, pneumothorax, secretion retention, or a combination of these	Transient fine rales; diminished breath sounds over affected lung segment; bronchial sounds over peripheral lung fields; decreased compliance; possible change in arterial blood gas (ABG) values	• Turn patient frequently. • Suction and hyperinflate patient's lungs periodically. • Use intermittent sighing. • Perform chest physiotherapy, as ordered. • Doctor may order bronchoscopy.	• Change patient's position every 1 to 2 hours and maintain good body alignment. • Give chest physiotherapy, and maintain good pulmonary hygiene. • Doctor may order PEEP. • Suction the patient, as needed. • Remember to sigh patient frequently. • Monitor the patient closely.
Cardiovascular impairment: Caused when positive intrathoracic pressure reduces venous return to heart's right side and compresses pulmonary blood circulation	Decreased blood pressure and cardiac output; possible decreased urinary output; increased central venous pressure and pulmonary artery pressure; increased heart rate	• Doctor may reduce intrathoracic pressure by decreasing PEEP, inspiratory flow rate, or tidal volume. • Doctor may order increased I.V. fluids or administration of plasma expanders such as albumin or colloidal substances.	• Monitor PaO_2 closely. It should not fall below 70 mm Hg. • Use PEEP only when necessary. • Shorten inspiration time to less than one half expiration time. • Maintain adequate blood volume.
Gastrointestinal complications such as GI bleeding, gastric distention, paralytic ileus, and stress ulcer: Caused by stress or swallowing air	Abdominal distention; steady decrease in hemoglobin and hematocrit measurement; positive hematest results on nasogastric drainage and stool; tarry stool	• As ordered, insert nasogastric tube for drainage. • Replace lost blood. • Use nasogastric tube to give antacids or other medication to decrease acid production.	• Avoid giving excessive positive pressure. • Reduce patient's psychological stress. • Give antacids and other medications to reduce acid production, as ordered.
Acid-base and fluid and electrolyte imbalance: Caused by positive water balance created by secretion of antidiuretic hormone (ADH). Also caused by reduced insensible losses from respiratory tract.	Probable change in blood gas measurements; decreased vital capacity; weight gain; ankle edema; moist rales in lungs' lower lobes; pulmonary edema confirmed by X-ray	• Doctor may restrict fluid intake and order diuretics. • Treat the patient for congestive heart failure (CHF), as ordered. • Apply rotating tourniquets to control pulmonary edema, as ordered. • Correct acid-base imbalance, as ordered. • Correct electrolyte imbalance, as ordered.	• Periodically obtain blood samples for ABG and electrolyte measurements. Monitor patient for hyperventilation or hypoventilation. • Monitor patient's fluid intake and output. • Weigh patient daily.
Tracheal trauma: Caused by constant pressure of cuffed endotracheal tube or nasal endotracheal tube on the patient's trachea	Decreased tidal volume from air leak; bleeding from trachea	• Depending on damage, the doctor may insert a new trach tube to change cuff's position and allow injured area to heal. • Give meticulous cuff care, using minimal leak technique, until tube can be removed.	• Give patient proper cuff care, using minimal leak technique when possible. • Doctor should use endotracheal or trach tubes with soft cuffs.
Respiratory infection: Caused when upper airway is bypassed, eliminating body's natural defense mechanisms against infection. Also caused by poor aseptic technique.	Elevated temperature and white blood cell count (WBC); increased amount of respiratory secretions, and change in their color and odor	• Notify doctor. • Change patient's position frequently and perform chest physiotherapy. • Use aseptic technique for trach care and for suctioning. • Administer prescribed antibiotics.	• Maintain good pulmonary hygiene by using aseptic technique and sterile equipment, changing ventilator tubing every 24 hours, and suctioning patient and hyperinflating his lungs as needed. • Turn patient frequently. • Perform chest physiotherapy. • Filter all inspired gas.
Oxygen toxicity: Caused by excessively high concentrations of oxygen (over 60%) administered over prolonged period (8 hours or more). May cause fibrotic tissue changes in lungs, possibly leading to death.	Retrosternal pain; sore throat; nasal congestion; burning chest pain on inspiration; dry, hacking cough; dyspnea; decreased compliance; decreased PaO_2 on the same oxygen concentration; decreased vital capacity; and X-ray changes	• Monitor oxygen levels carefully. Report signs of oxygen toxicosis immediately.	• Maintain good pulmonary hygiene so low oxygen concentrations are adequate. • Reduce oxygen concentrations as soon as possible. • Use PEEP to reduce oxygen concentration level, as ordered.

Respiratory support

Weaning: Determining the proper time

How long will your patient need mechanical ventilation? That decision rests with the doctor. But he'll need your assessment to help him determine when the patient's ready for weaning. To make an accurate assessment, check the patient's condition. Make sure you document all your observations in your nurses' notes.

You'll know your patient's ready if:
• the underlying disease process has been successfully controlled.
• he's awake, has good muscle strength, and has either an adequate natural airway or a functioning tracheostomy.
• he has a normal body temperature. (If his temperature's elevated, his oxygen requirements increase.)
• he has no life-threatening cardiac arrhythmias and requires little or no vasopressor medication.
• he can cough effectively enough to loosen and expel secretions.
• auscultation and X-ray reveal a reasonably clear chest.
• blood gas analysis shows that his PaO_2 is greater than 60 mm Hg when he's receiving less than 30% oxygen. Both $PaCO_2$ and pH should be within the normal range. However, blood gas measurements of a chronic obstructive pulmonary disease (COPD) patient need not be normal, but only typical for him in his chronic state. His $PaCO_2$ will probably be higher and his PaO_2 lower than those measurements for a non-COPD patient whose disease has been successfully controlled.
• his respiratory rate's less than or equal to 30 respirations per minute.
• he shows no symptoms of hypoxia or hypercarbia, such as confusion, dyspnea, cyanosis, or tachycardia.
• pulmonary function tests indicate: dead space to tidal volume ratio less than 0.55; vital capacity greater than 10-15 ml/kg of body weight and twice the spontaneous tidal volume; negative inspiratory pressure greater than 20 cm H_2O; respiratory minute volume (the volume that the patient inspires in one minute of breathing) less than 10 l/minute; $A-aDO_2$ gradient less than 350 mm Hg.

Weaning your patient from a ventilator

After the doctor has decided your patient can be weaned from the ventilator, you'll have to prepare her for what's ahead. Set up a weaning schedule that fits into the patient's daily routine. Take care not to schedule weaning periods when the patient may be fatigued from a bath or an X-ray examination, or immediately after a meal.

ment. Before each weaning period, draw arterial blood to obtain arterial blood gas (ABG) measurements. Suction the patient to clear her airways, and hyperinflate her lungs to expand the alveoli. Measure and record her tidal volume, vital capacity, and vital signs. Keep suctioning, oxygen-delivery, and ABG sampling equipment at the bedside.

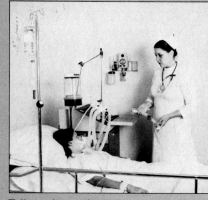

Talk to the patient
Consider her emotions. If she's been using a ventilator for a long time, she'll probably be afraid to leave it. To alleviate her fears, explain how weaning will help her breathe independently again. Tell her that you'll watch her carefully and will keep the ventilator nearby in case of trouble.

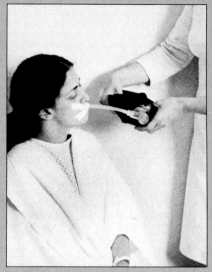

Initiate weaning from mechanical ventilation
Initiate weaning with one of the three weaning techniques discussed on page 54, according to doctor's orders. During the first few weaning periods, stay with your patient and offer her encouragement. Record her vital signs every 15 minutes at first, and then every half hour (provided she is showing signs of successful adjustment). When necessary, suction your patient and hyperinflate her lungs. However, don't do this immediately before you draw an arterial blood sample. Obtain the sample first, so you're sure of an accurate ABG measurement.

Nursing tip: If your patient has copious secretions, suction her, wait 20 minutes, and then draw arterial blood for ABG measurements. Otherwise her secretions may block her airway. The resulting hypoxia will affect her measurements.

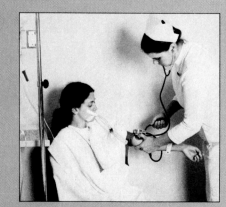

Prepare the patient physically
If possible, seat her in a chair to allow good chest and lung expansion. Or, raise her head as high as possible. Make sure she's in good body align-

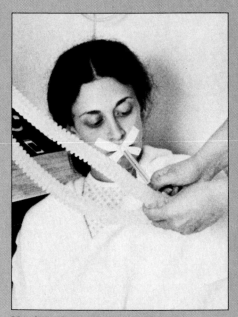

Monitor the patient closely
Watch for these signs of respiratory distress: labored breathing, increased respiratory rate, restlessness, confusion, blood pressure changes, tremors, tachycardia, or cardiac arrhythmias. If respiratory distress occurs, draw a sample of the patient's arterial blood immediately, and send it to the lab for ABG analysis. Reconnect the patient to the ventilator. Don't wait for a doctor's order to do so; call him afterward. Document the entire episode in your nurses' notes.

Your patient may also need to be reconnected to a ventilator if she complains that her chest muscles aren't working well. She could have diaphragm-intercostal muscle discoordination, a common problem for patients who've been on long-term mechanical ventilation. After you've reconnected the patient, notify the doctor. He'll probably want you to wean the patient using intermittent mandatory ventilation (IMV). This method allows for the gradual return of muscle coordination. (For information about IMV, see the following page.)

Remember, the weaning period may take as long as 3 weeks. Seeing the patient through will require much patience and encouragement on your part.

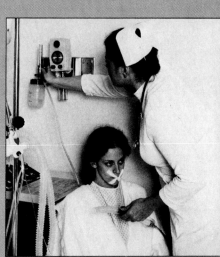

Wean the patient from oxygen
To wean her from oxygen, decrease the percentage she's receiving until she's breathing room air (21% oxygen), but maintaining a normal (or typical) PaO_2.

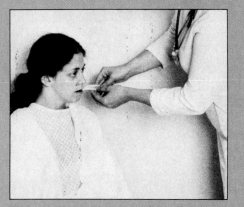

Remove the patient's endotracheal or trach tube
Do so after she's been off the ventilator for about 24 to 48 hours, as ordered. But first make sure she can cough up her own secretions and continues to breathe well on her own. If she can't do either because her secretions are copious and thick, leave the tube in place until her secretions have decreased.

Wean a patient with a tracheostomy in place by inserting an increasingly smaller-lumen trach tube each day. The stoma will begin to shrink, and eventually it will close completely as the patient resumes normal mouth and nose breathing.

Weaning your patient from positive end-expiratory pressure (PEEP)

If your patient's using PEEP, you must wean him from it before you can wean him from mechanical ventilation. If he's receiving a high level of PEEP, and a high oxygen concentration, gradually reduce the oxygen concentration to about 30%. Then, gradually decrease the PEEP level 2 cm H_2O. Continue to reduce the oxygen concentration and the PEEP level alternately. Never decrease them at the same time, because a decrease in PEEP level automatically results in a decrease in your patient's PaO_2. As you reduce PEEP levels, monitor the patient's vital signs carefully for increased cardiac output. (The increasing venous return from reduced PEEP levels could cause congestive heart failure [CHF].) After the patient's weaned from PEEP, continue to wean him from all mechanical ventilation.

Respiratory support

Three ways to wean effectively

Once the doctor's decided that your patient's ready for weaning, he may order one of the following methods. Here's how each works:

Conventional weaning

For this method, first record baseline measurements of your patient's respiratory rate, vital capacity, tidal volume, inspiratory force, heart rate, EKG reading, and blood pressure. Next, disconnect your patient's ventilator, and allow him to breathe spontaneously. At the same time, give him supplemental humidified oxygen through either a T piece or a trach collar. Keep him off the ventilator for 5 to 10 minutes. Before you reconnect him, repeat the measurements listed above and document them. Also, draw arterial blood to obtain arterial blood gas (ABG) measurements.

Continue the weaning process if tests show that the patient has satisfactory and stable ABG measurements, that he has an inspiratory force greater than -20 cm H_2O and that he has a tidal volume of at least 250 ml.

Note: Inspiratory force and tidal volume measurements may be less for a patient with lung disease.

Over the next 24 hours, take the patient off the ventilator for 5 to 10 minutes every hour during waking hours. Reconnect your patient at night so he can get adequate rest for the next day's weaning.

Remember: Your patient needs much emotional support. If he asks to be reconnected to the ventilator at any time during weaning, you should comply. Try not to show frustration with his level of progress. If you do so, you'll only increase his anxiety.

After the first day, increase his time off the ventilator by 5 to 10 minutes an hour each day, until he's able to stay off the ventilator completely. As he progresses, you can also gradually decrease the amount of time he spends on the respirator at night.

Temporarily discontinue the weaning process and reconnect your patient to the ventilator if any of these signs appear: a significant rise in blood pressure and pulse rate, a progressively decreasing tidal volume, unsatisfactory ABG measurements, increased fatigue, changed mental status, the appearance of previously unnoticed cardiac arrhythmias, or signs of poor chest muscle coordination.

Intermittent mandatory ventilation (IMV)

With this method, your patient remains on the ventilator, but receives only a set number of ventilator-controlled breaths per minute. The ventilator delivers a preset volume, but the patient's own unassisted breaths have a slightly lower volume. IMV works well for chronic lung disease patients who tend to be ventilator-dependent, because with IMV, weaning takes place very gradually. If the doctor orders IMV, you'll keep your patient on the ventilator at first, but gradually reduce the frequency of controlled breaths. Initially, set the respiratory rate for 1 to 2 breaths less than total controlled ventilation provides. Each day, reduce the rate by one to two breaths until the machine delivers fewer breaths than the patient draws unassisted. Continue this procedure until the patient can breathe on his own. Periodically check vital signs, vital capacity, tidal volume, and inspiratory force. Draw arterial blood for ABG measurements. Document all findings. When the patient's ready to be disconnected, the machine may be delivering as few as three breaths per minute.

Intermittent demand ventilation (IDV)

This method is sometimes called synchronized intermittent mandatory ventilation (SIMV). If the doctor orders IDV, you'll keep your patient connected to the ventilator. Set the ventilator on the assist mode, so that for a predetermined number of breaths per minute—for example, a ratio of one machine breath to five patient breaths—the patient triggers inspiration, but the machine completes the breath. During weaning, you'll gradually reduce the number of mechanically assisted breaths per minute. To compensate, your patient will begin increasing his breathing efforts until he eventually can breathe without the ventilator.

While the patient's gaining strength and confidence, offer your encouragement. Monitor his vital capacity, tidal volume, inspiratory force, and vital signs. Periodically draw arterial blood for ABG measurements.

Learning about the Ohio® Thoracic Drainage System

To save time and eliminate the risk of bottle breakage, many hospitals now use disposable, underwater-seal chest drainage systems. The photo at right shows the Ohio Thoracic Drainage System. As you can see, the system includes a disposable drainage unit and a reusable suction regulator. The drainage unit has a single collection receptacle and an underwater-seal chamber. When you depress the saline solution container at left, it releases saline solution into the underwater-seal chamber, creating the seal. You control suction with the regulator, which plugs into a wall vacuum outlet.

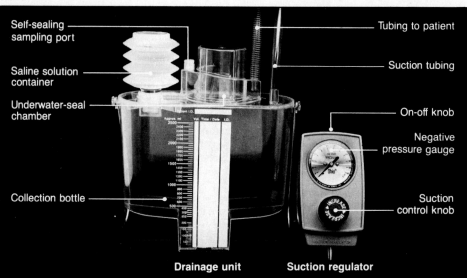

Self-sealing sampling port

Saline solution container

Underwater-seal chamber

Collection bottle

Tubing to patient

Suction tubing

On-off knob

Negative pressure gauge

Suction control knob

Drainage unit   **Suction regulator**

Using the Ohio Thoracic Drainage System

1 *Suppose your patient on a ventilator experiences pneumothorax. The doctor will insert a chest tube and connect it to a thoracic drainage system.*

To assist him, obtain a chest tube tray, a chest tube, and 1% lidocaine (Xylocaine*), povidone-iodine solution, a needle with a cutting edge (threaded with 2-0 silk), and sterile gloves. Also, obtain a disposable Ohio drainage unit and regulator, a 10 cc syringe, 22G and 25G needles, and rubber-shod clamps.

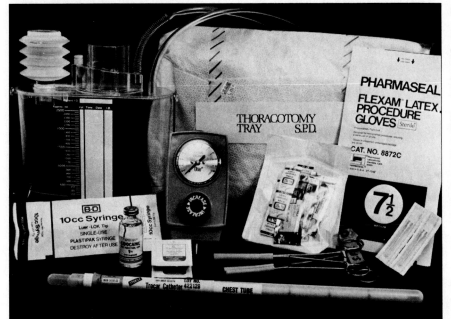

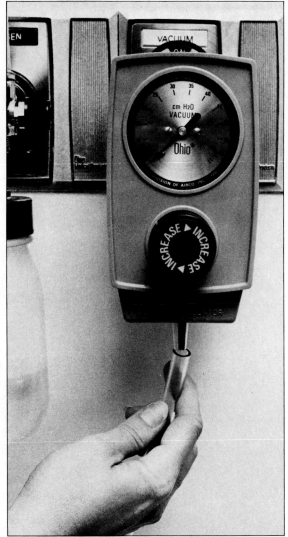

2 Make sure the patient or a family member signs a surgical consent form. Explain the procedure and answer any questions.

Wash your hands.

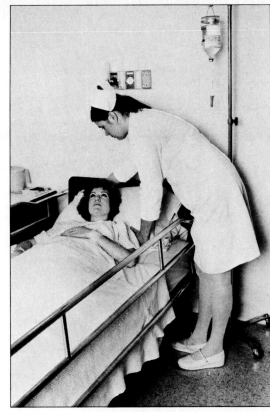

3 Unwrap the drainage unit carefully. If the doctor doesn't want suction used, clamp the end of the suction tubing and tape a gauze pad over it to keep it clean. If he does want suction, plug the suction regulator into the wall vacuum outlet. Then, attach the end of the tubing to the suction regulator, as shown here. But don't turn the regulator on yet.

*Available in both the United States and in Canada

Respiratory support

Using the Ohio Thoracic Drainage System continued

4 To activate the underwater seal, turn the saline solution container a half-turn to the right. Then, gently depress it. The saline solution will flow into the underwater-seal chamber.

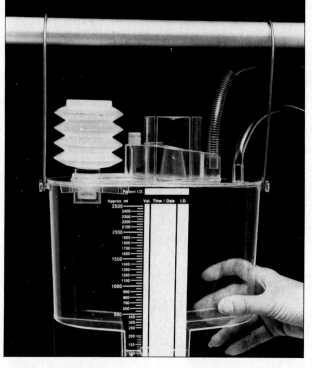

5 Hang the drainage unit on the bed railing.
At this point, the doctor will insert the chest tube. After cleaning the skin with povidone-iodine solution and anesthetizing the area, he'll make a small skin incision, dissect into the pleural space, and insert the tube. Then, he'll clamp the chest tube close to the chest wall. He'll suture the wound around the chest tube.

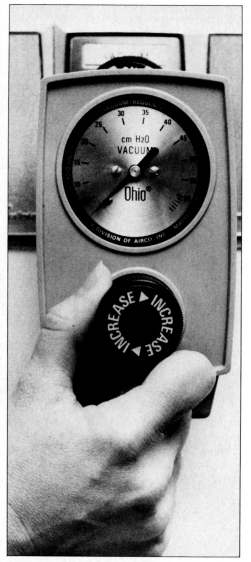

6 Assist the doctor in applying an airtight dressing around the insertion site. Then, hand him the drainage unit tubing, with the adapter on the end. He'll connect this to the patient's chest tube and unclamp the chest tube. To prevent air leaks and to keep the tubes securely connected, tape this junction as shown here.

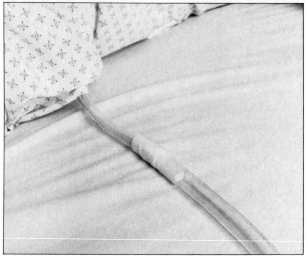

7 Now, turn on the suction regulator. Slowly increase the suction to the prescribed level of cm H_2O, by turning the suction control knob clockwise. The negative pressure gauge will indicate the cm H_2O level.

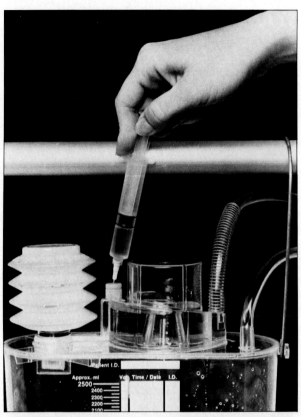

9 If you need a chest drainage specimen for analysis, aspirate it from the sampling port on the underwater-seal chamber. Use an 18G or 20G needle. Withdraw the desired amount, cap and label the syringe, and send it to the lab. Make sure the needle's securely attached to the syringe.

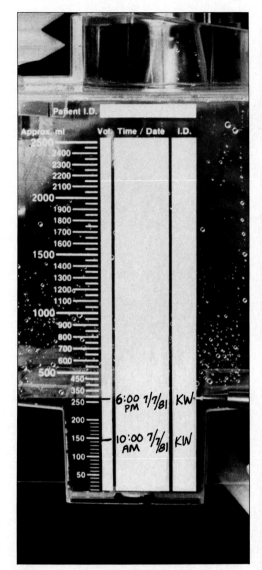

8 Every 8 hours, measure the drainage accumulated in the collection bottle. On the front panel of the unit, record the date and hour you measured the drainage. Also, record the amount, date, and time on the patient's intake and output record and in your nurses' notes.

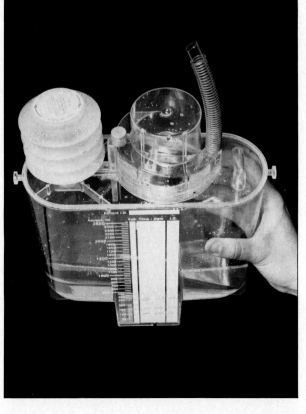

10 To dispose of the drainage after the collection bottle has filled, disconnect the suction tubing from the wall regulator. Then, clamp the chest tube and disconnect the bottle tubing from it. Immediately reconnect the chest tube to the tubing on a new drainage unit. Unclamp the chest tube.

Then, cut off the tubings, as shown here. Pour out the drainage and throw away the unit.

Important: If your patient has a contagious disease or a severe infection, don't empty the unit. Instead, clamp the tubings shut with disposable clamps, and discard the entire drainage unit, including contents.

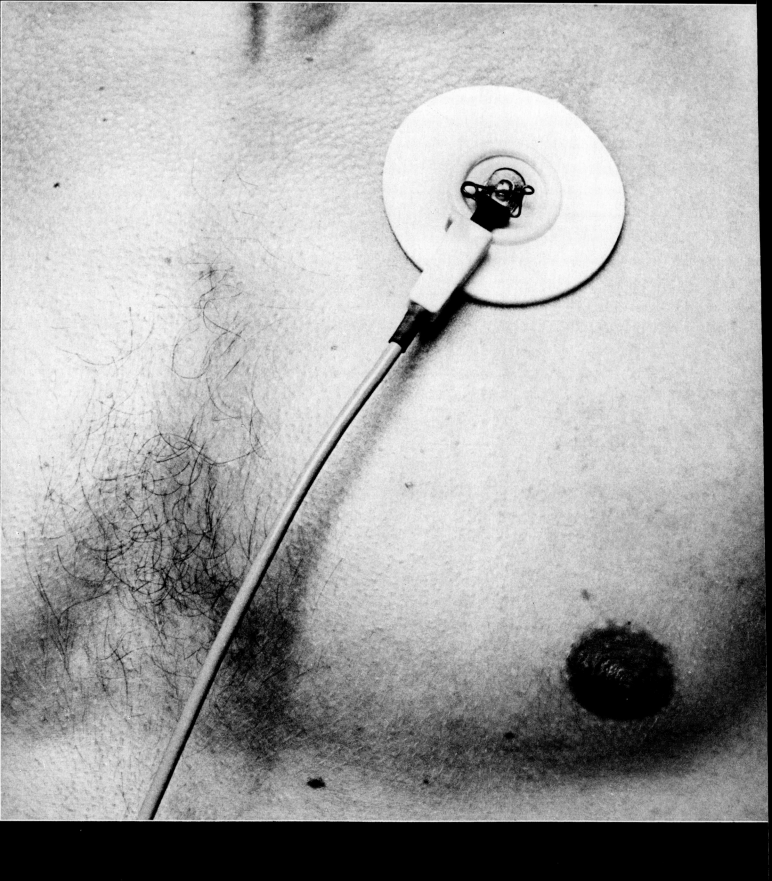

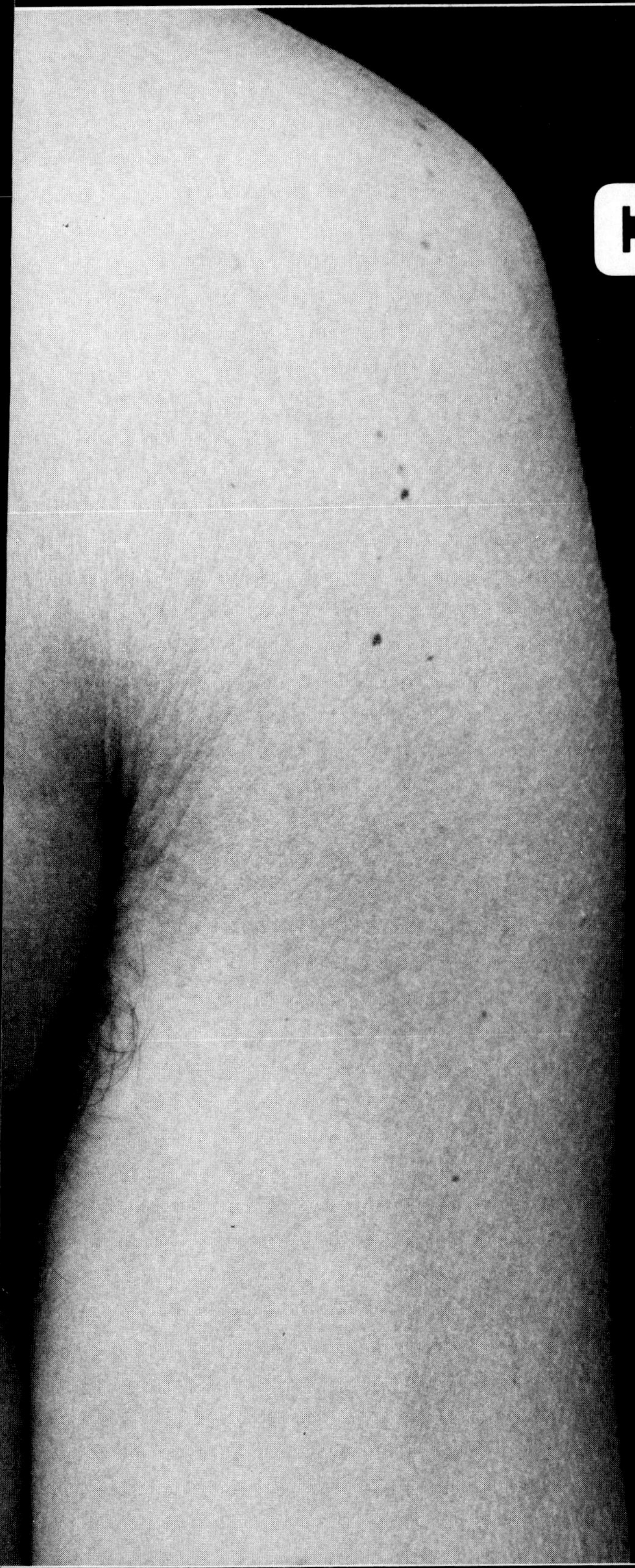

Caring for the Cardiovascular Patient

Cardiovascular basics
Cardiac monitoring
Hemodynamic monitoring
Cardiovascular emergencies
Cardiovascular disorders

Cardiovascular basics

Working in a coronary care unit (CCU)? Or in an ICU that includes cardiovascular patients? Every day, your patients rely on your cardiovascular nursing skills. Those skills begin with the basics: compiling the patient's personal and medical history, and assessing his physical condition. By becoming thoroughly acquainted with the patient, as well as with his condition, you can identify potential physical and psychological problems that may hamper his recovery. In the following pages, you'll learn what to look for.

But the basics don't stop with history-taking and physical assessment. Continuing care also depends on your skill in using one of the most basic tools of cardiovascular care: the 12-lead electrocardiogram (EKG). Can you set up the equipment correctly, run EKG strips, and interpret the results? If not, you'll find the information in this chapter invaluable.

Of course, your understanding of cardiac anatomy and physiology is essential. For that reason, we've begun with a brief review.

Reviewing the heart's anatomy

Even though you're already familiar with the heart's anatomy, use this frontal view as a handy map of its major anatomical structures and conduction system. Then, consider using it as an aid when you teach your patient or his family about cardiovascular disease.

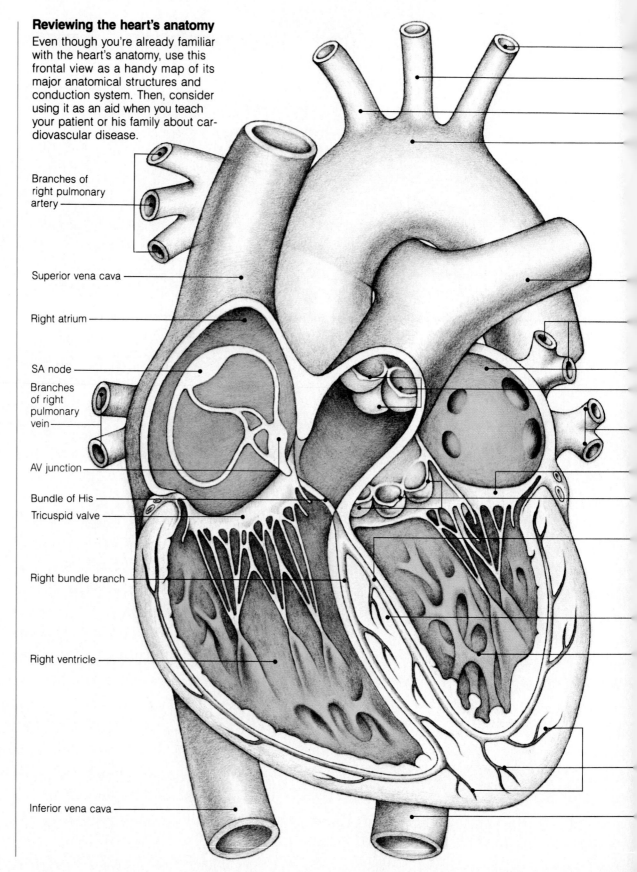

Branches of right pulmonary artery

Superior vena cava

Right atrium

SA node

Branches of right pulmonary vein

AV junction

Bundle of His

Tricuspid valve

Right bundle branch

Right ventricle

Inferior vena cava

Left subclavian artery

Left common carotid artery

Brachiocephalic artery

Aortic arch

Left pulmonary artery

ches of left pulmonary vein

Left atrium

Pulmonary valve

ches of left pulmonary vein

Mitral valve

Aortic valve

Left bundle branch

Septum

Left ventricle

Purkinje fibers

Descending aorta

Understanding the cardiac cycle

You can't understand your patient's cardiovascular problems without first understanding the cardiac cycle. Refer to the illustration on the preceding page as you review the basics. (For a detailed look at the cardiac cycle, see the NURSING PHOTOBOOK USING MONITORS.)

As you know, the cardiac cycle has two phases: diastole, when the heart's ventricles fill with blood from the atria; and systole, when the ventricles contract and eject the blood. During diastole, the right ventricle fills with venous blood from the right atrium. During systole, it ejects this blood into the pulmonary artery. The pulmonary artery then carries this blood to the lungs for oxygenation.

As the right ventricle fills with venous blood, the left ventricle fills with oxygenated blood returning from the lungs. During systole, the left ventricle ejects this oxygenated blood into the aorta, which distributes it to the rest of the body.

Understanding cardiac conduction

Your patient's life depends on conduction of electrical impulses through his heart. Any disturbance of cardiac conduction can be life-threatening. That's why understanding the basics of this process is vital.

The cardiac conduction system is made of highly specialized myocardial tissues: the sinoatrial (SA) node, the atrioventricular (AV) junction, the bundle of His, the right and left bundle branches, and the Purkinje fibers. These specialized tissues conduct electrical impulses much more quickly than other myocardial tissues. The electrical impulses conducted along their pathways trigger the mechanical events of the cardiac cycle. To see how, look at the illustration at left.

As you see, the SA node is located in the right atrial wall near the superior vena cava. Specialized pacemaker cells within the SA node, which function independently of the central nervous system, regularly generate electrical impulses. Each impulse is transmitted through the muscle fibers of the atria, causing them to contract.

Next, the electrical impulse travels to the AV junction, where it's delayed. This slowing-down process allows the heart's ventricles to fill with blood from the atria.

From the AV junction, the impulse travels down the bundle of His, the left and right bundle branches, and the Purkinje fibers. After the impulse stimulates the ventricles, they contract and eject blood into the pulmonary artery and the aorta. Finally, the cells in the ventricles repolarize.

If electrical impulses from the SA node are suppressed or blocked, the AV junction usually takes over and maintains a heart rate of 40 to 60 beats per minute. If the AV junction's impulses are also suppressed, ventricular cells initiate electrical conduction. However, the ventricular cells can maintain a heart rate of only 20 to 40 beats per minute.

To assess cardiac conduction, you'll run a 12-lead EKG. Beginning on page 67, we'll show you how to perform the procedure and interpret the results.

Cardiac care: Those critical early hours

In the ICU, you've probably cared for patients like George Klein, a 43-year-old bank executive. He began suffering severe pain in his left arm while playing golf. Fearing a heart attack, he asked his golf partner to drive him to the hospital. This quick action probably helped save his life.

Although some of your ICU patients have just had cardiovascular surgery, many, like Mr. Klein, enter the ICU after suffering a myocardial infarction (MI) or other cardiac emergency. Let's take a look at what happens to such a patient during his first hours at the hospital.

First stop: The emergency department
Chances are, a cardiovascular patient like Mr. Klein won't enter the ICU without first going through the emergency department (E.D.). The E.D. staff will do what they can to stabilize the patient's condition and perform an emergency assessment. Most likely, they'll take these steps:
• open the patient's airway (if necessary) and give oxygen
• take and record vital signs
• auscultate heart and lung sounds
• take a brief history of medications, chest pain, and allergies
• give nitroglycerine (as ordered) to relieve chest pain
• run a 12-lead EKG and/or connect the patient to a cardiac monitor
• start an I.V. with the appropriate solution (as ordered)
• give I.V. narcotic medication (such as morphine sulfate or Demerol*), as ordered, if chest pain persists despite nitroglycerine administration
• give antiarrhythmic drugs (if necessary), as ordered
• draw blood for stat lab tests; for example, electrolyte and cardiac enzyme studies.

Welcome to the ICU
Let's say that Mr. Klein's condition has stabilized. Now he's on his way to the ICU. What will you do for him when he arrives?
• First, reassure him that his condition is stable, and that you'll be watching him closely for any possible change. Remember, anxiety places an additional burden on his heart. Do your best to relieve his fears.
• Attach him to the ICU's cardiac monitor. (To see how, turn to page 76.) As you initiate monitoring, explain that the monitor allows you to watch his heart's rhythm and rate, even when you're at the nursing station.
• Check and record his vital signs.
• Administer medication (such as antiarrhythmics, analgesics, and oxygen), as ordered.
• Arrange for chest X-rays, as ordered.
• Take a complete nursing history. (For guidelines on taking a cardiovascular history, see the next page.)
• Do a complete cardiovascular assessment, and document your findings. Follow the guidelines outlined on page 63.

*Available in both the United States and in Canada

Cardiovascular basics

Taking a history

Documenting your patient's medical history is one of the most important parts of cardiovascular assessment. Not only will his history give you insight into his medical condition, it'll help you design a care plan suited to his unique needs.

Whenever possible, take a history before beginning your physical examination. The patient himself is your best source of information. But if he's unconscious, or too debilitated to talk to you, turn to his family or friends for the necessary information.

What do you need to know? First, record his name, sex, age, nationality, marital status, and his doctor's name. Then, begin gathering information, using the following questions as a guide. But remember, no matter what questions you ask, you're after more than just factual information. Read between the lines. Watch your patient's gestures and expressions for clues to his special fears and concerns. Keep in mind that the patient's religious beliefs, self-image, family life and personality type all affect how he'll respond to your care. Document these observations as carefully as you document the answers to these questions:

• What day was he admitted? What time? Note whether he walked in or entered on a stretcher or wheelchair.

• Why was he admitted? Encourage him to describe the circumstances, and document his own words.

• Has he experienced these symptoms before? If so, how many times? How long did they last each time? Find out if his present symptoms differ from past symptoms.

• Has he received medical treatment or been hospitalized in the past, for any reason? If so, when? Who was his doctor? How was he treated? Did he suffer any complications?

• Is he taking any medication, including over-the-counter drugs? Document usage and dosages.

• Does he have any allergies? If so, note them in red on the Kardex, and flag the patient's chart. Document the type and severity of past allergic reactions. Then place a drug allergy band on the patient's wrist.

• If your patient's a woman, has she ever taken birth control pills? They may contribute to coronary artery disease (CAD) or emboli.

• Do any of your patient's family members have heart disease, high blood pressure, or any other serious illness? Document the age and health status of close family members. In addition, note the cause of death of any immediate family member.

• Is he a high school or college graduate? Noting his level of education will help you tailor your patient teaching to his level of understanding.

• Does he ever experience shortness of breath, nocturnal dyspnea, or orthopnea? Ask how many pillows he sleeps on at night. In addition, ask if he feels more comfortable sleeping in a chair than in a bed.

• Is the patient generally active, or sedentary? Ask if his symptoms limit his activity.

• Does he have any problems with incontinence, nocturia, or dysuria?

• Does he have any problems with constipation or diarrhea? Ask if he's noticed any recent changes in his bowel habits.

• Is the patient on a special diet; for example, a low sodium or low cholesterol diet? Ask him to describe his eating habits, including salt usage.

• Has he experienced any significant weight loss or gain lately? Has he noticed any swelling, especially of his hands, feet or ankles?

• Does he smoke cigarettes? How many packs per day? If he quit smoking, note how long ago, and how many packs he smoked before quitting. If he smokes a pipe or cigars, ask him if he inhales.

• Does he drink alcoholic beverages? If so, what kind? Ask him to describe his drinking habits.

• Is he currently working? Document his job and note whether it's stressful or physically demanding.

• Does he live alone? Does he have children living with him?

• Does he wear contact lenses or dentures? If he wears dentures, note whether they're partial or full, upper or lower.

• Does he use a hearing aid or prosthesis?

Document all findings in your nurses' notes.

Watching for telltale signs

You'll learn a great deal about your patient's condition from his history and your physical assessment. But your own observations can be just as revealing. Take a close look at your patient. As this chart shows, his general appearance can provide valuable clues to cardiovascular disease.

If you notice:	Consider this possible cause:	If you notice:	Consider this possible cause:
Central cyanosis	• Hypoxia caused by heart and/or lung disease	Cool, moist skin	• Vasoconstriction • Anxiety
Cold extremities and weak or absent pulses, with or without peripheral cyanosis or cyanotic nailbeds	• Peripheral vascular disease • Decreased cardiac output	Pretibial edema and pedal edema	• Vascular disease (edema without pitting) • Congestive heart failure (edema with pitting)
Pallid nailbeds	• Vasoconstriction	Diagonal earlobe crease (McCarthy's sign)	• Coronary artery disease
Clubbed fingers	• Chronic hypoxemia • Congenital heart disease	Subtle up-and-down movements of head synchronized with heart beat (Musset's sign)	• Aortic aneurysm • Aortic insufficiency
Thick fingernails	• Peripheral vascular disease, causing impaired oxygen delivery to the extremities	Greyish-white ring at junction of iris and sclera (corneal arcus)	• Atherosclerosis
Cool, dry skin	• Vascular insufficiency	Pulsations in aorta	• Aortic aneurysm

Performing a cardiovascular assessment

Like a medical history, a complete cardiovascular assessment provides the basis for ongoing care. By frequently updating your assessment, you can evaluate your patient's progress. Use this systematic approach:

Palpate the patient's arteries, and assess his arterial pulses. For details on interpreting your findings, read the chart on page 64.

Measure his arterial blood pressure. To take a noninvasive blood pressure reading, place the cuff over the patient's brachial artery, about 1" (3 cm) above his antecubital fossa. If possible, take a pressure reading from each arm. (*Remember:* Never take a cuff reading from an arm with an I.V. or an arterial line in place.) Next, if the patient's condition permits, take readings while he's lying down, and when he's sitting up. If the patient's blood pressure changes when his position changes, alert the doctor. Such changes in blood pressure may be caused by the patient's medication, or may indicate decreased cardiac output, incompetent heart valve function, cardiac tamponade, or constrictive pericarditis.

Suppose you hear diastolic sounds until the cuff is completely deflated (0 mm Hg pressure). Carefully document these three points: when you first hear systolic sounds; when the sounds become less audible or muffled; and when they

disappear. For example, you might document a reading like this: 180/70/0. Such a reading may suggest aortic regurgitation or thyrotoxicosis.

If your patient has an arterial line in place, take a pressure cuff reading and compare it to the monitor's reading. (The monitor's blood pressure reading will probably show a higher systole and a lower diastole than your cuff pressure reading.) If the readings vary significantly, recalibrate the monitoring equipment. Then, if the monitor's reading still varies significantly from the pressure cuff reading, notify the doctor.

Check his central venous pressure. If your patient has a pulmonary artery (PA) line in place, document the monitor's digital pressure reading. But if he doesn't have a PA line in place, evaluate his venous pressure this way: First, elevate him to a 45° angle. If his external jugular veins remain flat and barely visible, his venous pressure's normal. But if they clearly pulsate above his sternal angle, his venous pressure's abnormally high.

To observe internal jugular pulsations, shine a flashlight across your patient's lower neck at a tangential angle. The internal jugular vein, which lies beneath the sternocleidomastoid muscle, will cast a slight shadow. If venous pressure's elevated, the internal jugular vein will cast a shadow *above* the sternal angle. Elevated

venous pressure may indicate congestive heart failure (CHF), cardiac tamponade, or superior vena cava obstruction.

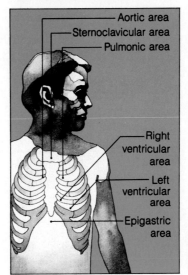

Inspect and palpate the chest area over his heart. Use the illustration above as a guide.

Examine his thorax and lungs. To see how, review the information on pages 22 and 23.

Percuss his heart to learn its size and precise location. Find the heart's left sternal border at the left midclavicular line, 5th intercostal space. Begin percussing the area just to the left of this landmark and move across his chest. When the percussion sound changes from dull to resonant, you have crossed the cardiac border and begun percussing lung tissue. Percuss along the cardiac

border until you can visualize the position of the entire left border.

Locating the right border is more difficult, because it lies under the sternum. But you can estimate the right ventricle's size by percussing the sternum. Begin at the top of the sternum and move down. If you begin hearing dull sounds, instead of the flat sound normally associated with bone percussion, suspect an enlarged right ventricle.

Auscultate his heart. If necessary, review the cardiac auscultation areas shown in the illustration below.

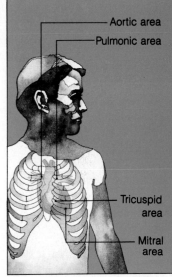

Document your findings. Consider clear, complete documentation an essential component of cardiovascular assessment.

MINI-ASSESSMENT

Assessing pulse amplitude

To accurately gauge your patient's pulse amplitude, use this standard scale:
0: pulse is not palpable.
+1: pulse is thready, weak; difficult to find; may fade in and out; and disappears easily with pressure.
+2: pulse is constant but not strong; light pressure must be applied or pulse will disappear.

+3: pulse considered normal; is easily palpable; and does not disappear with pressure.
+4: pulse is strong, bounding; and does not disappear with pressure.

Compare each artery's measurement with that of the artery that corresponds bilaterally, and document your findings in your nurses' notes.

Cardiovascular basics

Interpreting arterial pulses

Your patient's arterial pulses reflect changes in his left ventricle; a weak or absent arterial pulse may signal an arterial obstruction, injury, or disorder. To assess your patient's arterial pulses, palpate each of these major arteries: carotid, brachial, radial, femoral, popliteal, posterior tibial, and dorsalis pedis. *Important:* For accuracy, measure pulse rate for exactly 1 minute.

Arterial wall
Normal condition
• Soft and pliable
Abnormal condition
• Tortuous and ropelike
Possible cause
• Atherosclerosis

Pulse rate
Normal condition
• 50 to 100 beats per minute
Abnormal condition
• Bradycardia (less than 50 beats per minute)
• Tachycardia (more than 100 beats per minute)
• Pulse deficit (peripheral and apical rates differ)
Possible cause
• Sinoatrial (SA) node disease, hypothyroidism
• Fever, hemorrhage, shock, anxiety
• Cardiac arrhythmia, atrial fibrillation

Pulse rhythm
Normal condition
• Regular
Abnormal condition
• Irregular
Possible cause
• Arrhythmias, such as premature contractions or atrial fibrillation

Pulse amplitude
Normal condition
• Strong, easy to detect (+ 3)
Abnormal condition
• Weak, faint, or not palpable
• Pulsus alternans (one weak beat/one strong beat)
• Pulsus paradoxus (change in amplitude during respiration)
• Plateau pulse (small amplitude, slow rise, sustained summit, gradual fill)
• Pulsus bisferiens (double beat at summit)
• Corrigan's or water-hammer pulse (bounding; abrupt rise and fall back to diastolic level)
Possible cause
• Partial occlusion of artery, heart disease, shock
• Left ventricular failure
• Severe lung disease, cardiac tamponade, advanced heart failure
• Aortic stenosis
• Aortic insufficiency

Equality of bilateral pulses
Normal condition
• Equal
Abnormal condition
• Unequal
Possible cause
• Obstructive arterial disease, dissecting aneurysms

Interpreting your inspection and palpation findings

Inspection and palpation area	Possible observations	Possible abnormalities
Sternoclavicular	• Abnormally strong pulsation	• Aortic aneurysm
Aortic	• Abnormally abrupt pulsation	• Rheumatic heart disease • Systemic hypertension
	• Thrill	• Aortic stenosis
Pulmonary	• Abnormally abrupt pulsation	• Essential pulmonary hypertension
	• Thrill	• Pulmonic stenosis
	• Abnormally strong or forceful pulsation	• Emphysema, mitral stenosis • Extensive pneumonia • Pulmonary embolism
Right ventricular	• Thrill	• Ventricular septal defect
	• Heave and lift with each heartbeat	• Right ventricular hypertrophy • Pulmonic stenosis • Systemic hypertension • Emphysema, mitral stenosis • Extensive pneumonia
Left ventricular	• Thrill	• Mitral stenosis
	• Gallop	• Ischemia • Injury • Myocardial infarction
	• Impulse far to the left or low	• Aortic regurgitation • Aortic stenosis • Left ventricular hypertrophy • Systemic hypertension
	• Impulse covering a large area	• Aortic regurgitation • Aortic stenosis • Left ventricular hypertrophy • Systemic hypertension
	• Impulse long in duration and/or abnormally strong	• Aortic regurgitation • Aortic stenosis • Left ventricular hypertrophy • Systemic hypertension
Epigastric	• Abnormally strong pulsation	• Aortic aneurysm

Nurses' guide to heart sounds

Can you identify and interpret the heart sounds you hear during auscultation? Can you distinguish normal sounds from abnormal ones? If not, study this chart carefully. (For a review of cardiac auscultation areas, see the illustration on page 63.) *Note:* Unless otherwise indicated, auscultate heart sounds with the diaphragm of your stethoscope.	**S₁** **Timing in cardiac cycle** Beginning of systole **Physiology** Mitral and tricuspid valves close almost simultaneously, producing a single sound. S₁ corresponds to the carotid pulse. **Indication** • Normal **Where to auscultate** Mitral area (apex) or fifth left intercostal space **What you'll hear** **Lub**-dup *Also described:* **Lub**-dub	**Split S₁** **Timing in cardiac cycle** Beginning of systole **Physiology** Mitral valve closes slightly before the tricuspid valve. **Indication** • Normal, in most cases • Right bundle branch block (wide splitting of S₁) **Where to auscultate** Begin at mitral area and move toward tricuspid area, where you will hear the split S₁ sound. **What you'll hear** **Thrup**-dup *Also described:* **T-lub**-dub	**S₂** **Timing in cardiac cycle** Beginning of diastole **Physiology** Pulmonic and aortic valves close almost simultaneously. **Indication** • Normal **Where to auscultate** Aortic and pulmonic areas (base). Heard best at aortic area. **What you'll hear** Lub-**dup** *Also described:* Lub-**dub**	**Physiologic split S₂** (S₂ is split on inspiration but not split on expiration.) **Timing in cardiac cycle** End of systole **Physiology** During inspiration, the pulmonic valve closes later than the aortic valve. (Pulmonic valve closure is normally delayed during inspiration. Inspiration draws more blood into the right side of the heart, delaying right-sided systole.) **Indication** • Normal; a physiologic S₂ split corresponds to the respiratory cycle. **Where to auscultate** Aortic and pulmonic areas. Heard best at pulmonic area. **What you'll hear** Lub-**thrup** (during inspiration) Lub-**dup** (during expiration) *Also described:* Lub-**T-dub** (during inspiration) Lub-**dub** (during expiration)
Persistant (wide) split S₂ (S₂ split on both inspiration and expiration, but more widely split on inspiration.) **Timing in cardiac cycle** End of systole **Physiology** Pulmonic valve closes late, or (less commonly) the aortic valve closes early. **Indication** *Late pulmonic valve closure:* • Complete right bundle branch block, which delays right ventricular contraction. As a result, the pulmonic valve closes later. • Pulmonary stenosis, which prolongs right ventricular ejection *Early aortic valve closure:* • Mitral insufficiency • Ventricular septal defect **Where to auscultate** Aortic and pulmonic areas **What you'll hear** Lub-**thurup** (during inspiration) Lub-**thrup** (during expiration)	**Fixed split S₂** (S₂ is equally split on inspiration and expiration.) **Timing in cardiac cycle** End of systole **Physiology** Pulmonic valve closes later than aortic valve. **Indication** • Severe right ventricular failure, which prolongs right ventricular systole • Atrial septal defect, which causes the right ventricle to eject more blood than the left • Pulmonic stenosis **Where to auscultate** Aortic and pulmonic areas **What you'll hear** Lub-**thrup** (during inspiration and expiration) *Also described:* Lub-**T-dub**	**Paradoxical (reversed) S₂ split** (S₂ is widely split on expiration.) **Timing in cardiac cycle** End of systole **Physiology** Aortic valve closes after the pulmonic valve, due to delayed or prolonged left ventricular systole. **Indication** • Left bundle branch block (most common cause) • Aortic stenosis • Patent ductus arteriosus • Right ventricular ectopy • Severe hypertension • Left ventricular failure, disease, or ischemia **Where to auscultate** Aortic area **What you'll hear** Lub-**thrup** (during expiration) *Also described:* Lub-**T-lup**	**S₃** (ventricular gallop) **Timing in cardiac cycle** Early diastole **Physiology** The ventricles fill early and rapidly. (S₃ may occur on either side of the heart.) **Indication** • Early congestive heart failure • Ventricular aneurysm • Atrioventricular valve incompetence • Thyrotoxicosis anemia • Atrial septal defect • Aortic, mitral, or tricuspid valve regurgitation **Where to auscultate** Mitral area and right ventricular area, using stethoscope bell. Place patient on his left side. **What you'll hear** Lub-dup**a**	**S₄** (atrial gallop) **Timing in cardiac cycle** Late diastole **Physiology** The atrium makes an extra effort to fill a diseased ventricle. (S₄ may occur on either side of the heart.) **Indication** • Acute myocardial infarction or ischemia • Angina pectoris • Chronic coronary artery disease • Aortic stenosis • Pulmonic stenosis • Pulmonary artery hypertension **Where to auscultate** Left or right side of the heart (usually at mitral area), using stethoscope bell **What you'll hear** **Ta**-lub-dup

Cardiovascular basics

Assessing your patient's chest pain

When your patient complains of chest pain, you must first identify the type of pain he's experiencing. This chart will tell you how to assess his chest pain, and how to relieve it.

Type and location	Signs and symptoms	Nursing intervention
Angina Substernal or retrosternal pain or discomfort spreading across chest; may radiate to inside of either or both arms and shoulders, or to neck or jaw	• Sudden onset • Squeezing, burning, heavy-pressure pain; or milder feelings of distress in upper body • Patient may describe pain as feeling like indigestion; he may locate it by clenching his fist over his sternum. • Pulse rate and blood pressure may rise or fall. • Pain usually subsides within 10 minutes after treatment.	• Instruct patient to lie down, or place him in semi-Fowler's position, if that's more comfortable for him. • Administer a coronary vasodilator such as isosorbide dinitrate (Isordil*) or nitroglycerine, as ordered. • Administer a beta-adrenergic blocking agent (such as Inderal*) as ordered, if nitrites or nitroglycerine do not provide relief. • Administer sedative, as ordered.
Myocardial infarction (MI) Substernal or precordial pain, or pain in arm, neck, or jaw; may radiate from chest, or remain isolated in chest, arm, neck, or jaw.	• Sudden onset • Crushing, viselike, sometimes burning pain • Patient may describe pain as feeling like indigestion. • More severe and prolonged than anginal pain • May be accompanied by shortness of breath, nausea, vomiting, perspiration, weakness and fatigue, feelings of impending doom, headache, falling blood pressure, tachycardia, and peripheral cyanosis	• Administer oxygen and morphine, as ordered. • Administer atropine sulfate, as ordered, for bradyarrhythmias associated with falling blood pressure. • If premature ventricular contractions (PVCs) are present, administer lidocaine hydrochloride (Xylocaine Hydrochloride*), as ordered.
Pericardial chest pain Substernal or left of sternum; may radiate to neck, arms, or back	• Severe, sudden onset • Sharp, intermittent pain (accentuated by swallowing, coughing, inspiration, or lying in a supine position); or continuous, low-level ache • May occur intermittently over several days	• Instruct patient to bend forward (or help him to assume any position that's comfortable). • Administer analgesics, as ordered. • Administer anti-inflammatory drugs, as ordered, to reduce cardiac inflammation. • Administer oxygen, as ordered.
Pulmonary origin (pleuritis, pulmonary embolism [PE]) Inferior portion of the pleura; may radiate to costal margins or upper abdomen	• Sudden onset • Shortness of breath • Stabbing, knifelike pain (accentuated by respirations) • May last a few days	• Administer codeine or morphine sulfate for pain, as ordered. • Administer antibiotic for infection, as ordered. • Administer anticoagulant for PE, as ordered. • Administer oxygen, as ordered. *Important:* If the doctor orders arterial blood gas measurements, obtain an arterial blood sample before giving oxygen.
Esophageal pain Substernal; may radiate around chest to shoulders	• Sudden onset • Burning, knotlike pain (simulating angina) • Usually subsides within 15 to 20 minutes after treatment	• Administer antacids, as ordered. • Instruct patient to sit upright.
Chest wall pain Costochondral or sternocostal junctions; does not radiate	• Often begins as dull ache, increasing in intensity over a few days; aching pain or soreness • Usually long-lasting	• Administer muscle relaxants and analgesics, as ordered. • Doctor may inject a local anesthetic for pain at affected costal junction.
Anxiety Left chest (variable); does not radiate	• Sudden onset • Sharp and stabbing pain, or vague discomfort • May last less than a minute or for several days	• Instruct patient to lie down and breathe normally. • Administer sedatives, as ordered.

*Available in both the United States and in Canada

Placing chest electrodes correctly

In the photostory beginning on the next page, you'll learn how to run a 12-lead electrocardiogram (EKG). During the procedure, you must place the chest electrode in different positions for each of the six chest leads (leads V_1 through V_6). This illustration shows the exact location of each position.

V_1: Fourth intercostal space to right of sternum

V_2: Fourth intercostal space to left of sternum

V_3: Halfway between V_2 and V_4

V_4: Fifth intercostal space at midclavicular line

V_5: Anterior axillary line (halfway between V_4 and V_6)

V_6: Midaxillary line, level with V_4

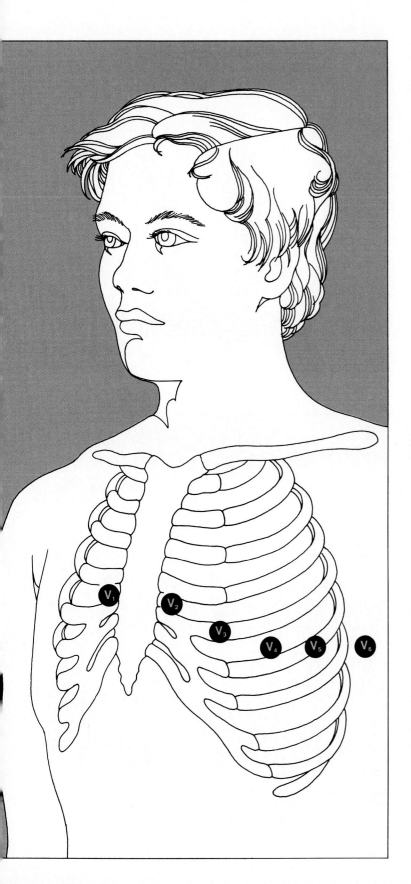

Running a 12-lead electrocardiogram (EKG)

You're caring for Charles Bakey, a 54-year-old salesman who's recovering from an inferior wall myocardial infarction (MI). His doctor's ordered you to run daily 12-lead EKGs on your patient, even though he's undergoing continuous monitoring. Do you know why?

Unlike a three-electrode cardiac monitor, the 12-lead EKG examines the heart's electrical activity from 12 different views. Because it provides a more complete view of the heart's activity, it provides a more accurate picture of the patient's condition. The EKG not only helps the doctor pinpoint trouble spots in the heart, it helps him evaluate how well the patient's responding to treatment.

Consider 12-lead EKGs essential to ongoing assessment. Make sure you can do the procedure correctly by studying the following photostory.

1 First, gather the equipment you'll need: an EKG machine with five lead wires, four limb lead electrodes with rubber straps, one suction cup chest electrode, conductive jelly, alcohol pads, and 4"x4" gauze pads.

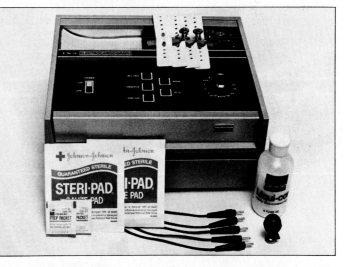

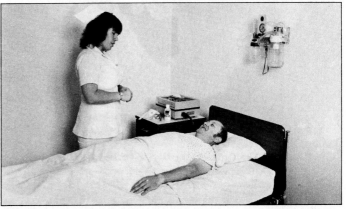

2 Place Mr. Bakey flat on his back, and make sure his feet don't touch the bed's footboard. Explain the procedure to him and ask him to lie quietly while you work. Assure him that the procedure's painless. Then, remove his gown and expose his arms and lower legs. (Cover him with the sheet until you apply the chest electrode.)

Cardiovascular basics

Running a 12-lead electrocardiogram (EKG) continued

3 To apply limb lead electrodes to the patient's arms, first select a flat, fleshy site. Avoid bony or muscular areas. Then, place a small dab of conductive jelly on the site. (If conductive jelly isn't available, use a presoaked alcohol swab or a gauze pad soaked with normal saline solution.)

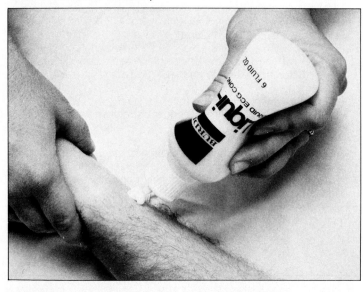

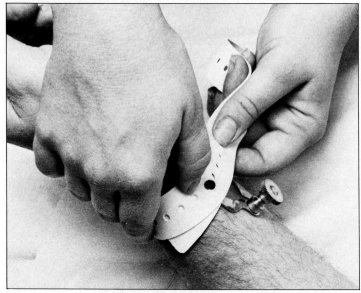

4 Place one of the limb lead electrodes on top of the jelly. Firmly secure the electrode with a rubber strap, as shown here.
Note: Avoid pulling the rubber strap too tight. Doing so may cause muscle spasms that will distort the EKG readings.

Follow the same procedure to apply a limb lead electrode at a corresponding point on the other wrist.

Then, choose a flat, fleshy site on one of the patient's legs and repeat the procedure. Apply the fourth limb lead electrode to a corresponding point on the patient's other leg, using the same procedure.

Nursing tip: Place the leg electrodes so their lead wire connectors point up the leg. This way, you can connect the lead wires to them without bending or straining the wires.

5 Connect each limb lead wire to the appropriate electrode. (Lead wires are coded by initials and/or colors.) Plug the lead wire prong into the electrode's lead wire connector. Secure it by turning the electrode screw, as shown here.

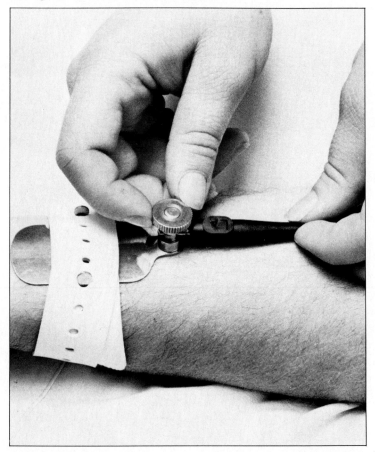

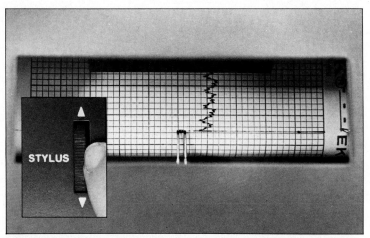

6 To turn on the EKG machine, depress the POWER switch. Then, make sure the stylus rests in the center of the EKG paper, as shown here. If it doesn't, adjust the STYLUS wheel, as shown in the inset.

If everything's OK, press the RECORD button. The stylus will draw a straight baseline on the middle of the EKG paper.

7 To standardize (calibrate) the EKG machine, turn the lead selector to ST'D (standardize); then, press the ST'D button, as shown in the inset photo. As shown in the larger photo, you'll see a square wave that's 1 millivolt high (the height of two large squares on the EKG paper). To provide a consistent frame of reference throughout the procedure, standardize the machine after you run each lead.

Note: The machine used here automatically standardizes itself. If the one you're using doesn't, you must adjust it so the square wave is 1 millivolt high. To learn how, check the operator's manual.

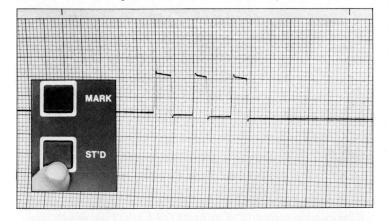

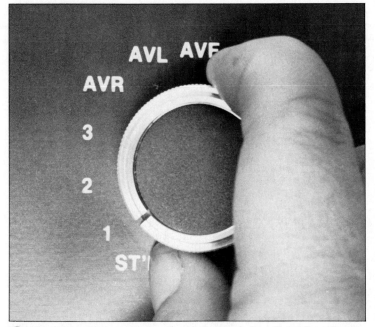

8 To run lead I, turn the lead selector knob to 1 (lead I) and run a 6-second strip.

Note: If ectopic beats or rhythm changes appear, the doctor may ask you to run longer strips.

As the strip runs, press the MARK button to mark the strip with the correct code. (If you're not sure how to code the strips, check the manufacturer's instructions or your hospital's policy.)

Now, press the AMP OFF button to stop the strip. Turn the lead selector to 2 (lead II). Then, run and mark another strip. Repeat this procedure until you've run and marked strips for leads III, AVR, AVL, and AVF.

9 Now, you're ready to apply the suction cup chest electrode. Expose Mr. Bakey's chest and place a dab of conductive jelly at the V_1 position (see page 67). Attach the chest lead wire to the chest electrode. Squeeze the electrode's rubber bulb and place the electrode on his chest, as the nurse is doing here.

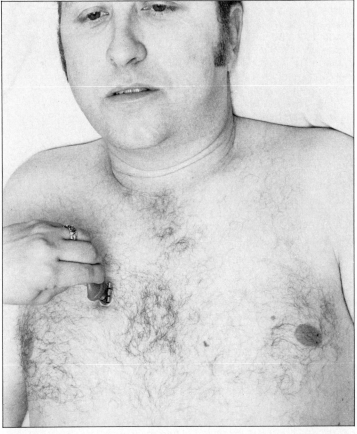

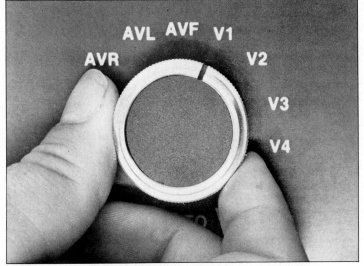

10 To run the first lead, set the lead selector on V_1, as shown here. Repeat the procedure you used to run the first six leads.

Cardiovascular basics

Running a 12-lead electrocardiogram (EKG) continued

11 To run each of the five remaining chest leads, first press AMP OFF to stop the strip. Then, reposition the chest electrode at the appropriate location, and run and mark another strip. (If the electrode won't adhere firmly, apply more conductive jelly. Or, use two fingers to hold the rubber bulb in place. To avoid causing irregularities on the strip, take care to hold your hand steady.)

After you've run all six chest leads, remove the electrodes from the patient's skin, and disconnect the lead wires from the electrodes.

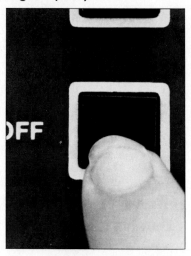

12 Using 4"x4" gauze pads, clean the conductive jelly from Mr. Bakey's skin. Help him into a gown, and position him comfortably.

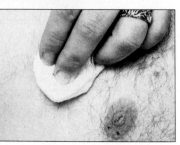

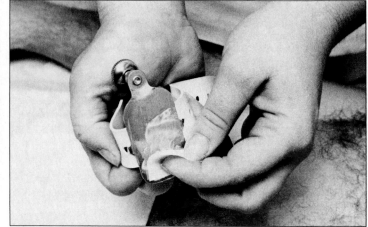

13 Use alcohol pads to clean the limb lead electrodes, as shown here. To clean the chest electrode, hold it under running water; then dry it thoroughly. Return the electrodes to the proper drawers.

Finally, document the entire procedure. On the back of each EKG strip, write the patient's name and room number, his age, the date and time of the procedure, the doctor's name, and your initials. Note whether the patient is receiving antiarrhythmic or other cardiac drugs, since they may affect heart rate or conduction intervals. In addition, write any other relevant information; for example, whether the patient was experiencing chest pain during the procedure. Then, mount the EKG strip on his chart.

Recognizing EKG waveforms

When you run a 12-lead EKG, you'll notice that each lead's waveform is distinctive. The reason, of course, is that each lead reflects the heart's electrical activity from a different view.

These illustrations show typical waveforms for each of the 12 leads. Notice that leads AVR, V_1, V_2, and V_3 show strong negative deflections; that is, deflections *below* the baseline. This is normal for those leads. Negative deflections simply show that the electrical current's flowing away from the positive electrode. Likewise, positive deflections (deflections *above* the baseline) show that the electrical current's flowing toward the positive electrode.

Take special note of the lead II waveform. Because it most clearly depicts the heart's rhythm, it's sometimes called the *rhythm strip*.

LEAD I	LEAD AVR	LEAD V₁	LEAD V₄
LEAD II	LEAD AVL	LEAD V₂	LEAD V₅
LEAD III	LEAD AVF	LEAD V₃	LEAD V₆

EKG interpretation: The basics

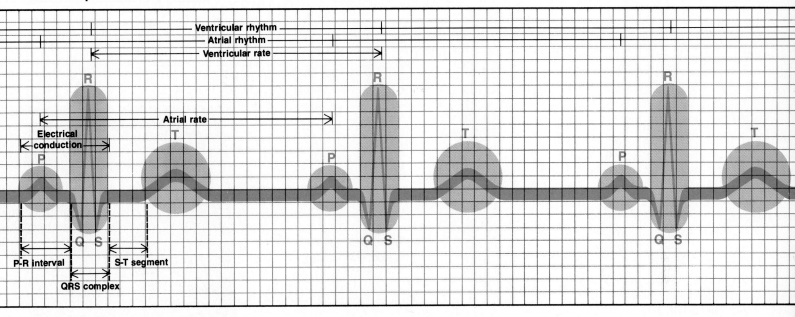

To read an EKG correctly, you must first examine the waveform to gather some basic information from it. Do you know what this basic information is? Read what follows:
● *Heart rhythm.* You can determine whether or not your patient's heart rhythm is regular or irregular by measuring the distance between each wave in a series. To determine atrial rhythm, measure the distance between two P waves, using calipers or a piece of paper. Tighten the calipers, or mark the piece of paper to indicate this distance. Then, using this marked-off distance, compare it with the distances between other P waves on the EKG strip. If the distance between each wave is exactly the same or varies less than 0.12 seconds, your patient's atrial rhythm is regular. If the distance varies slightly, his atrial rhythm's slightly irregular. If it varies markedly, his atrial rhythm is considered markedly irregular.

To determine your patient's ventricular rhythm, repeat the entire measuring procedure, using the QRS complexes. Measure from R wave to R wave.
● *Heart rate.* As you probably know, you're measuring only your patient's ventricular heart rate when you take his pulse. But you can measure both his ventricular and atrial heart rates from his EKG. If your patient's heart rhythm is *regular,* follow these steps:

Since the P wave represents atrial activity, you'll use this wave to determine your patient's atrial heart rate. Study two consecutive P waves. Select identical points on each; for example, the waves' starting points or their apex. Then, count the number of squares between these two points.

Each square represents 0.04 seconds. That means that 1,500 squares equal 1 minute. Since you want to find the atrial heart rate per minute, divide 1,500 by the number of squares you counted between P waves. The quotient is your patient's atrial heart rate.

Now, repeat the procedure with the QRS complex, measuring from R to R. This will tell you your patient's ventricular heart rate.

If your patient's heart rhythm is *irregular,* follow this procedure instead:

To determine the atrial heart rate, count the number of P waves within the space of 30 large blocks. Since each small block is equal to 0.04 seconds, and it takes five small blocks to make up one large block, each large block equals 0.2 seconds. Thirty large

blocks, therefore, equal 6 seconds. Take the number of P waves you counted within 30 large blocks (6 seconds), and multiply it by 10 to get your patient's atrial rate for 1 minute.

To determine ventricular rate for the patient with an irregular rhythm, repeat the same calculations, this time counting QRS complexes instead.
● *Electrical conduction.* Conduction refers to the time it takes for an electrical impulse originating in the heart's sinoatrial node to stimulate ventricular contraction. To determine conduction time, measure the P-R interval and the duration of the QRS complex.

To measure the P-R interval, count the squares between the beginning of the P wave and the beginning of the R wave. Then, multiply this number by 0.04 seconds. The sum represents how long it took an electrical impulse to travel from the heart's sinoatrial node through the atrium to the ventricles. The normal time is 0.12 to 0.2 seconds.

Follow the same steps to find the duration of the QRS complex. Count the squares between the beginning of the Q wave and the end of the S wave. Multiply this number by 0.04 seconds to find out how long it took an electrical impulse to pass through the heart's ventricles. The normal time is 0.04 to less than 0.12 seconds.
● *Configuration and location.* Ask yourself these basic questions to determine the configuration and location of the wave pattern: Are all the P waves the same size and shape? Do they point in the same direction? Do they precede QRS complexes? Are they all the same distance from the T waves that precede them? Are all the QRS complexes the same shape and size? Do they point in the same direction? Do they follow a P wave? Do they precede T waves? Are they all the same distance from the T waves that follow them? Are the S-T segments above or below the baseline? Do they line up with the P-R intervals? Are T waves present? Are all the T waves the same shape and size? Do they all point in the same direction?

Knowing how to gather this basic information will help you learn how to read an EKG. You'll need this same information when you use a cardiac monitor. To learn about cardiac monitoring, read the following pages.

Cardiac monitoring

Like the 12-lead electro-cardiogram (EKG), a cardiac monitor helps you assess your patient's heart conduction. But a monitor has one big advantage over the EKG—it lets you assess heart conduction *continuously.* As a result, it can warn you of cardiac problems while there may still be time to manage them successfully.

Continuous cardiac monitoring is designed with the patient's comfort in mind. Instead of applying metal electrodes to the patient's arms and legs (as you do to run a 12-lead EKG), you'll apply lightweight, comfortable disposable electrodes to his chest. These electrodes are specially designed to minimize artifact from patient movement—a must for continuous, long-term monitoring.

Can you position the electrodes correctly? Set up and operate the monitoring system? Interpret waveforms? Troubleshoot problems? For guidance, read the next few pages.

Understanding your cardiac monitor

A cardiac monitor can look intimidating. Take this central console as an example. Because it can monitor four patients at once, it has a large instrumentation panel. (A bedside monitor is less complicated.)

Examine this monitor's panel closely, so you can quickly identify its components. Chances are, the cardiac monitor in your unit is similar. *Important:* Always review the operator's manual before using any equipment.

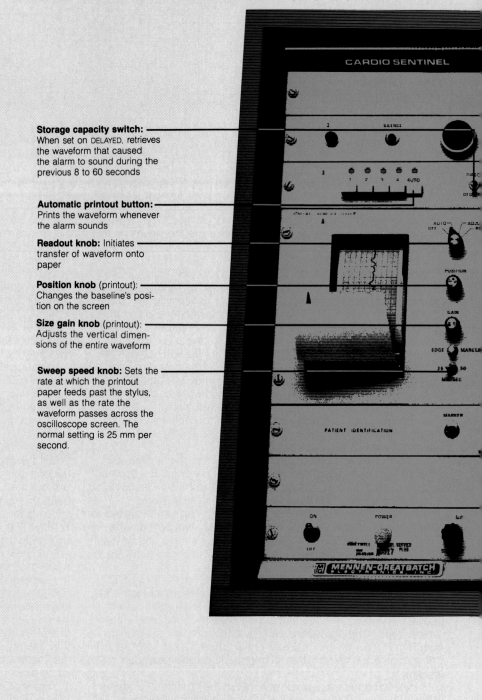

Storage capacity switch: When set on DELAYED, retrieves the waveform that caused the alarm to sound during the previous 8 to 60 seconds

Automatic printout button: Prints the waveform whenever the alarm sounds

Readout knob: Initiates transfer of waveform onto paper

Position knob (printout): Changes the baseline's position on the screen

Size gain knob (printout): Adjusts the vertical dimensions of the entire waveform

Sweep speed knob: Sets the rate at which the printout paper feeds past the stylus, as well as the rate the waveform passes across the oscilloscope screen. The normal setting is 25 mm per second.

Low alarm slide tab: Sets the alarm to sound when the patient's heartbeat drops below the allowable per minute setting

High alarm slide tab: Sets the alarm to sound when the patient's heartbeat rises above the allowable per minute setting

Rate meter: Displays the setting for the following: maximum and minimum numbers of heartbeats per minute allowable for your patient, and the actual number of heartbeats per minute your patient has

Alarm light: Flashes when the alarm goes off

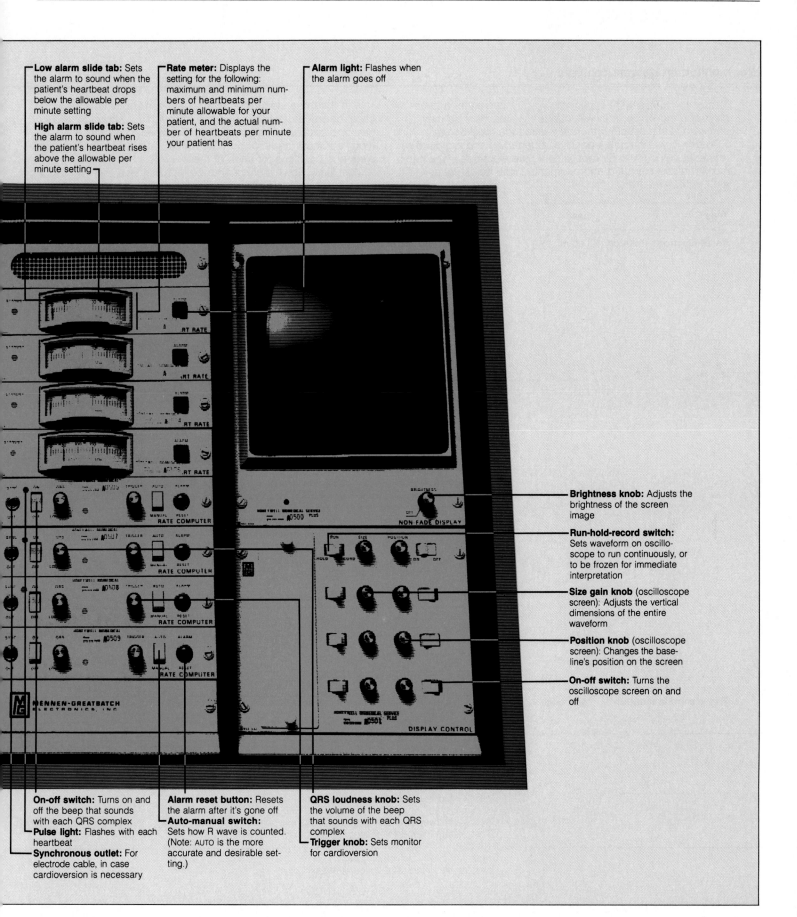

Brightness knob: Adjusts the brightness of the screen image

Run-hold-record switch: Sets waveform on oscilloscope to run continuously, or to be frozen for immediate interpretation

Size gain knob (oscilloscope screen): Adjusts the vertical dimensions of the entire waveform

Position knob (oscilloscope screen): Changes the baseline's position on the screen

On-off switch: Turns the oscilloscope screen on and off

On-off switch: Turns on and off the beep that sounds with each QRS complex

Pulse light: Flashes with each heartbeat

Synchronous outlet: For electrode cable, in case cardioversion is necessary

Alarm reset button: Resets the alarm after it's gone off

Auto-manual switch: Sets how R wave is counted. (Note: AUTO is the more accurate and desirable setting.)

QRS loudness knob: Sets the volume of the beep that sounds with each QRS complex

Trigger knob: Sets monitor for cardioversion

Cardiac monitoring

How monitoring systems compare

To monitor your patient continuously, you'll use either a three-electrode monitor or a five-electrode monitor. How do they compare? Let's consider the three-electrode monitor first.

To use it, you'll apply a positive, a negative, and a ground (or reference) electrode. By repositioning the electrodes, you can monitor all six standard and augmented limb leads (leads I, II, III, AVR, AVL, AVF).

With the three-electrode monitor, you can't obtain the six chest or precordial leads (leads V_1 through V_6). However, you can *approximate* leads V_1 and V_6. To do so, you'll use the modified chest leads, abbreviated MCL_1 and MCL_6. The correct electrode positions for each of these leads are shown below.

Most likely, you'll monitor your patient with lead II, lead MCL_1, or lead MCL_6. (That's why we've illustrated electrode placement

Type	Lead	Electrode placement	
Three-electrode monitor	Lead II	Positive (+): left side of chest, lowest palpable rib, midclavicular Negative (−): right shoulder, below clavicular hollow Ground (G): left shoulder, below clavicular hollow	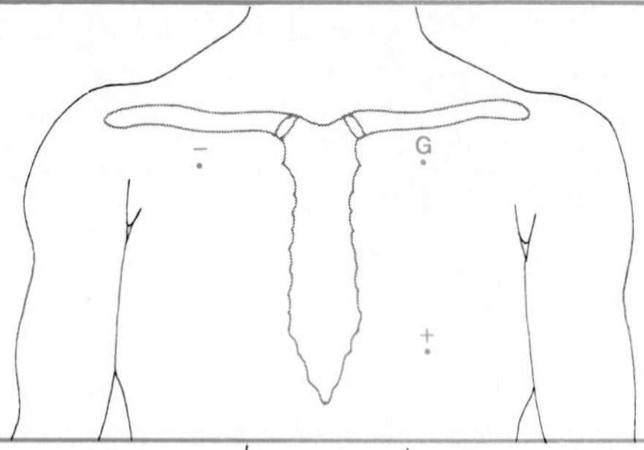
	MCL_1	Positive (+): right sternal border, lowest palpable rib Negative (−): left shoulder, below clavicular hollow Ground (G): right shoulder, below clavicular hollow	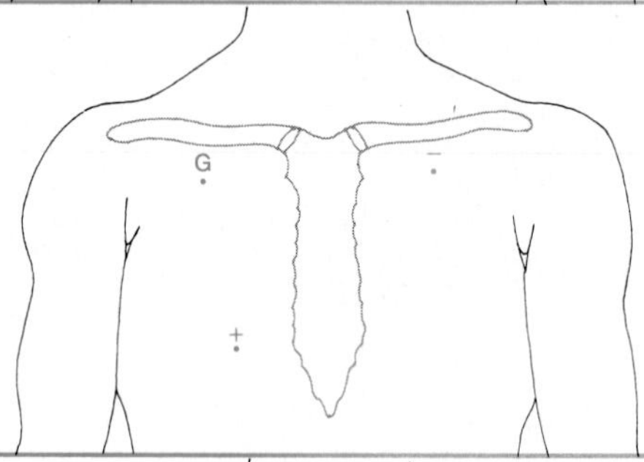
	MCL_6	Positive (+): left side of chest, lowest palpable rib, midclavicular Negative (−): left shoulder, below clavicular hollow Ground (G): right shoulder, below clavicular hollow	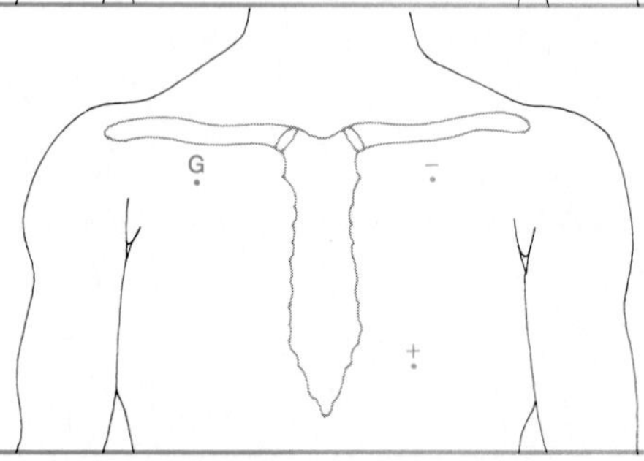
Five-electrode monitor	V_1 through V_6	Left leg (LL): left side of chest, just below lowest palpable rib Right arm (RA): right shoulder, midclavicular Ground (G): right side of chest, just below lowest palpable rib Left arm (LA): left shoulder, midclavicular Chest V_1: fourth intercostal space to right of sternum Chest V_2: fourth intercostal space to left of sternum Chest V_3: halfway between V_2 and V_4 Chest V_4: fifth intercostal space, midclavicular, left side Chest V_5: halfway between V_4 and V_6 Chest V_6: fifth intercostal space at midaxillary line	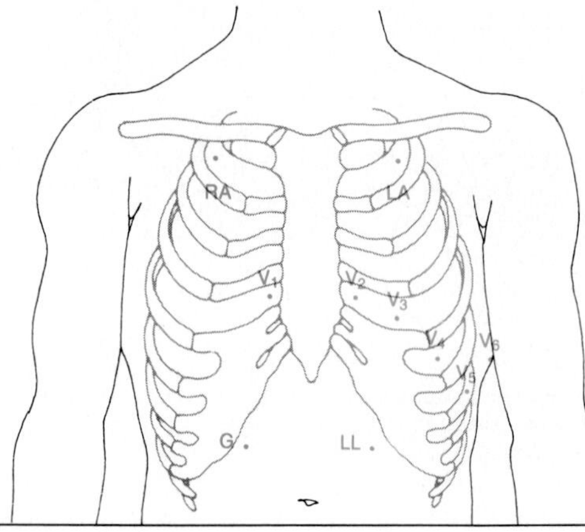

for these three leads.) The doctor will choose the lead depending on the part of the heart he wants to monitor. To change from one lead to another, you must reposition the electrodes.

The five-electrode system is more versatile: It can monitor all 12 leads, just like the 12-lead EKG. The four basic electrodes are the right arm (RA), left arm (LA), right leg (RL), and left leg (LL). The right leg electrode is always the ground. Once these four electrodes are in place, you can monitor each of the first six standard and augmented limb leads by simply changing the monitor's lead selector switch.

Now, how about the six chest leads? As with a 12-lead EKG, you'll position the fifth electrode at a different location for each of the six chest leads. (See the fourth drawing on page 74.)

Read this chart to learn more about these two systems.

Purpose	Advantages	Disadvantages	Waveform
• Identifies atrial and some ventricular arrhythmias • Detects hemiblocks	• Clear P wave • Tall, distinct R wave	• Can't distinguish between right or left bundle branch blocks	
• Identifies atrial and ventricular arrhythmias • Identifies complete and incomplete right bundle branch blocks • Identifies ventricular conduction	• Positive electrode placement doesn't interfere with auscultation or defibrillation • Detects left bundle branch block or left ventricular hypertrophy	• R wave depressed or of insufficient voltage	
• Identifies ventricular arrhythmias • Detects left bundle branch block • Replaces MCL₁ if that arrangement can't be used	• Tall, distinct R wave • Detects right bundle branch block	• Poor visualization of atrial and arrhythmic activity	
• Obtains a precise, multiplaned view of the heart's activity • Detects ventricular hypertrophy	• Standard and augmented leads obtained by turning a monitor switch, instead of moving an electrode	• Two more electrodes are attached to the patient's chest	

Cardiac monitoring

Initiating continuous monitoring

1 *Doris Samuels, a 73-year-old retired professor, has suffered a myocardial infarction. One of the first things you do when she enters the ICU is to begin continuous cardiac monitoring. In this photostory, you'll see how to set up a three-electrode monitor.*

First, gather this equipment: three disposable electrodes, an alcohol swab, a sterile 4"x4" gauze pad, three lead wires, and a lead wire receptacle. (If your patient's a man, you may also need a razor to shave his chest hair before applying the electrodes.) If your ICU is like most units, a cardiac monitor is permanently installed at bedside.

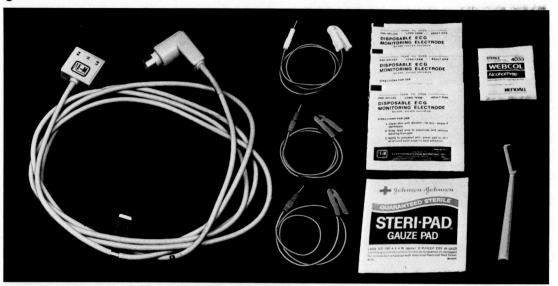

2 Explain the procedure to Mrs. Samuels. Assure her that although the equipment is electrical, it won't cause an electrical shock. In addition, explain the monitor's alarm system, so she won't panic if an alarm sounds. Answer all her questions before proceeding.

Let's say the doctor's chosen lead II for monitoring Mrs. Samuels. The chart on page 74 shows you where to apply the electrodes for that lead. At each location, clean the skin with an alcohol swab, and abrade the skin slightly with the gauze pad. (Some disposable electrodes are designed with a rough patch for this purpose.)

Nursing tip: If your patient's diaphoretic, try spraying a little antiperspirant at the site to prevent electrode slippage.

3 Then, peel off the electrode's paper backing, as shown here, and place the electrode on the intended site with the adhesive side down. Ensure a good seal by applying pressure, beginning at the center of the electrode and moving outward. This way, you're unlikely to force out any of the conductive jelly.

Important: For better conduction, try to avoid placing electrodes directly over bones.

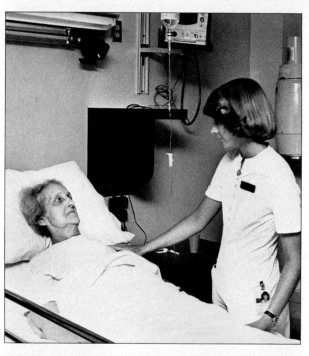

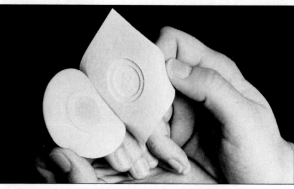

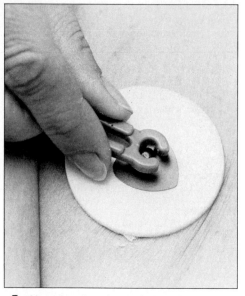

4 Now that the electrodes are in place, how can you tell which lead wire to attach to which electrodes? If your lead wires are marked +, −, or G, just attach them to their corresponding electrodes, as labeled in the chart on page 74.

But, what if your lead wires are coded RA, LA, LL, and (with five-electrode monitors) RL? Mentally divide your patient's chest into quadrants. Attach the RA lead wire to the electrode positioned nearest the patient's right arm. Attach the RL lead wire to the electrode nearest the patient's right leg, and so on. (The fifth lead wire of the five-electrode monitor attaches to the fifth electrode on the patient's chest.)

If your lead wires are color coded, consult the operator's manual for instructions.

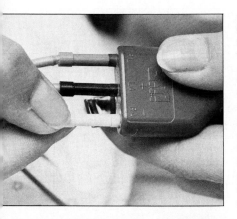

5 Attach the other ends of the lead wires to the lead wire receptacle. How can you tell which lead wires attach to which electrode outlets? The electrode outlets will be marked either with +, −, G symbols; RA, LA, RL abbreviations; or colors. Know your system's markings.

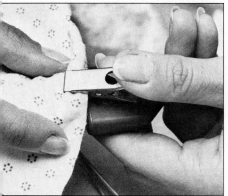

6 Fasten the lead wire receptacle to the patient's gown. This prevents undue stress on the lead wires when the patient moves.

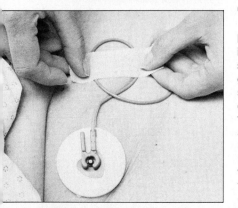

7 Form a stress loop in each lead wire, and tape it to the patient's skin with nonallergenic tape, as shown here. Leave enough slack between the electrode and the stress loop to allow for patient movement without straining the electrode connection.

8 Plug the lead wire receptacle cable into the bedside monitor.

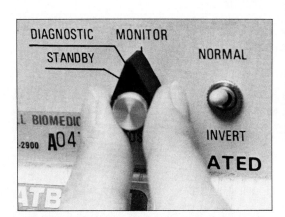
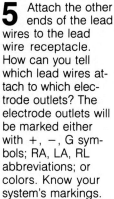

9 Turn the HOLD-RUN-RECORD switch to RUN.
Then, turn the mode switch from STANDBY to MONITOR, as shown. Expect a tracing to appear in about 20 seconds.

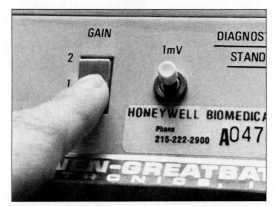

10 How tall is the QRS complex you're getting? It must be tall enough for the monitor to record each beat. But don't make it so tall that it barely fits on the oscilloscope screen.
If you want to enlarge the QRS complex, set the GAIN switch at 2. If you want to decrease it, set the GAIN switch at 1.

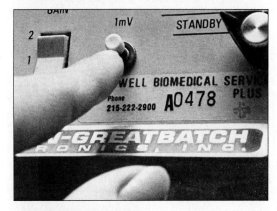

11 Next, calibrate the monitor by pressing the button marked 1mV or CAL, (depending on the equipment). This will produce a 1 millivolt high waveform on the oscilloscope. If the R wave of the patient's QRS complex isn't higher than the 1 millivolt waveform, adjust the GAIN setting so it is.

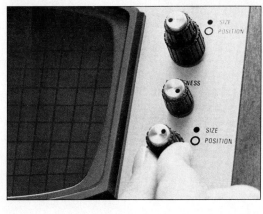

12 Then, if necessary, turn the position knob to center the waveform on the oscilloscope.

Cardiac monitoring

Initiating continuous monitoring continued

13 Most likely, your monitoring system has a central console, like this one. Find the group of controls on the console's front panel that corresponds to the controls on the bedside monitor. Touch only these controls.

If you're using a self-contained bedside monitor, continue the procedure there.

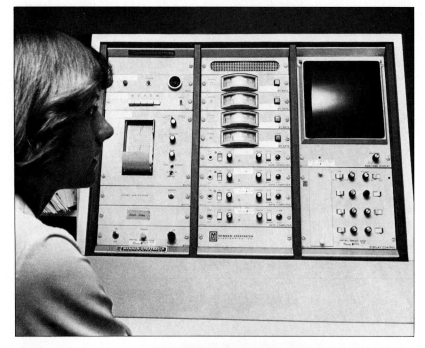

14 Set the HIGH alarm at 120 beats per minute (BPM) and the LOW alarm at 50 BPM, unless the doctor orders otherwise.

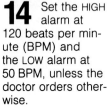

15 Set the heart rate alarm to AUTO, so it'll sound whenever the patient's heart rate goes above or below the limits you've set.

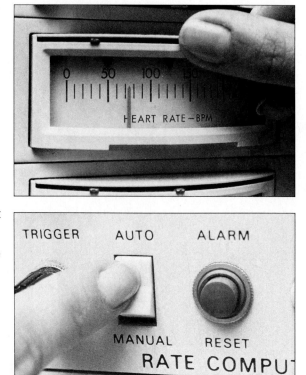

16 Now, check to see if each QRS complex on the oscilloscope is being counted by the monitor. First, turn on the audible QRS signal. It will sound with each QRS complex counted. You can also tell if they're counted by watching the rate light. If the audible alarm doesn't sound, or the rate light doesn't blink with each complex, increase the GAIN setting until the QRS complex is tall enough to trigger these signals every time.

Note: When you're using a central console, don't make the QRS complex so tall that it interferes with other waveforms on the console's oscilloscope.

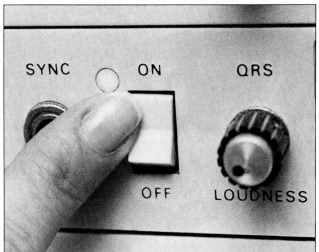

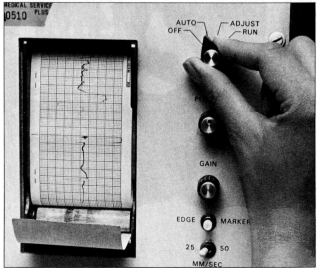

17 Turn the recorder to AUTO and the SWEEP to 25 mm/sec. With these settings, if the patient's heart rate sets off the alarm, the recorder will print as fast as the oscilloscope shows the waveform.

Finally, check the paper in the recorder. If necessary, add more paper, following the instructions in the operator's manual.

Now that you've initiated continuous monitoring, you can readily evaluate Mrs. Samuels' heartbeat throughout her hospitalization.

Troubleshooting cardiac monitors

This chart shows you how to troubleshoot the common problems you're apt to encounter while working with a cardiac monitor. Keep in mind that no matter what problem arises with the equipment, always examine your patient first.

Problem	Possible causes	Solution
Skin excoriation under electrode	• Patient allergic to the electrode adhesive	• Remove electrodes and apply nonallergenic electrodes and nonallergenic tape.
	• Electrode left on skin too long	• Remove electrode, clean site, and reapply electrode at new site. *Note:* Do this every 2 or 3 days to avoid the problem.
Broken lead wires or a broken cable	• Stress loops not used on lead wires	• Replace lead wires and retape them, using stress loops.
	• Cables and lead wires cleaned with alcohol or acetone, causing brittleness	• Clean cable and lead wires with soapy water instead of alcohol or acetone. *Important:* Do not get cable ends wet.
Wandering baseline	• Patient restless	• Encourage patient to relax.
	• Chest wall movement during respiration	• Tighten electrode connections.
	• Improper application of electrodes; electrode positioned over bone	• Check electrodes and reapply them, if necessary. Place electrodes on fleshy, not bony areas.
	• Use of nonpolarized electrodes	• Replace electrodes with polarized ones.
Straight line on monitor (not caused by asystole)	• Improper connection of lead wire to either electrode or cable	• Check cable and electrode connections and adjust them, if necessary.
Fuzzy baseline (60- or 50-cycle interference)	• Electrical interference from other equipment in the room	• Make sure all electrical equipment is attached to the patient's common ground. Check three-pronged plugs to make sure none of the prongs are loose.
	• Improper grounding of patient's bed	• Make sure the bed ground is attached to the room's common ground.
Artifact (waveform interference)	• Patient experiencing seizures, chills, or anxiety	• Notify doctor if the patient's having seizures, and treat patient, as ordered. Keep patient warm and reassured. Spend time with him, and discuss his fears.
	• Patient restless	• Encourage patient to relax.
	• Dirty or corroded connections	• Replace dirty or corroded wires.
	• Improper application of electrodes	• Check electrodes and reapply them, if necessary. Take care to clean the patient's skin thoroughly, because skin oils and dead skin cells interfere with conduction. • Check electrode jelly. If the jelly's dry, apply new electrodes.
	• Electrical short circuit in lead wires or cable	• Replace broken equipment. Use stress loops when applying lead wires.
	• Electrical interference from other equipment in the room	• Make sure all electrical equipment is attached to a common ground. Check three-pronged plugs to make sure none of the prongs are loose.
	• Static electricity interference, from decrease in room humidity.	• Regulate room humidity to 40%, if possible.
Double-triggering (P wave and QRS complex, or QRS complex and T wave, are of equal height)	• GAIN setting too high, particularly with MCL$_1$ setting	• Reset GAIN. If possible, monitor patient on MCL$_6$ or another available lead.
Alarm sounds, but you see no evidence of arrhythmia	• Improper application of electrodes	• Reapply electrodes.
	• QRS complex too small to register	• Reset GAIN so that the height of the complex is greater than 1 millivolt.
	• QRS complex not registering because of axis shift	• Try monitoring patient on another lead.
	• HIGH alarm set too low, or LOW alarm set too high	• Set alarm limits according to patient's heart rate.
	• Artifact (waveform interference)	• Check electrodes and reapply them, if necessary.
	• Wire or cable failure	• Replace faulty wire or cable.
	• Voltage too high or too low	• Adjust GAIN on bedside monitor.

Cardiac monitoring

Nurses' guide to cardiac arrhythmias

Suppose you're caring for a cardiovascular patient. Suddenly, his cardiac monitor's oscilloscope screen begins displaying one of the waveforms shown below. Can you tell what's happening? Do you know what nursing actions to take? Read this chart for details. Of course, you'll administer drugs and treatments according to the doctor's orders. But you're also responsible for understanding each drug's effects. To help, we've provided information on what drugs the doctor's likely to order, and why. For more information about drug dosages and side effects, see the NURSE'S GUIDE TO DRUGS™ or the NURSE'S DRUG HANDBOOK.

Arrhythmia	Description	Possible cause	Nursing intervention
Sinus bradycardia 	• 50 beats per minute (BPM) or less • Regular rhythm • Normal waveform configuration and electrical conduction	• Increased intracranial pressure • Vagal stimulation • Sick sinus syndrome • Hypothyroidism • Hypothermia • Sleep • Treatment with beta-blockers and sympatholytic drugs • Treatment with morphine sulfate *Note:* Sinus bradycardia may be normal in an athlete.	• Treat only if patient is symptomatic. • Give at least 0.5 mg atropine sulfate I.V., and repeat every 5 minutes, up to 2 mg, to treat low cardiac output, dizziness, weakness, altered level of consciousness, or low blood pressure. (Less than 0.5 mg atropine sulfate may cause paradoxical slowing of impulses generated by the sinoatrial [SA] node.) • Elevate legs to increase venous return. • If atropine sulfate isn't effective, the doctor may insert a temporary pacemaker. Or, the doctor may give isoproterenol hydrochloride (Isuprel*).
Sinus tachycardia 	• 100 to 180 BPM • Regular rhythm • Normal waveform configuration and electrical conduction	• Congestive heart failure • Myocardial infarction • Cardiac tamponade • Anemia • Hyperthyroidism • Hypovolemia • Pulmonary embolism • Myocarditis • Hypoxia or hypercapnia • Vagolytic, sympathomimetic drugs or bronchodilators *Note:* Sinus tachycardia may be a normal response to fever, anxiety, or pain.	• If patient is symptomatic, give propranolol hydrochloride (Inderal*) to increase cardiac output. • Administer sedatives to control anxiety. • Administer analgesics for pain and antipyretics to reduce fever.
Wandering pacemaker 	• 60 to 100 BPM • Variable rhythm • Variable P-R intervals (but no more than 0.2 seconds) • Irregular P waves, indicating that they're not all from the SA node or a single atrial focus and that some isolated beats are controlled by the atrioventricular (AV) junction • P wave for each QRS complex • Normal QRS complexes	• Inflammation of the SA node caused by pancarditis • Ischemia of SA node • Digitalis toxicity • Sick sinus syndrome • Pressure on carotid artery • Administration of phenylephrine hydrochloride (Neo-Synephrine*), causing reflex vagal stimulation	• Discontinue digitalis or other drugs that may cause wandering pacemaker, as ordered.
Premature atrial contractions (PACs) 	• Variable rate • Irregular rhythm, due to premature P waves • P waves may be inverted or irregularly-shaped • P wave may appear or may be buried in the preceding T wave • P-R intervals may be extended because of premature P waves • QRS complexes follow P waves, except in very early or blocked PACs • QRS complex usually normal	• Vagal stimulation • Congestive heart failure • Hyperthyroidism • Rheumatic valvular disease • Electrolyte imbalance • Ischemic heart disease • Cor pulmonale • Acute respiratory failure • Atrial disease or enlargement • Chronic obstructive pulmonary disease • Treatment with digitalis, aminophylline, or sympathomimetic drugs such as dextroamphetamines, which increase neuromuscular activity • Anxiety • Excessive caffeine consumption	• If PACs appear more than six times a minute, and the patient shows signs of compromised cardiac function (such as decreased cardiac output), give digitalis to increase myocardial contractility and decrease impulse conduction through the AV node to slow heart rate. • If digitalis alone isn't effective, give it with quinidine or procainamide hydrochloride (Pronestyl*). *Note:* Occasional PACs may be normal and are not treated unless the patient is symptomatic.

*Available in both the United States and in Canada

Arrhythmia	Description	Possible cause	Nursing intervention
Paroxysmal atrial tachycardia (PAT) 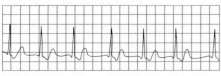	• 150 to 250 BPM • Regular rhythm • P wave abnormal or inverted, but shape stays constant • P wave sometimes merges with T wave • P-R interval may (rarely) be prolonged • QRS complex normal *Note:* Onset and termination of arrhythmia occur suddenly.	• Intrinsic abnormality of AV conduction system • Congenital accessory atrial conduction pathway • Physical or psychological stress • Hypoxia • Hyperthyroidism • Hypokalemia • Digitalis toxicity • Excessive use of caffeine, alcohol, or tobacco • Rheumatic heart disease • Hypertension • Mitral valve prolapse • Coronary artery disease • Cor pulmonale	• Have patient perform Valsalva maneuver. • Instruct patient to sit and lean forward with head down or to lie prone with head lower than trunk. • Perform carotid artery massage if hospital policy allows. *Important:* Massage only one artery at a time for no longer than 5 seconds. If PATs don't stop within 5 seconds, consider the massage ineffective and stop. • Administer cardiac glycosides such as digoxin (Lanoxin*), to decrease heart rate and increase cardiac output. (Don't give digitalis if cardioversion is planned.) • Administer antiarrhythmic drugs, such as procainamide hydrochloride, (Pronestyl*), disopyramide phosphate (Norpace*), phenytoin sodium (Dilantin*), or propranolol hydrochloride (Inderal*) to restore normal sinus rhythm. • Administer sympathomimetics such as phenylephrine hydrochloride (Neo-Synephrine*) to increase heart rate and ventricular contractility. • Stimulating the patient's gag reflex also provides vagal stimulation, which can convert PAT to normal sinus rhythm. • Doctor may perform elective cardioversion if drug therapy fails.
Atrial flutter	• Atrial rate from 250 to 350 BPM; ventricular rate variable (usually 60 to 100 BPM) • Atrial rhythm regular; ventricular rhythm variable • QRS complexes uniform in shape • QRS complex follows flutter (F) wave, but not all flutter waves are followed by QRS complex • F waves have sawtooth shape	• Congestive heart failure • Coronary artery disease • Valvular heart disease (such as rheumatic heart disease) • Myocardial infarction • Pulmonary embolism • Hyperthyroidism • Hypertension • Wolff-Parkinson-White (WPW) syndrome (also called preexcitation syndrome)	• Give digitalis, propranolol hydrochloride (Inderal*), quinidine gluconate, or procainamide hydrochloride (Pronestyl*). • Don't give digitalis if atrial flutter is caused by WPW syndrome. Instead, give quinidine gluconate or propranolol hydrochloride (Inderal*). • Doctor may perform cardioversion and insert an atrial pacemaker. • If digoxin and quinidine ordered, give digoxin first to delay conduction.
Atrial fibrillation	• Atrial rate 350 to 600 BPM; ventricular rate variable • Irregular rhythm • P waves absent • P-R intervals can't be measured • QRS complexes uniform in shape, but irregular in rate • P wave indistinct and may appear as wavy baseline • A ventricular response of 100 beats or less is called controlled atrial fibrillation.	• Coronary artery disease • Rheumatic heart disease • Hypertension • Hyperthyroidism • Pericarditis • Pulmonary embolism • Mitral stenosis • Cardiomyopathy • Myocardial infarction	• Administer digitalis and quinidine gluconate for rapid ventricular rate. • Administer quinidine gluconate to restore normal sinus rhythm. • Give diuretics for congestive heart failure. • Doctor may perform elective cardioversion, if drug therapy fails. • Administer quinidine gluconate, propranolol hydrochloride (Inderal*), and procainamide hydrochloride (Pronestyl*), in addition to digitalis.
Junctional rhythm (nodal rhythm)	• 40 to 60 BPM • Regular rhythm • P wave, if present, is inverted; may precede, follow, or be hidden in QRS complex • QRS complex usually normal	• Digitalis toxicity • Inferior wall myocardial infarction or ischemia • Sick sinus syndrome • Hypoxia • Vagal stimulation • Acute rheumatic fever • SA node dysfunction	• Give atropine sulfate to correct slow heart rate. • If patient is taking digitalis, discontinue it. • Treat only if patient is symptomatic.

*Available in both the United States and in Canada

Cardiac monitoring

Nurses' guide to cardiac arrhythmias continued

Arrhythmia	Description	Possible cause	Nursing intervention
Premature junctional contractions (PJCs)	• Variable rate • Irregular rhythm • Premature P waves shorten P-R intervals; premature P waves may follow or be hidden in QRS complexes • QRS complex uniform in shape, but irregular in rhythm • No P wave or inverted P wave before, in, or following QRS	• Myocardial infarction or ischemia • Sick sinus syndrome • Digitalis toxicity • Congestive heart failure • Excessive use of caffeine or tobacco	• Give quinidine gluconate to decrease cardiac excitability. • If patient is taking digitalis, discontinue it. Note: PJCs are not treated unless the patient is symptomatic.
Premature ventricular contractions (PVCs)	• Variable rate; QRS complex premature and usually followed by a complete compensatory pause after PVC • Irregular pulse • QRS complex wide and distorted; QRS complex usually premature in relation to prevailing rhythm • S-T segment and T wave usually in opposite direction of QRS complex. Note: PVCs can occur singly, in pairs, or in groups of three or more. They may alternate with normal beats, and are considered most ominous when clustered and multifocal with R wave on T pattern.	• Coronary artery disease • Congestive heart failure • Myocardial infarction • Cardiomyopathy • Hypoxia • Drug toxicity (digitalis, aminophylline, tricyclic antidepressants, beta-adrenergics) • Hypokalemia • Psychological stress • Hypercalcemia • Rheumatic heart disease • Hypertension • Hyperthyroidism	• Cautiously give lidocaine hydrochloride (Xylocaine*) I.V. bolus and by drip infusion or procainamide hydrochloride (Pronestyl*) I.V. Note: PVCs may trigger ventricular fibrillation. • If PVCs are caused by digitalis toxicity, discontinue drug. • If PVCs are caused by hypokalemia, give potassium chloride I.V. • Give phenytoin sodium (Dilantin*) to decrease conduction velocity through the AV conduction system, and to decrease ventricular automaticity. • Give atropine sulfate or isoproterenol hydrochloride (Isuprel*) to increase heart rate. Doctor may insert a pacemaker. • Give quinidine gluconate to depress myocardial excitability, conduction velocity, and contractability.
Ventricular tachycardia (VT)	• Ventricular rate 100 to 270 BPM; atrial rate variable • Regular atrial rhythm; ventricular rhythm may be regular • P wave normal when visible; P wave relationship to QRS complex variable • P-R interval variable	• Myocardial infarction, myocardial ischemia or ventricular aneurysm • Ventricular irritation, such as that caused by ventricular catheter • Digitalis or quinidine toxicity • Hypokalemia or hyperkalemia • Hypercalcemia • Adams-Stokes syndrome • Wolff-Parkinson-White (WPW) syndrome	• Initiate cardiopulmonary resuscitation (CPR), if necessary. • Give lidocaine hydrochloride (Xylocaine*) I.V. bolus and by drip infusion to decrease ventricular excitability. • Give bretylium tosylate (Bretylol) to treat recurrent episodes. • Give procainamide hydrochloride (Pronestyl*) or quinidine gluconate, except with heart block or Adams-Stokes syndrome. In those cases, give isoproterenol hydrochloride (Isuprel*). • Give potassium chloride, if VTs are caused by digitalis toxicity. • Initiate emergency cardioversion, according to hospital policy. • Doctor may insert an artificial pacemaker to treat drug-resistant ventricular tachycardia.
Ventricular fibrillation	• Very rapid chaotic ventricular rate with undeterminable atrial rate • No visible P waves • P-R interval undeterminable • QRS complexes wide and irregular Note: Ventricular fibrillation causes loss of consciousness with no pulses, blood pressure, audible heart sounds, or respirations; possible seizures; and death (if uncorrected).	• Myocardial ischemia or infarction • Untreated ventricular tachycardia • Electrolyte imbalance • Digitalis, procainamide hydrochloride, or quinidine toxicity • Electric shock • Hypothermia • Left ventricular failure • Hypoxia • Pacemaker malfunction	• Initiate CPR. • Initiate defibrillation. Prior administration of epinephrine hydrochloride (Adrenalin Chloride) improves the heart's response to defibrillation. • Give lidocaine hydrochloride (Xylocaine*) to restore normal rhythm, or bretylium tosylate (Bretylol) I.V. to treat recurrent episodes. • Give sodium bicarbonate to correct lactic acidosis. • Give lidocaine hydrochloride (Xylocaine*) to prevent further ventricular fibrillation.

*Available in both the United States and in Canada

Arrhythmia	Description	Possible cause	Nursing intervention
Ventricular standstill (asystole)	• Regular P waves, no QRS complexes	• Myocardial infarction or ischemia • Ruptured ventricular aneurysm • Aortic valve disease • Hyperkalemia • Acute respiratory failure	• Initiate CPR. • Give epinephrine hydrochloride (Adrenalin Chloride) and calcium gluconate (to restore myocardial contractability) and sodium bicarbonate (to correct lactic acidosis). *Note:* Do not give calcium gluconate if patient's taking digoxin. • Doctor may insert a temporary pacemaker.
First degree AV block	• Variable rate (usually 60 to 100 BPM) • Regular rhythm • P waves normal • P-R interval prolonged (greater than 0.2 seconds) • QRS complex normal	• Inferior or anterior wall myocardial infarction or ischemia • Hypothyroidism • Digitalis, quinidine, or procainamide hydrochloride toxicity • Hyperkalemia • Rheumatic heart disease	• If patient's taking digitalis, discontinue it as ordered. • Be alert for increasing block. • Give atropine sulfate to accelerate AV conduction. • Give isoproterenol hydrochloride (Isuprel*) if atropine sulfate fails to increase cardiac output. • Doctor may insert a transvenous pacemaker, if drug therapy's unsuccessful. *Note:* First degree AV block usually doesn't require special treatment, unless the patient develops symptoms.
Second degree AV block (Wenckebach or Mobitz Type I)	• Variable heart rate (atrial rate greater than ventricular rate) • Irregular ventricular rhythm; regular atrial rhythm • P-R interval becomes progressively longer with each consecutive cycle until QRS complex disappears (dropped beat). After a dropped beat, P-R interval shortens; then becomes gradually longer until another beat is dropped. • P waves usually precede QRS complex, but QRS complex may not follow each P wave • QRS complex usually normal	• Inferior wall myocardial infarction • Digitalis, quinidine, or procainamide hydrochloride toxicity • Vagal stimulation • Rheumatic heart disease	• Give atropine sulfate to accelerate AV conduction. • Give isoproterenol hydrochloride (Isuprel*) to increase heart rate. • If patient is taking digitalis (or another drug that may cause block), discontinue it. *Note:* If block is above the bundle of His, the patient's heart rate is probably adequate, and no therapy is needed.
Second degree AV block (Mobitz Type II)	• Variable heart rate (atrial rate greater than ventricular rate) • P-R interval usually normal, consistent with QRS complex • QRS complex may not follow each P wave • Ventricular rhythm may be irregular with pause caused by missing QRS complex. (Two identical P-R intervals precede a dropped QRS complex.) • QRS complex usually wide, with bundle branch configuration	• Degenerative disease of conduction system • Ischemia of AV node caused by anterior myocardial infarction • Digitalis toxicity	• Give isoproterenol hydrochloride (Isuprel*) to increase conduction through AV node. • If patient is taking digitalis, discontinue it. • Doctor will insert temporary or permanent pacemaker.
Third degree AV block (complete heart block)	• Regular rhythm • Regular atrial rate; slow, regular ventricular rate (usually 20 to 45 BPM) • Atrial and ventricular rates and rhythms are independent of each other • No relationship between P waves and QRS complexes • No constant P-R interval • QRS complex normal (junctional pacemaker), or wide and bizarre (ventricular pacemaker)	• Digitalis toxicity • Myocarditis • Cardiomyopathy • Myocardial infarction or ischemia • Hypoxia	• Give epinephrine hydrochloride (Adrenalin Chloride) to restore myocardial activity, or isoproterenol hydrochloride (Isuprel*) to increase cardiac output. • Doctor will insert a temporary pacemaker. Later, he will probably insert a permanent pacemaker.

*Available in both the United States and in Canada

Hemodynamic monitoring

Accurate hemody-namic measurements remain one of the best—and earliest—indicators of changes in your patient's con-dition. Without ques-tion, your skill at taking accurate mea-surements is crucial.

In the ICU, you may monitor the blood pressure in your patient's peripheral arteries invasively or noninvasively. In the following pages, we'll show you how to do both.

In addition, we'll introduce you to the balloon-tipped pulmo-nary artery (PA) cath-eter that's threaded through the heart's right chambers. When your patient has a PA catheter in place, you can directly mea-sure hemodynamic pressures inside his heart.

Like any equipment, hemodynamic moni-toring equipment can be temperamen-tal. To help you solve problems you may occasionally encoun-ter, we've also pro-vided two pages of troubleshooting tips.

How blood pressure varies among arteries

As you know, you may take a blood pressure reading from more than one artery. But have you ever considered how your choice of an artery affects the reading? As you see in this illustration, diastolic pressure and mean arterial pressure (MAP) decrease slightly as blood travels from the heart. Sys-tolic pressure, on the other hand, in-creases. In fact, systolic pressure usually registers 20 to 30 mm Hg higher in a patient's lower legs than in his forearms.

Why? Because arteries in the extremities are narrower and less elastic than arteries closer to the patient's heart. As a result, resistance to blood flow increases as blood travels away from the heart.

In addition, blood is reflected at branches where two arteries meet (anastomoses). The backward pressure exerted by this re-flected blood also increases resistance and adds pressure to the systolic pulse.

Now, suppose your patient has an arterial line in place. How does the catheter's location affect the waveform displayed on the monitor's oscilloscope screen? Look at the illustrations below. If the catheter rests in a small artery far from the heart (such as the dorsalis pedis or radial artery), the waveform's systolic peak is narrow and pointed. As the illustrations indicate, the dicrotic notch disappears from the wave-form, but a prominent diastolic hump develops.

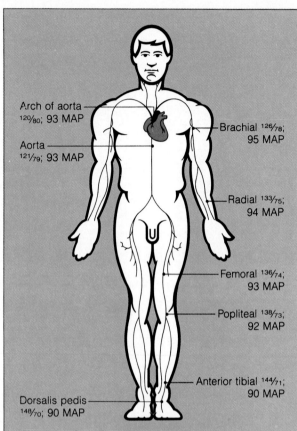

Arch of aorta ${}^{120}/_{80}$; 93 MAP

Aorta ${}^{121}/_{79}$; 93 MAP

Brachial ${}^{126}/_{78}$; 95 MAP

Radial ${}^{133}/_{75}$; 94 MAP

Femoral ${}^{136}/_{74}$; 93 MAP

Popliteal ${}^{138}/_{73}$; 92 MAP

Anterior tibial ${}^{144}/_{71}$; 90 MAP

Dorsalis pedis ${}^{148}/_{70}$; 90 MAP

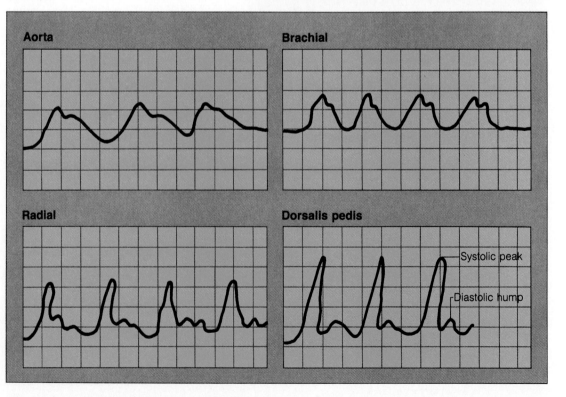

Aorta

Brachial

Radial

Dorsalis pedis

Systolic peak

Diastolic hump

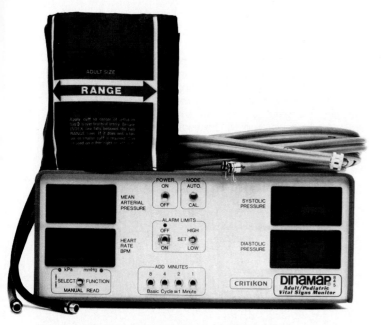

Noninvasive blood pressure monitoring

If your patient needs frequent blood pressure monitoring, but doesn't have an arterial catheter in place, you may use a noninvasive blood pressure monitor, like the Critikon Dinamap® 845 shown here. After automatically inflating an ordinary pressure cuff, the monitor provides highly accurate blood pressure and heart rate measurements.

Unlike an arterial line, this monitor can't provide *continuous* monitoring. However, it can provide *frequent* monitoring at intervals as brief as 1 minute. In addition, it eliminates the risks of invasive monitoring.

The Dinamap monitor operates by the oscillometric method. In simple terms, it detects pressure pulsations (oscillations) as the cuff deflates. It does this with a transducer located inside the monitor itself— not the pressure cuff. The placement of the precalibrated transducer inside the monitor contributes to the system's accuracy.

In addition to providing systolic, diastolic, and heart rate measurements, the monitor provides mean arterial pressure (MAP) readings after each inflation. Since MAP indicates the pressure available for tissue perfusion, it's a valuable indicator of your patient's condition.

Examine the Dinamap's front and back panels, shown above and below. Then, read the following photostory to see how to operate this monitor.

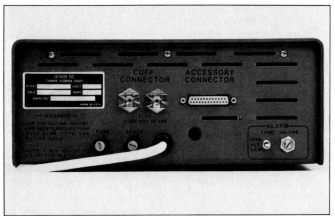

Using a Critikon Dinamap® monitor

1 *Let's say the doctor wants you to monitor your patient's blood pressure at 6-minute intervals. Because your unit has a Critikon Dinamap blood pressure monitor, you'll follow these steps to initiate monitoring:*

First, obtain the monitor, dual air hose, and a specially-fitted pressure cuff. Take care to choose the correct pressure cuff size, because a cuff that's too large or too small will distort your readings. Use a cuff that's ⅖ wider and ⅕ longer than the circumference of the limb being monitored.

Place the monitor on a firm, immobile surface near the patient's bed, as shown here. Make sure the back of the monitor's unobstructed to permit heat dissipation.

Don't proceed without first telling the patient what the monitor's for and how it works. Explain the alarm system to her, so she won't be frightened if she hears an alarm.

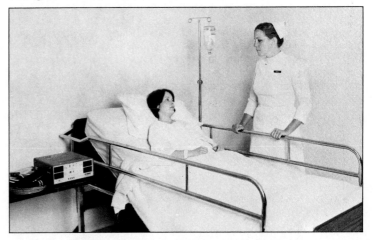

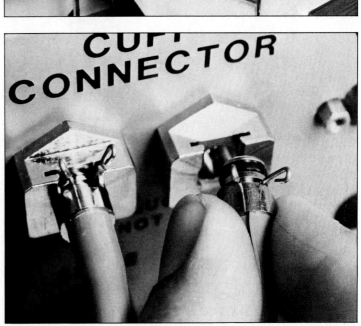

2 Make sure the POWER switch is off; then, plug the monitor into a properly-grounded wall outlet. Next, connect the dual air hose to the hose connector sockets on the back of the monitor, as the nurse is doing here. Secure the air hose by squeezing the two thin metal prongs on each metal tip, and pressing the tip firmly into the socket.

Hemodynamic monitoring

Using a Critikon Dinamap® monitor continued

3 Now, screw the pressure cuff's tubing into the other ends of the dual air hose. Turn each screw tightly to prevent air leaks.

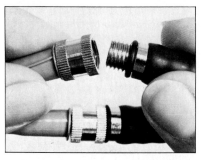

4 Squeeze all air from the cuff. Then, wrap it around the patient's limb. In most cases, you'll wrap it around the patient's upper arm, to monitor blood pressure in her brachial artery.

But, you may use her wrist, ankle, calf, or thigh instead. *Note:* Consecutive measurements taken on a leg may cause venous congestion, soreness, or emboli. Also, never apply a pressure cuff to a limb with an I.V. line in place.

Apply the pressure cuff snugly, but not too tightly. Make sure you can just insert two fingers under it, as shown here. *Note:* Place the air hoses out of the patient's way, so they don't become occluded when she moves.

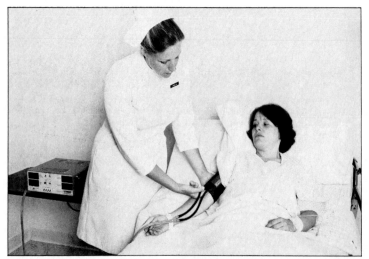

5 Now, make sure the MODE switch is in the AUTO position. (You'll use the CAL mode only to verify the monitor's calibration, as described on page 88.)

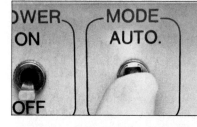

6 Place the ALARM LIMITS OFF/ON switch in the ON position. This ensures an audible alarm when the monitor detects mean arterial pressure (MAP) that's either too high or too low. (We'll show you how to set the alarm limits in frame 8.)

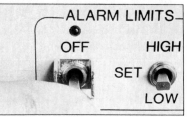

7 Now, set the interval for cuff inflations. Take a look at the ADD MINUTES toggle switches at the bottom of the monitor panel. When all four switches are down, the monitor will inflate the cuff and take readings once each minute. You can lengthen this interval by raising any combination of ADD MINUTES switches.

Because the doctor's ordered pressure readings every 6 minutes, lift switches 1 and 4, as shown here. This adds 5 minutes to the basic 1-minute cycle, for a total of 6 minutes.

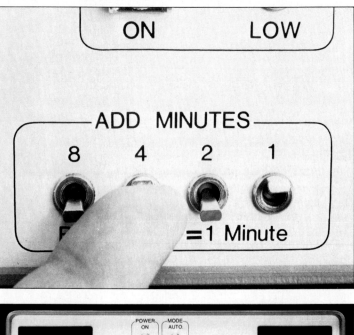

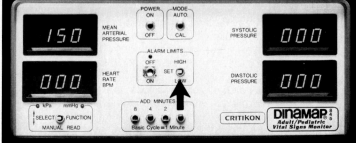

8 Place the POWER switch in the ON position. Then, adjust the monitor's alarm limits, if necessary. The monitor is preset to sound an alarm if the patient's MAP falls below 50 mm Hg or rises above 140 mm Hg. But you can raise either or both of these limits if your patient's condition requires. For example, if your patient is hypertensive, her MAP may normally be above 140 mm Hg. In this case, the doctor may ask you to reset the high alarm limit to 150 mm Hg.

Here's how: Hold the switch marked ALARM LIMITS HIGH/LOW up, toward HIGH (see arrow). For about 1 second, the MAP display window will show the preset high limit: 140 mm Hg. If you release the switch immediately, this limit will not change. But if you continue to hold the switch up, the high alarm limit will begin to rise in increments of 5 mm Hg. When it reaches 150, as shown here, release the switch. The high alarm limit is now reset.

To raise the low alarm limit, hold the HIGH/LOW switch down, toward LOW, and follow the same procedure. To return the monitor to its preset limits, just turn the monitor's POWER switch off, then on again.

9 Next, check SELECT FUNCTION at the lower left of the monitor's panel. If the light labeled *kPa* is lit, hold the SELECT FUNCTION switch up momentarily; then release it. You'll see the light labeled *mm Hg* come on, indicating that all readings displayed by the monitor are represented in millimeters of mercury. (The initials kPa stand for kilopascals, a European standard of measurement.)

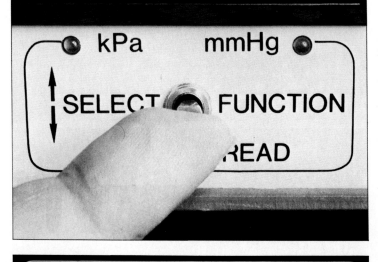

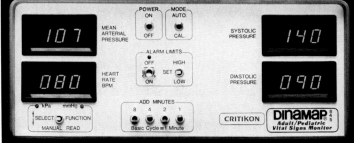

10 About 20 seconds after you flip on the POWER switch, the monitor will begin inflating the cuff. (You'll see a small red light on the left side of the MEAN ARTERIAL PRESSURE display window as the cuff inflates.) For the first inflation, the monitor inflates the cuff to 160 mm Hg. Then, it deflates the cuff in increments of about 6 mm Hg. As it does, it detects systolic, mean arterial, and diastolic pressure.

After deflating the cuff, the monitor displays the patient's systolic, diastolic, and mean arterial pressures, and his heart rate, as shown here.

Each subsequent inflation will be 35 mm Hg above the previous systolic reading. But suppose the patient has a sudden, steep rise in blood pressure. Then, the cuff inflation pressure may not be strong enough to occlude the artery. If it isn't, the monitor can't obtain a systolic reading on that inflation, although it will display a mean arterial pressure. On its next inflation, it'll inflate the cuff to 50 mm Hg above the last MAP reading, up to a maximum pressure of 250 mm Hg.

Between cuff inflations, the MEAN ARTERIAL PRESSURE window will alternately display the patient's MAP, and the number of minutes since the last inflation. For example, if the MEAN ARTERIAL PRESSURE window alternately displays 56 and 4, you know that the patient's MAP was 56 mm Hg at the last reading, and that the last reading occurred 4 minutes ago.

11 What if you want to take blood pressure and heart rate readings immediately, without waiting for the next cuff inflation? Simply depress the MANUAL READ switch, as the nurse is doing here. The monitor will immediately inflate the cuff and take readings. Then, it will continue to take readings at the intervals you've already set.

Document your patient's blood pressure and heart rate at regular intervals. *Important:* Regularly check the patient's hand and arm below the cuff. Short-interval cuff inflations may cause blanching and loss of sensation. If this occurs, remove the pressure cuff and notify the doctor.

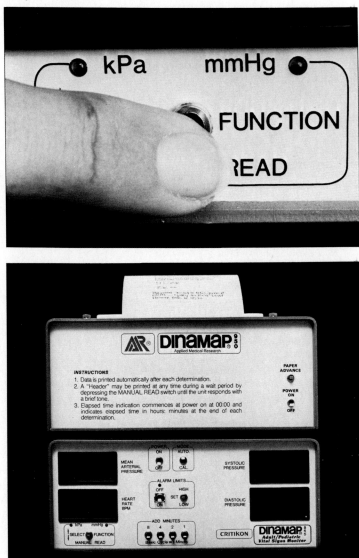

12 For automatic recordings of the Dinamap monitor's readings, use this Dinamap printer. Simply set it on top of the monitor, as shown here, and plug its grey INTERFACE cord into the receptacle on the monitor's back panel. Then, plug its POWER cord into a wall outlet. As you see, operating instructions appear on the printer's front panel. For more details (including how to use the specially-designed printout strip to determine MAP and heart rate trends), read the operator's manual.

Hemodynamic monitoring

Checking Dinamap accuracy

If you ever question the Dinamap monitor's accuracy, follow this simple procedure:

• Turn off the monitor and remove the pressure cuff from the patient's arm. Unscrew one of the air hoses from the pressure cuff, and squeeze the air from the cuff.

• Flip the MODE switch to the CAL position, and turn the monitor back on.

• Watch the four display windows. About 20 seconds after you turn on the power, the windows will display the same number, which is usually between 005 and 025. If the number's not in this range, call a qualified technician to recalibrate the monitor. (*Note:* Immediately after you turn on the monitor, you'll see a sequence of three numbers in each window. These numbers aren't significant when you're checking calibration.)

To learn how to check the monitor's integral voltage, and how to check its gain with a mercury manometer, read the operator's manual.

Invasive hemodynamic monitoring: Pros and cons

Invasive hemodynamic monitoring poses risks for your patient. But for your critically ill patient, the advantages may outweigh the disadvantages. Here are the pros and cons you should know:

Advantages

• Permits accurate, continuous blood pressure readings, even when your patient's in shock and noninvasive methods of pressure monitoring fail

• Reveals subtle changes in your patient's cardiovascular system that may be undetectable by noninvasive methods

• Reflects your patient's immediate response to medication, therapy, or stress

Disadvantages

• Increases the risk of complications for the patient; for example, infection, bleeding, embolism, and tissue or blood vessel damage. In addition, the introduction of a pulmonary artery catheter may cause cardiac arrhythmias.

• Requires specialized training to use. Otherwise, you may not recognize (or know how to correct) possible errors or inaccuracies in the monitoring system.

• May give you a false sense of security. Remember, monitoring is only one part of complete nursing care.

Balancing and calibrating pressure monitoring equipment

1 *Most invasive hemodynamic monitoring systems consist of a monitor, a pressure transducer, a disposable transducer dome, and a fluid-filled line to the patient. To ensure accurate pressure readings, first balance (or zero) the transducer to atmospheric pressure. Then, to make sure that the monitor correctly interprets the transducer's signals, calibrate the monitor to the transducer. Do these procedures whenever you set up a hemodynamic line, and repeat them once every 8 hours during monitoring (or as often as necessary).*

In the following photostory you'll see how to balance and calibrate equipment made by Gould, Inc. (For more details on balancing and calibrating, see the NURSING PHOTOBOOK USING MONITORS.)

To balance a standard-sized transducer, first mount it on an I.V. pole, using a transducer holder. Plug the transducer into the monitor, and turn on the monitor. Allow about 3 minutes for the monitor and transducer to warm up. (Some types of equipment take longer. Check the operator's manual for details about any equipment you use.).

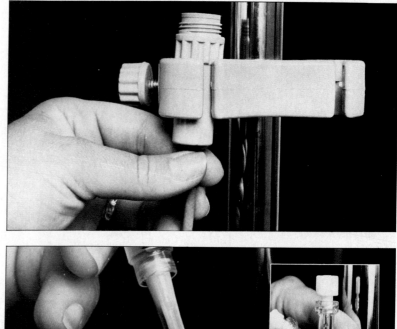

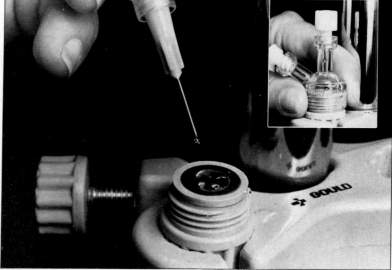

2 Next, put several drops of sterile water on the transducer diaphragm. Then, securely screw the dome onto the transducer (inset). Sterile water should completely cover the diaphragm.

Important: Take care not to trap air bubbles between the dome and transducer. Doing so will cause a damped waveform.

3 Consider the dome's upright arm to be the balancing port. Position the balancing port (*not* the transducer itself) level with the patient's right atrium, (approximately midway between the patient's back and sternum, at the fourth intercostal space, midaxillary). Mark this point with a small piece of tape. Then, maintain the balancing port at this level throughout monitoring.

Note: If your patient can't tolerate lying flat, clearly document what his position was when you balanced and calibrated the equipment. The patient must remain in the same position when you take readings. If his position changes, balance and calibrate again.

Then, uncap the balancing port to expose the transducer diaphragm to atmospheric pressure.

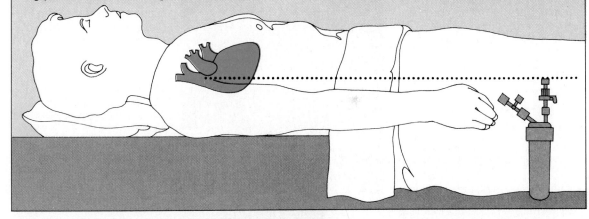

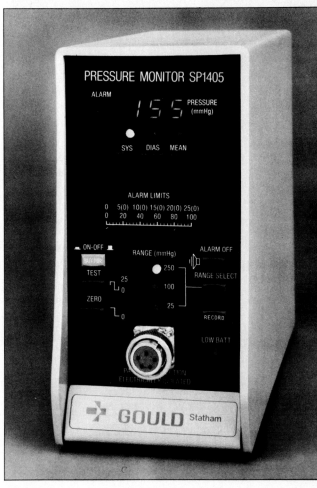

4 Depress the automatic ZERO button located at the lower left of the monitor's front panel. The monitor's digital reading will be 000 or 001, indicating that the transducer's balanced.

Note: If your monitor doesn't have an automatic ZERO button, balance the transducer manually by turning the monitor's ZERO knob until the digital reading's zero.

Complete the balancing procedure by capping the balancing port.

Now what about calibration? The Gould monitor featured here is precalibrated, so you needn't take any further steps. *Note:* You can verify calibration by depressing the TEST button. You'll also use the TEST button to calibrate the monitor to a recorder, if you use one. (For details, read the operator's manual.)

However, your monitor may require you to determine its cal factor, and then calibrate it manually. To learn how, see the NURSING PHOTOBOOK USING MONITORS, or check the operator's manual.

When your equipment's balanced and calibrated, open the line between the patient and the transducer, and begin monitoring. *Important:* Calibration ensures only that the monitor's reading corresponds to the transducer's sensitivity. To ensure that the pressure reading itself is accurate, periodically use a mercury sphygmomanometer to apply a known pressure to the transducer, and calibrate the monitor to that pressure.

Assembling your equipment

When you set up an arterial line (or *any* invasive hemodynamic monitoring line), consider this equipment essential:
• Pressure bag: Because the blood flow in a patient's arteries and central veins exerts such strong pressure, you must infuse I.V. flush solution under pressure (usually 300 mm Hg).
• I.V. flush solution (either sterile normal saline solution, or 5% dextrose in water).
• Heparin: To reduce risk of clotting at catheter tip, inject heparin directly into the flush solution (1 to 2 units heparin per ml of solution).
• Rigid pressure tubing between the catheter and the transducer: Regular I.V. tubing will expand under high hemodynamic pressures, distorting readings.
• Continuous flush device (for example, the Sorenson Intraflo® or the Gould Critiflo™ Diaphragm Dome): This device helps keep the line patent by maintaining a continuous flow rate of 3 to 4 ml per hour. In addition, it allows safe, fast flushing.

Hemodynamic monitoring

Setting up equipment for an arterial line

1 *Let's say the doctor's planning to insert an arterial catheter in your patient's radial artery for continuous blood pressure monitoring. Can you set up the necessary equipment? Read this photostory to learn how. Important: Before the doctor inserts the catheter, assess the blood supply to your patient's hands by performing the Allen's test (see the* NURSING PHOTOBOOK PROVID-ING RESPIRATORY CARE.) *If blood supply to either hand is impaired, tell the doctor. He'll choose another insertion site.*

First, obtain a monitor, I.V. pole, sphygmomanometer, leveling arm, and transducer holder. Then, wash your hands and gather the equipment shown below: pressure bag, 500 ml bag normal saline solution, label, transducer, transducer dome, 3 cc syringe and 1½" needle, syringe (with needle) filled with 1,000 units heparin, alcohol swab, two-way stopcock, two three-way stop-cocks, male adapter plug, microdrip I.V. pressure tubing, 4' pressure tubing, 6" pressure tubing, continuous flush device, and sterile water. (If the doctor wants you to apply a dressing, you'll need antimicrobial ointment, an adhesive bandage strip, a splint, and 2" wide adhesive tape.) Maintain aseptic technique throughout the procedure.

Turn on the monitor and plug in the transducer, so they can warm up while you work. *Note:* Replace vented stopcock caps with closed ones before you begin.

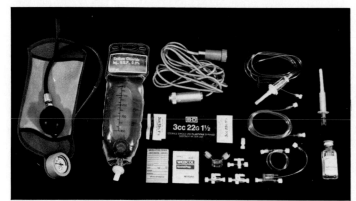

2 Label the I.V. saline solution bag with the patient's name and hospital number, the time and date, your initials, and the amount of heparin you'll inject. Then, spike and invert the bag, and squeeze out all the air through the drip chamber, as shown here. Close the line's flow clamp, and hang the bag on the I.V. pole.

[Inset] Inject hep-arin into the I.V. bag.

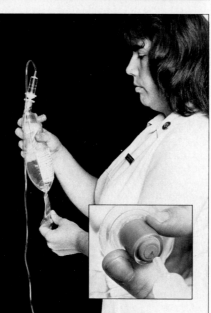

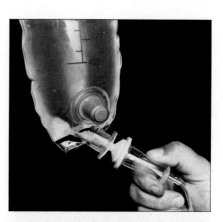

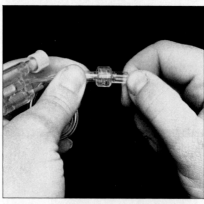

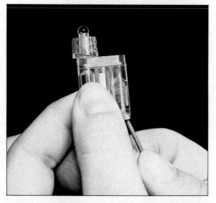

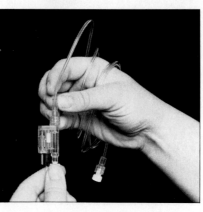

3 Gently squeeze the drip chamber until it's half full. *Nursing tip:* As you squeeze, tilt the drip cham-ber sideways. This helps pre-vent air bubbles from forming as the drip chamber fills.

Now, open the line's flow clamp, and prime the tubing until all air bubbles are flushed from the tubing. Close the clamp. *Important:* Always take care to eliminate air bubbles at every step of the procedure.

4 Next, attach a continu-ous flush device to the line, and screw it on *tightly.*

Important: Always tighten connections securely. A disconnection in an arterial line can cause serious, possibly fatal, bleeding.

5 To flush the air from the continuous flush device, uncap the Luer-Lok port and hold it upright. Open the flow clamp, and pull the pigtail on the continuous flush device until the saline solution runs out the Luer-Lok port. Release the pigtail.

6 Next, attach the 4' pres-sure tubing to the Luer-Lok port, as the nurse is doing here.

7 Uncap the Luer-Tip port and hold it upright. As shown here, pull the pigtail until saline solution runs out the port. Hold the pigtail taut until all air bubbles are expelled. Cap the Luer-Tip port.
Nursing tip: Expel stubborn air bubbles by flicking the continuous flush device with your finger. When the air bubbles rise to the top, pull the pigtail to flush them out.

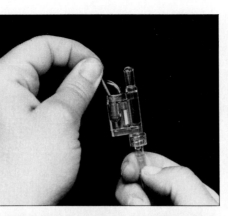

8 Uncap the 4' pressure tubing, and pull the pigtail to flush it, as the nurse is doing here.

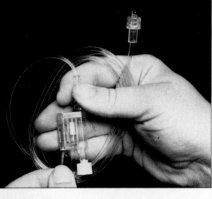

9 When the 4' pressure tubing has been completely flushed, attach a three-way stopcock to the end of it. For easy reference, we'll call this Stopcock #1.

10 Attach the 6" pressure tubing to Stopcock #1, as shown here.

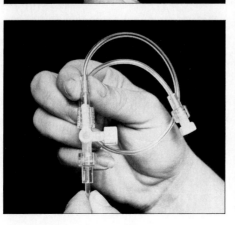

11 Turn Stopcock #1 off to the middle port, and uncap the 6" pressure tubing. Holding its end upright, flush the 6" pressure tubing by pulling the pigtail. When you're sure all the air's expelled, cap the end of the line.

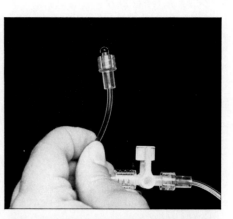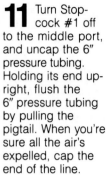

12 Turn Stopcock #1 off to the 6" pressure tubing. Now the line's open between the bag and the stopcock's middle port. Remove the cap from the middle port, and pull the pigtail until saline solution runs out the port and all the air's expelled.

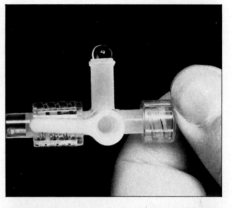

13 When you're sure the air's out, cap the port with a male adapter plug (injection nipple).

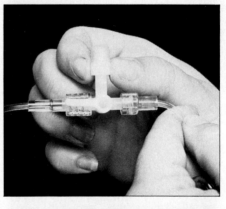

14 Uncap the Luer-Tip port of the continuous flush device, and attach a second stopcock (Stopcock #2). Although some nurses don't use a stopcock at this juncture, we recommend it. It permits you to isolate the transducer from the line.

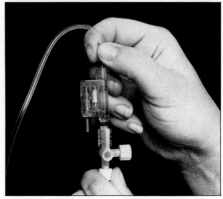

Hemodynamic monitoring

Setting up equipment for an arterial line continued

15 Turn Stopcock #2 off to its lateral port. Hold the middle port upright and uncap it. Pull the pigtail to flush the middle port, as shown here. When all the air's expelled, cap the port.

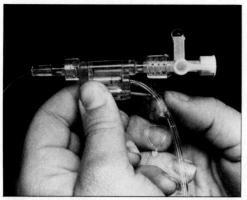

16 Turn Stopcock #2 off to its middle port, and follow the same procedure to flush its lateral port. Remember to hold the lateral port upright.

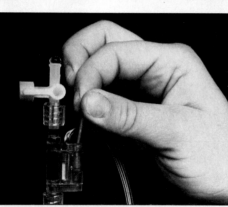

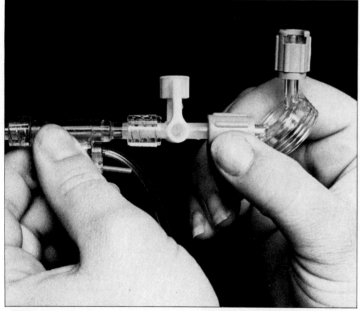

17 Screw one arm of the transducer dome onto the lateral port of Stopcock #2. This leaves the other arm of the dome free for balancing.
  The holder made for this particular transducer allows you to mount the transducer at an angle, so the balancing arm's upright and level. But if the dome you're using has a side arm and an upright arm, leave the *upright* arm free for balancing.

18 Next, place a two-way stopcock (Stopcock #3) on the other arm of the transducer dome. Open the line to the top port. (Remember, the handle position of a two-way stopcock points to an *open* line, not a closed line.)
  Hold Stopcock #3 vertically, and remove the cap from its top port. Then, pull the pigtail, as shown, and flush the dome with saline solution. The air will escape through the top port of Stopcock #3. When the dome and Stopcock #3 are free of air, cap Stopcock #3. (If you use a three-way stopcock, make sure you flush all its ports.)

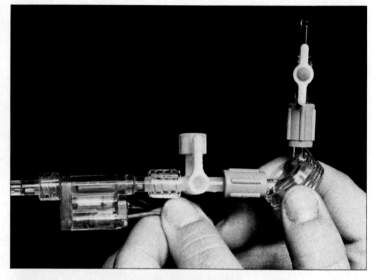

19 Now, attach the dome to the transducer, as shown on page 88. Mount the transducer on the I.V. pole.

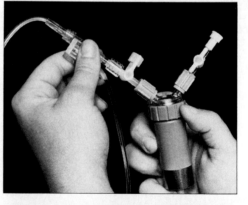

20 Now, place the I.V. bag inside a pressure bag. (Make sure the flow clamp's closed.) Pump up the pressure bag until its gauge shows a pressure of 300 mm Hg.

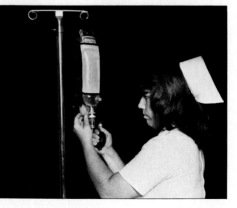

21 After the doctor has sutured the catheter to the patient's skin, apply antimicrobial ointment to the insertion site, and cover it with an adhesive bandage strip. Then, place a strip of 2" wide tape over the adhesive bandage strip and around the patient's wrist. (These precautions temporarily stabilize the catheter while you work. Later, tape the catheter more securely.)

Now, get ready to start the infusion. To prevent blood backflow in the catheter, *gently* press down on the artery, just beyond the tip of the catheter, as shown here. Or, apply a sphygmomanometer's pressure cuff to the patient's arm.

Then, quickly connect the end of the 6" pressure tubing to the patient's catheter, open the line's flow clamp, and begin the infusion. *Important:* As the I.V. bag empties, check the pressure gauge frequently to make sure the pressure remains constant at 300 mm Hg. Too little pressure permits blood backflow. But too *much* pressure may loosen the connections.

24 When the catheter's secure, balance and calibrate the equipment (for guidelines, see pages 88 and 89). Then, open the line between the patient and the monitor, and begin monitoring your patient's arterial blood pressure.

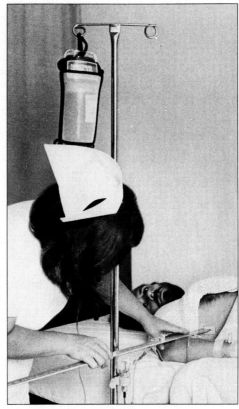

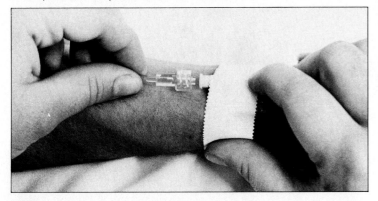

22 Turn the two-way stopcock (Stopcock #3) so it's off to its top port. Then, gently pull the pigtail to flush the line. As you do, watch the drip chamber. If the solution flows steadily and rapidly, the catheter's patent and properly positioned. Release the pigtail. The drip rate should be 3 to 4 ml/hour.

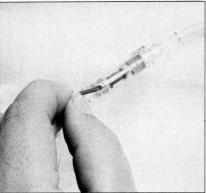

23 When the infusion's flowing properly, finish taping the catheter. If the catheter's inserted in the radial artery, apply a short splint (armboard) to your patient's arm. Label the dressing. Leave the stopcock and all connections exposed, so you can examine them easily.

Label the tubing as an arterial line, as shown here, so no one mistakes it for an I.V. line.

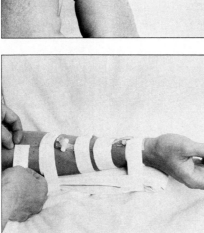

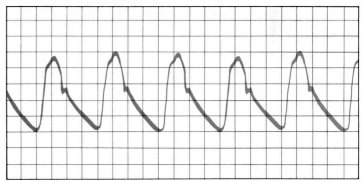

25 Check the waveform on the oscilloscope screen or readout strip. Expect it to be well defined, with a visible dicrotic notch, like the one shown here. If it isn't, see the troubleshooting tips on pages 98 and 99.

Next, check your patient's blood pressure with a sphygmomanometer. (Apply the cuff to the arm without the catheter.) Keep in mind that the monitor's blood pressure reading will probably show a higher systole and a lower diastole than your cuff blood pressure reading. Document both readings in your nurses' notes. Then, document the entire procedure.

Finally, double-check all connections to make sure they're secure. At least once each hour, check the pulse, color, sensation, and mobility of your patient's hand or foot to ensure adequate circulation. To maintain catheter patency, use the pigtail to flush the catheter once each hour and whenever you draw a blood sample.

Important: Change the dressing, tubing, and flush solution every 24 to 48 hours, according to hospital policy.

Hemodynamic monitoring

Looking at the pulmonary artery catheter

As you probably know, a balloon-tipped pulmonary artery (PA) catheter can provide highly accurate information about your patient's progress. Take a look at the PA catheter shown here. It's designed to measure pulmonary artery pressure (PAP), pulmonary artery wedge pressure (PAWP), central venous pressure (CVP), and cardiac output. On the following pages, we'll show you how to set up a PA line, and how to measure PAWP. For more details on PA lines, consult the NURSING PHOTOBOOK USING MONITORS.

Note: Keep in mind that PA catheters vary. Some, for example, have fewer lumens than this one. Check the manufacturer's instructions before using any PA catheter.

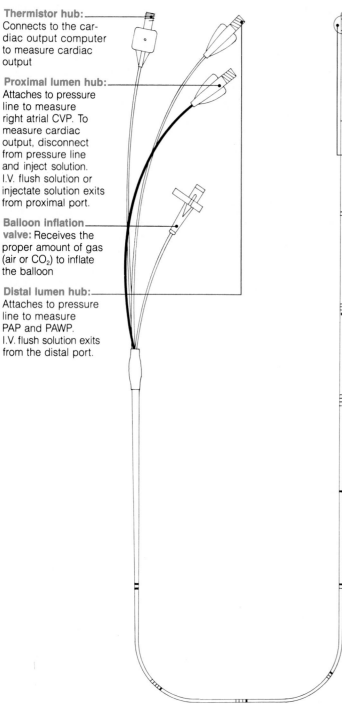

Thermistor hub: Connects to the cardiac output computer to measure cardiac output

Proximal lumen hub: Attaches to pressure line to measure right atrial CVP. To measure cardiac output, disconnect from pressure line and inject solution. I.V. flush solution or injectate solution exits from proximal port.

Balloon inflation valve: Receives the proper amount of gas (air or CO_2) to inflate the balloon

Distal lumen hub: Attaches to pressure line to measure PAP and PAWP. I.V. flush solution exits from the distal port.

Distal lumen port: Rests in the pulmonary artery

Thermistor: Detects blood temperature changes used to measure cardiac output. Located about 1½" (3.8 cm) from the catheter tip

Balloon: Expands around catheter, when inflated, without occluding distal port

Proximal lumen port: Rests in the right atrium

How to set up equipment for a pulmonary artery (PA) catheter

If the doctor's planning to insert a pulmonary artery (PA) catheter in your patient, he'll expect you to set up the monitoring equipment. Start by following the same procedure you used for a peripheral arterial line (see pages 90 to 93). Then, when the tubing, transducer dome, and stopcocks are completely flushed, set up the line in one of the ways shown at right. Which setup you choose depends on the number of pressures the doctor wants to monitor.

As you set up the equipment, explain the procedure to your patient. Remember, he's probably apprehensive, so do your best to reassure him.

Let's imagine the doctor wants to monitor your patient's pulmonary artery pressure (PAP) and pulmonary artery wedge pressure (PAWP). To do so, he'll insert a PA catheter with only one lumen hub. In the first illustration to the right, you see a setup for this PA catheter.

But suppose the doctor also wants to monitor right atrial (RA) pressure (also called central venous pressure, or CVP). In that case, he'll insert a PA catheter with *two* lumen hubs. As you see in the illustration on the far right, you'll need a Y connector between the I.V. bag and the transducer.

Mount a double stopcock manifold on the I.V. pole above the transducer, and connect each line's continuous flush device to a stopcock. To measure PAP or PAWP, turn the stopcock controlling the RA line off to the transducer and open the PAP line to the transducer, as shown here. To monitor RA pressure (CVP), reverse this procedure.

Important: As soon as you take an RA reading, close the RA line and reopen the PAP line. The doctor will expect you to monitor PAP continuously.

Can your monitor display two pressures at once? To get two pressure readings, you'll have to use two transducers. Connect the second transducer to the RA line.

If your patient has a peripheral arterial line in place (in addition to his PAP and RA lines), use a triple stopcock manifold. You'll use a three-way connector between the I.V. bag and the transducer, instead of a Y connector.

Important: No matter which setup you use, you must level each transducer's balancing port with the patient's right atrium.

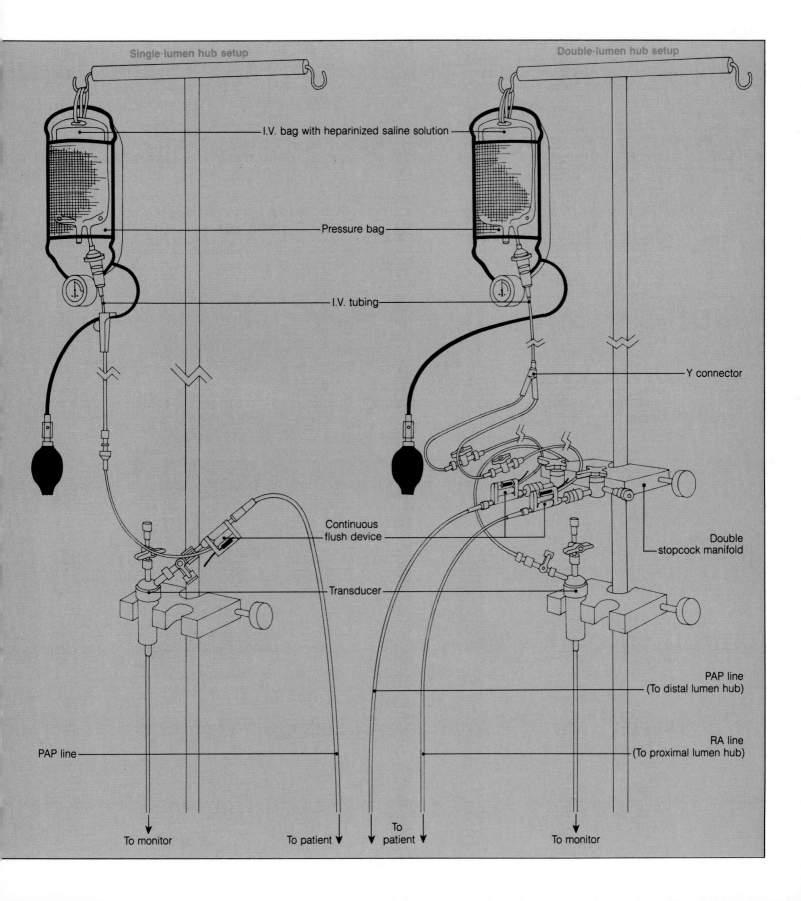

Single-lumen hub setup

Double-lumen hub setup

I.V. bag with heparinized saline solution

Pressure bag

I.V. tubing

Y connector

Continuous flush device

Double stopcock manifold

Transducer

PAP line (To distal lumen hub)

PAP line

RA line (To proximal lumen hub)

To monitor

To patient

To patient

To monitor

Hemodynamic monitoring

Measuring your patient's pulmonary artery wedge pressure (PAWP)

When the pulmonary artery (PA) catheter tip is positioned properly in your patient's artery, you can inflate its flexible latex balloon to measure her pulmonary artery wedge pressure (PAWP). Here's what happens:

The inflated balloon floats into a pulmonary artery branch, occluding it. Then, the catheter's distal lumen, located in front of the balloon, registers left heart pressure. After you deflate the balloon, the catheter tip floats back into the main branch of the pulmonary artery, and normal circulation's restored. A PAWP measurement reflects left ventricular function and may provide an early indication of pulmonary congestion.

In the following photostory, you'll see how to take a PAWP measurement. For most patients, the only special equipment you'll need is a tuberculin (TB) syringe; you'll use room air to inflate the balloon.

Important: If air bubbles escaping from a ruptured balloon might enter your patient's arterial circulation (for example, if she has a suspected right to left intracardiac shunt), don't inflate the balloon with air. Instead, use CO_2. Unlike air, a CO_2 bubble will probably dissolve in the patient's blood before it causes an embolism.

1 First, wash your hands thoroughly. Then, place your patient flat on her back or in semi-Fowler's position. Explain the procedure.

If necessary, balance and calibrate the equipment.

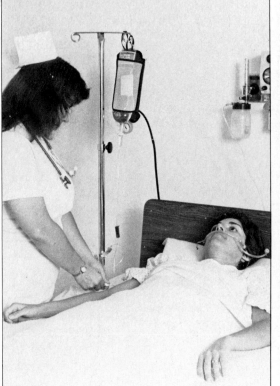

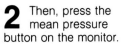
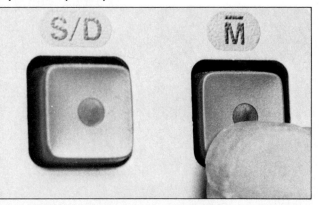

2 Then, press the mean pressure button on the monitor.

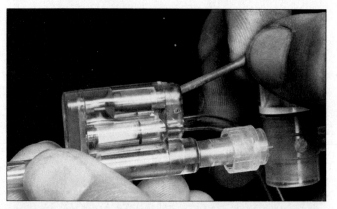

3 Pull the pigtail on the continuous flush device to flush the line. If the line doesn't flush properly, locate and correct the problem. (For troubleshooting tips, see page 99.)

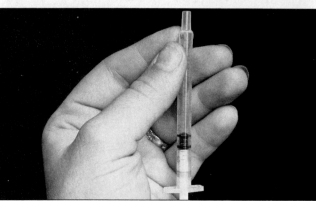

4 Next, check the side of the catheter for the *maximum* amount of air recommended by the manufacturer to inflate the balloon.

Then, draw 0.3 to 0.5 cc *less* than that amount into the syringe.

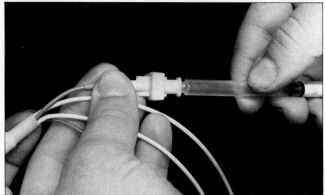

5 Make sure the balloon inflation valve on the PA catheter is open, and attach the syringe to it.

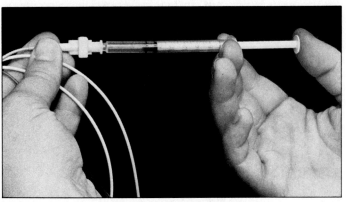

6 To inflate the balloon with air, slowly and carefully depress the syringe plunger. Expect to feel slight resistance. *Important:* If you don't feel resistance, suspect a ruptured balloon. Stop the procedure at once, and notify the doctor.

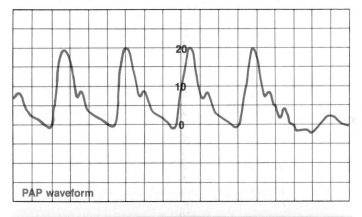

PAWP waveform

7 As you inflate the balloon, watch the oscilloscope screen closely. Stop injecting air as soon as the pulmonary artery pressure (PAP) waveform changes to the PAWP waveform shown here. Record the reading.

Then, immediately release the syringe's plunger: Prolonged wedging may cause pulmonary infarction. All the air you inserted should return to the syringe. If it doesn't, suspect a ruptured balloon. (Never aspirate the air, or you may rupture the balloon.)

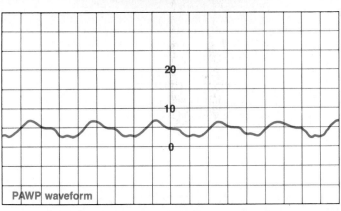

PAP waveform

8 When the balloon's completely deflated, the PAP waveform will return, as shown here. If the PAWP waveform remains, the balloon may still be inflated, or the catheter tip may be wedged in a small pulmonary capillary. Ask the patient to cough, deep breathe, or change position, which may jolt the catheter free. If a clear PAP waveform doesn't return, notify the doctor at once, and prepare the patient for a chest X-ray.

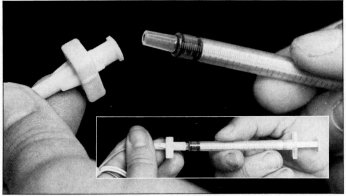

9 When the balloon's completely deflated, remove the syringe, as shown here. Depress its plunger to expel the air. Then, reattach the syringe to the balloon inflation valve, as shown in the inset photo. This precaution ensures that no one will mistake the balloon inflation valve for an injection hub.

Document the entire procedure. Measure and record PAWP every 4 hours, as ordered.

Measuring cardiac output

As you know, the term cardiac output indicates the amount of blood ejected from the heart each minute. At rest, a healthy heart ejects from 4 to 6 liters each minute.

If your patient's pulmonary artery (PA) catheter has a thermistor, you can measure his cardiac output with a special computer, using the thermodilution technique. These measurements help you assess left ventricular and valve functions.

The thermodilution technique works like this: First, you'll obtain a predetermined amount of either normal saline solution or 5% dextrose in water. This solution must be cooler than the patient's blood. (The computer's temperature probe measures the solution's exact temperature.) Then, you'll inject the solution into the patient's cardiovascular system through the proximal lumen.

This solution then mixes with the blood of the superior vena cava or right atrium (depending on the catheter's exact location) and lowers the temperature of the blood in the heart. When this cooler blood flows past the thermistor embedded in the distal end of the PA catheter, the thermistor detects the temperature drop and sends a signal back to the computer. Finally, the computer analyzes this information and records the patient's cardiac output.

For a step-by-step demonstration of the thermodilution technique, refer to the NURSING PHOTOBOOK USING MONITORS.

Hemodynamic monitoring

Troubleshooting a damped waveform

You probably know what damped waveforms look like. Unlike the sharply defined waveforms you expect to see, damped waveforms lack definition. They're smooth and wavy in appearance, and abnormally low. But do you know how to correct them, as well as how to prevent them from occurring? Read this chart to find out.

Problem	Nursing action	Prevention
Air bubbles somewhere in line; for example, tubing, transducer dome, or stopcocks	• Check stopcocks and make sure they're positioned correctly. • Check the line for leaks. Then, replace the line, if necessary. • Check for loose connections, especially dome connections, and tighten them, if necessary. • Take care to flush out air bubbles through an open stopcock port.	• Flush all air from line when setting up equipment. • Avoid rapid, repeated pulling of the pigtail on the fast flush valve. This causes turbulence in the flushing solution, which in turn produces air bubbles. • Make sure the drip chamber is at least half-full at all times. Avoid use of microdrip tubing.
Blood clot in catheter or stopcock	• Pull the pigtail on the fast flush valve to flush catheter. *Important:* Never flush any hemodynamic line with a syringe. You may cause an embolus. • Try to aspirate the clotted blood with a syringe. • If the catheter remains clotted, notify the doctor and prepare to replace the line.	• Maintain adequate flow rate of heparinized flush solution (3 to 4 ml per hour). • Use the fast flush valve to flush the catheter after drawing blood samples.
Arterial catheter pulled out of blood vessel or pressed against vessel wall	• Pull the pigtail on the fast flush valve. • Attempt to aspirate blood to confirm proper placement in vessel. • If you can't aspirate blood, notify doctor and prepare to replace the line. *Note:* Bloody drainage at the insertion site may indicate catheter displacement. Notify the doctor at once.	• Tape the catheter securely. • Stabilize the insertion site with a splint.
Pulmonary artery (PA) catheter pressed or wedged against blood vessel wall	• Deflate balloon on PA catheter completely. • Ask patient to cough. This may jolt the catheter free. • Fast flush the catheter, using the fast flush valve. This also may jolt it free. • Notify the doctor, so he can reposition the catheter, if necessary. • Prepare the patient for a chest X-ray to confirm correct catheter placement.	• Make sure the catheter is securely sutured and taped. • Observe PA waveforms closely. • Make sure the balloon's *completely* deflated after each use.
Regular I.V. tubing used between catheter and transducer	• Replace I.V. tubing with rigid pressure tubing.	• Always use rigid pressure tubing between the catheter and the transducer. Regular I.V. tubing expands under pressure, causing damped waveforms.
Transducer not balanced properly	• Check transducer cable for occlusion or compression. • Level the transducer's balancing port with the patient's right atrium, and balance the transducer to atmospheric pressure. • Recalibrate the monitor with the transducer. (For details on balancing and calibrating, see pages 88 and 89.)	• Keep transducer cable off the floor so it isn't damaged. • Reposition the transducer whenever the patient's position changes. Remember, its balancing port must always be level with the patient's right atrium. • Rebalance and recalibrate equipment if the room temperature changes significantly. • Rebalance and recalibrate equipment routinely, at least once every 8 hours. 📠 *Nursing tip:* When using a standard-sized transducer, avoid putting more than two or three drops of sterile water between the transducer and the dome. Too much fluid can dampen the waveform.
Blood backup in line	• Check stopcock positions and make sure they're correct. • Check for loose connections and tighten them, if necessary. • Use the fast flush valve to flush blood from catheter. • Replace dome if blood backs up into it.	• Maintain 300 mm Hg of pressure in the pressure bag at all times.

Troubleshooting other common hemodynamic pressure monitoring problems

On the preceding page, you learned how to troubleshoot a damped waveform. By reading this chart, you'll learn how to recognize and deal with some other common hemodynamic monitoring problems.

Problem	Possible causes	Nursing action
No waveform	• Power supply off	• Check power supply.
	• Oscilloscope's pressure range set too low	• Reset oscilloscope's pressure range higher, if necessary. Then, rebalance and recalibrate the equipment.
	• Loose connection in line • Transducer's stopcock off to patient	• Tighten any loose connections, and position stopcocks correctly.
	• Catheter occluded or out of blood vessel	• Use fast flush valve to flush line. • Try to aspirate blood from the catheter. If the line still won't flush, notify the doctor and prepare to replace the line.
Drifting waveforms	• Monitor and transducer not warmed up properly	• Allow monitor and transducer to warm up 10 to 15 minutes.
	• Monitor's electrical cable compressed	• Place monitor's cable where it can't be stepped on or compressed.
	• Temperature change in room air or I.V. flush solution	• Remember to routinely rebalance and recalibrate 30 minutes after setting up the equipment. This gives the I.V. fluid sufficient time to warm to room temperature.
Line won't flush	• Stopcock positioned incorrectly	• Check stopcocks to make sure they're positioned correctly.
	• Inadequate pressure from pressure bag	• Check pressure bag to make sure pressure reads 300 mm Hg.
	• Kink in pressure tubing or blood clot in catheter	• Check pressure tubing for kinks. • Try aspirating blood clot with a syringe. • If the line still won't flush, notify the doctor and prepare to replace the line. *Important:* Never use a syringe to flush any hemodynamic line.
Artifact (waveform interference)	• Patient movement	• Wait until the patient's quiet before taking a reading.
	• Catheter fling (tip of pulmonary artery [PA] catheter moving rapidly in large blood vessel or heart chamber)	• Notify doctor of catheter fling. He may try to reposition the catheter.
	• Electrical interference	• Make sure electrical equipment's connected and grounded correctly.
False high readings	• Transducer's balancing port positioned below the patient's right atrium	• Position the transducer's balancing port level with the patient's right atrium.
	• Transducer unbalanced	• Rebalance and recalibrate the equipment. • Check transducer's cable, and make sure it's not kinked or occluded.
	• Flush solution flow rate too fast	• Check flow rate of flush solution. Maintain it at 3 to 4 ml per hour.
	• Catheter fling	• Notify doctor of catheter fling. He may try to reposition the catheter.
False low readings	• Transducer's balancing port positioned above the patient's right atrium	• Position transducer's balancing port level with right atrium.
	• Loose connection in line	• Check all connections and tighten them, if necessary.

Cardiovascular emergencies

Code! Remember how you felt the first time someone shouted that word? No matter how many times you've heard it, it's always frightening. You know that someone's life is at stake—and that your quick action may help him survive.

As an ICU nurse, what's your function during a code? The photostory in this section will show you. We've also provided a look at a typical crash cart, guidelines for lending emotional support to those affected by the code, and information on essential cardiac emergency drugs.

What's on the crash cart?

When a code's called in your unit, the code team will bring a crash cart to the patient's bedside. Do you know what's included on a hospital crash cart? You should. When seconds count, you must be able to find what you need without delay.

Take the time to carefully examine one of your unit's crash carts. Go over its equipment, item by item, until you know what everything's for and where to find it.

Although crash carts vary from hospital to hospital, a typical cart includes the following equipment: defibrillator with paddles, conductive jelly, and saline pads; a CPR board; oxygen cylinder (D size) with O_2 tubing and masks; a suction machine with suction catheters; a hand-held resuscitator; a laryngoscope tray with blades and endotracheal tubes; assorted oral and nasal airways, stylet, and padded tongue depressors; a cutdown tray; assorted I.V. solutions, tubing, catheters and needles, additive labels, armboard, and tourniquets; an arterial blood sampling kit, assorted syringes and needles, including intracardiac and spinal needles; a trach tray; a nasogastric tube with bulb syringe; a CVP manometer; disposable scalpels; hemostats; 4"x4" and 2"x2" sterile gauze pads; adhesive tape, alcohol swabs; assorted sutures; and sterile gloves.

The crash cart also contains emergency drugs. For a review of some of the first-line drugs you're likely to find on a crash cart, see the chart on page 105.

Important: To ensure cleanliness, keep your unit's crash cart covered when not in use. Assign someone to check the cart each shift (and after each code) to restock supplies and to test the defibrillator. Also, check the expiration dates on drugs, and trach and cutdown trays. Replace them, if necessary.

Your role during a code

During a code, events occur quickly. When a patient suffers cardiac arrest in the ICU, the entire code team must assemble at his bedside within 1 minute. So the team can work smoothly, each member must know his own job—and understand other team members' jobs, as well.

As an ICU nurse, you must be trained in cardiopulmonary resuscitation (CPR). Whenever you discover a patient in cardiac arrest, consider yourself part of the code team. Initiate CPR at once and remain with the patient throughout the crisis (unless the doctor coordinating the code team directs otherwise). However, if resuscitation efforts are prolonged, ask someone to relieve you before you become exhausted. The doctor will decide when to discontinue CPR.

In the following photostory, you'll see one possible sequence of events during a code. Of course, each code is different, depending on the patient's condition and on how well he responds to treatment. Nevertheless, by understanding how events are likely to unfold, you'll be better prepared to help the team function efficiently.

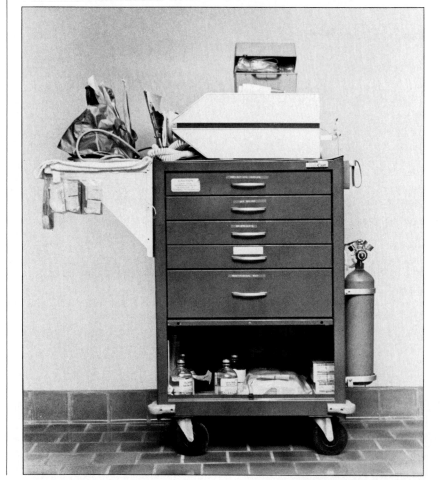

Calling a code

1 *You hurry to check Mr. Stout as soon as his cardiac monitor alarms. You discover him apparently unconscious, and the monitor's oscilloscope indicates he's in cardiac arrest. Here's what you do next:*

To make sure the patient's not sleeping, shake his shoulder and call his name. Look and listen for breathing. If he doesn't respond, and isn't breathing, call a code.

Since your patient's in the ICU, a loud call to the nurses' station is probably the best way to call for help. To avoid alarming the other patients, use your hospital's code word or phrase for cardiac arrest. Some hospitals use Code 99 or Doctor 99; others use CR (cardiac resuscitation) unit. Your hospital may have some other code. *Important:* If your hospital's code phrase eludes you, don't waste time trying to think of it. Instead, immediately call out, "Cardiac arrest!" Getting prompt help for the patient is top priority.

Never leave your patient's bedside before help arrives.

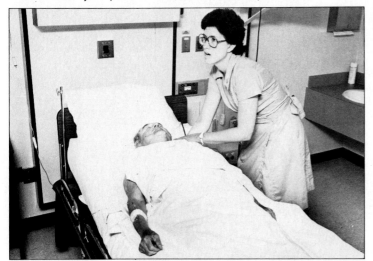

2 Now that you've alerted the nurses' station to the emergency, depend on others to summon the code team. In the meantime, you must begin CPR. As you know, the first step is to clear the patient's airway, as the nurse is doing here.

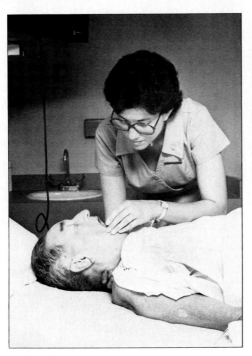

3 When you're sure his airway's open, hyperextend his neck and ventilate his lungs with four quick, full breaths. Then, feel for a carotid pulse.

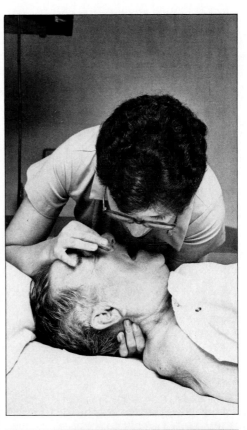

4 If you feel no pulse and the patient still isn't breathing, position your shoulders directly over his sternum. Your arms should be straight and at a 90° angle to his chest. If necessary, kneel on the bed frame, as the nurse is doing here. Then, interlock your fingers, position your hands over the patient's sternum, and begin chest compressions.

Never delay chest compressions, even if the patient isn't lying on a firm surface. Expect someone to bring a crash cart, which contains a board.

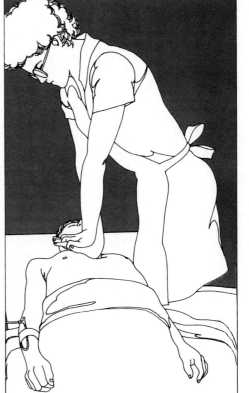

Cardiovascular emergencies

Calling a code continued

5 When another nurse arrives with the crash cart, help her slide the board under the patient. As you do so, remain poised to ventilate the patient as soon as the board's in place. When the board's in place, the second nurse will lower the bed, if necessary, so the patient's lying flat.

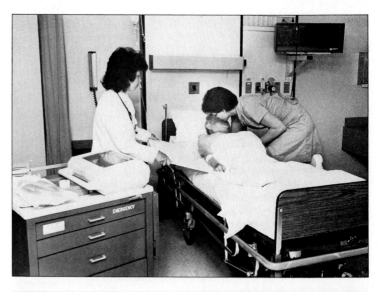

6 By now, the entire code team should be assembled. In addition to you and another nurse, code team members will include a doctor, who directs medication administration; an anesthesiologist or nurse anesthetist; and a respiratory therapist. In addition to the crash cart, code team members will bring a defibrillator (if it's not on the crash cart), and a ventilator. (Since this patient is already being monitored, an EKG machine isn't necessary. However, for the patient who isn't being monitored, the team would bring an EKG machine, attach limb leads, and run rhythm strips.)

While you continue chest compressions, the anesthetist inserts an endotracheal tube. The respiratory therapist begins ventilating the patient with a hand-held resuscitator.

While performing a quick assessment, the doctor feels for the patient's femoral artery pulse. Meanwhile, the second nurse begins assembling prefilled syringes of first-line drugs (see page 105).

Note: Most drugs will be administered I.V., for fast effect. Because this patient already has an I.V. in place, the doctor does not need to perform venipuncture.

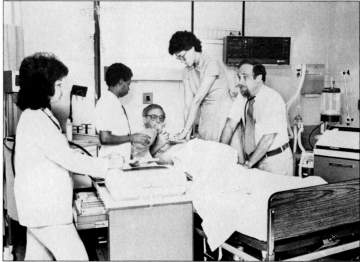

7 While the doctor administers drugs, the second nurse will turn on the defibrillator and apply conductive jelly to the paddles. At the doctor's direction, she'll set the electrical charge on the defibrillator control panel (usually at 400 watt-seconds) and charge the paddles.

Then, the doctor places the paddles at the correct position on the patient's chest, orders everyone to stand clear of the bed, and discharges an electrical shock to the patient. *Note:* In some hospitals, defibrillation is a nursing responsibility.

As you see in this photo, the second nurse is documenting events. She is responsible for noting the patient's condition at each step of the code, as well as what drugs were given at what time, who gave them, and what other treatment (such as defibrillation) was given.

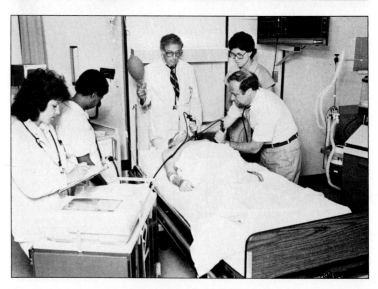

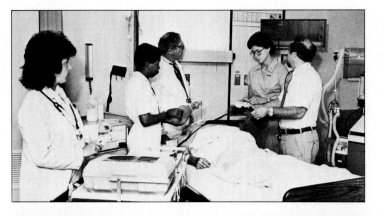

8 After defibrillation, the doctor looks at the cardiac monitor screen to see if the heart's rhythm has been restored. Meanwhile, you prepare a syringe for withdrawing an arterial blood sample.

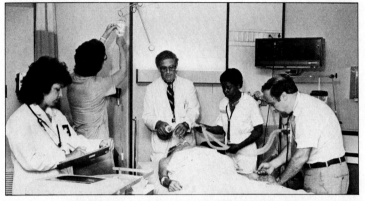

9 The patient's heart rhythm is restored. While the doctor withdraws an arterial blood sample for an arterial blood gas (ABG) analysis, the respiratory therapist connects the ventilator to the patient's airway. You hang and label the I.V. medication that the doctor's ordered, while the second nurse continues to document.

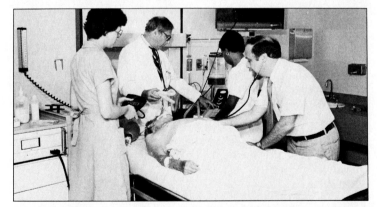

10 Now, the anesthetist and respiratory therapist make sure the ventilator's set properly and that the patient's being ventilated adequately. The doctor's auscultating the patient's heart. In the meantime, you prepare to take the patient's blood pressure with a sphygmomanometer. Later, the doctor may insert an arterial line for continuous blood pressure monitoring.

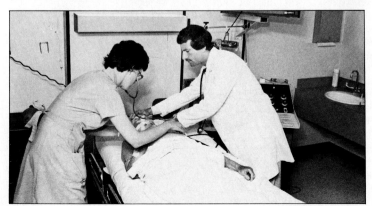

11 After the code, the cardiac resident, or the patient's own doctor, will examine the patient and prescribe further treatment. When the patient's stable, document the code by mounting the CPR record sheet on the patient's chart. Document the code in your nurses' notes, too. Then, send a duplicate of the CPR record sheet or appropriate requisition forms to the pharmacy so the drugs used during the code can be replaced and properly charged.

Note: Don't forget to check the patient's chest for possible burns caused by the defibrillator paddles. Document burns and treat them appropriately.

Cardiovascular emergencies

Providing emotional support

If your patient suffers cardiac arrest (or another crisis that requires calling a code), your first thought is saving his life. But providing emotional support for those affected by the code—the patient's family, other patients who witnessed the event, and the patient himself, if he survives—is an equally important task.

Family in crisis

Consider this situation: Mr. Volpe goes into spontaneous ventricular fibrillation while his family is visiting. Within seconds, the code team is assembled and working intently to save his life. A nurse escorts Mr. Volpe's terrified family out of the ICU and asks them to wait in the lounge. Then, preoccupied with the emergency, she rushes back to the ICU. In all the excitement, no one thinks of the family for another half hour.

To the family, this half hour seems like an eternity. Don't leave them alone while they wait. If everyone on the ICU staff is busy, ask the ward secretary to call a hospital social worker, clergyman, or other designated person to wait with them. Remember to give them regular reports of the patient's condition, especially if the code is prolonged. If you suspect the patient won't survive, prepare the family with gentle frankness. For example, say something like this: "His condition hasn't changed, but the doctors and nurses are still treating him. I'll be back in 5 minutes to tell you how he's doing." Then, keep your promise.

Suppose Mr. Volpe dies? His family needs your support more than ever. Take them to a private place where the doctor can explain what happened. Don't be afraid to show your compassion by putting your arm around a family member's shoulder, or by crying. Offer to perform small services, such as making phone calls.

Unless the family objects, arrange for them to see the patient's body. For many people, this is an important step toward accepting death.

If Mr. Volpe's family wasn't at the hospital during the code, the doctor should call them as soon as possible. If he's unable to do so, call them yourself.

If the patient has died, don't inform the family over the phone. Instead, tell them that his condition has worsened, and ask them to come to the hospital. If necessary, arrange for someone to accompany them. *Important:* Try to avoid panicking them. Otherwise, they may have an accident in their rush to the hospital.

For more guidelines on helping the family deal with a crisis, review pages 14 and 15.

How other ICU patients react

Because ICU patients have limited privacy, they may all be unwilling witnesses to a code. If possible, close the door or pull the bedside curtain around the patient being resuscitated.

How do other patients feel about witnessing a resuscitation effort? Expect to hear remarks like these:
● "I was just talking to Joe this morning. He seemed fine. Could the same thing happen to me?" A patient may become anxious and fearful after watching a code. After all, he, too, is in the ICU with a serious condition. Watching a code may make him wonder if he'll be the next victim of a life-threatening crisis.

● "Why did we all have to watch that? Couldn't you have pulled the curtain sooner?" Don't be surprised if a patient seems angry. This may be his way of coping with fear and anxiety.
● "I was impressed with how efficiently everyone worked." A patient may be reassured by watching the code team in action. He may now feel he can trust the team to make the same effort to save him, if necessary.

How can you ease post-code trauma in the ICU? Spend time discussing the event with each witness. If someone seems anxious, take care to stress the differences between his condition and the condition of the patient who experienced the code. No matter how obvious this reassurance may be, most patients find it comforting.

The code survivor: A special patient

Let's say you've helped to resuscitate a patient who suffered cardiac arrest. Even though his condition's now stable, your job hasn't ended. A survivor of cardiac arrest may suffer long-term emotional effects, such as anxiety, depression, and recurring nightmares. The patient may resume life feeling that he's different from other people; that in a sense, he's returned from the dead. These feelings of separateness, anxiety, and depression are called the Lazarus complex.

To minimize post-code emotional suffering for your patient, follow these guidelines:
● Tell the patient exactly what happened. If his condition permits, you (or the doctor) should do this within a day of the code. Don't delay this important task. Even if the patient has no memory of events surrounding the code, he'll know that *something* happened to him. Wondering about the details will only increase his anxiety.
● Assure the patient that just because he needed resuscitation, his condition isn't necessarily worsening. The resuscitation, in itself, does not reduce his long-term chance for recovery. If the conditions which led to the cardiac arrest have improved, offer this information to relieve his fear that another cardiac arrest is imminent.
● Encourage him to discuss his feelings—as well as any memories or dreams he had during the code—with you, a family member, or a clergyman. Most patients have no specific memory of code events. However, they may report vivid dreams, or surrealistic, out-of-body experiences. A patient who's had an out-of-body experience may recall watching the code team work to revive his body, seeing deceased relatives, or having a profound religious experience.

A few patients apparently remain conscious throughout resuscitation. They may recall, for example, the pain of defibrillation.

No matter what memories your patient reports, take care to be accepting and nonjudgmental—regardless of your own beliefs. Your support can help him successfully adjust to this traumatic event.

Important: You and the other health care professionals involved in the code may experience some of the same strong emotions felt by patients and their families. Consider organizing informal support groups to share thoughts and feelings about resuscitation events.

Emergency drug guide ◆

Drug
atropine sulfate
bretylium tosylate (Bretylol)
dopamine hydrochloride (Intropin*)
epinephrine hydrochloride (Adrenalin Chloride)
isoproterenol hydrochloride (Isuprel*)
lidocaine hydrochloride (Xylocaine*)
sodium bicarbonate

Indications and dosage	Selected undesirable effects	Special considerations
Severe nodal or sinus bradycardia, atrioventricular (AV) block, junctional or escape rhythms: Bolus: 0.5 to 1 mg I.V. May repeat every 5 minutes up to 2 mg.	• Tachycardia; palpitations; confusion; coma; urinary retention	• Watch heart rate and rhythm to determine drug effects. • Don't use in patients with tachycardia. • Store in a light-protective container. *Note:* Doses less than 0.5 mg may cause paradoxical slowing of heart rate.
Ventricular fibrillation: Bolus: 5 to 10 mg/kg I.V. Repeat every 15 to 30 minutes up to 30 mg/kg. *Maintenance:* I.V.: 500 mg in 500 ml of 5% dextrose in water or normal saline solution, at 1 to 2 mg/min. I.M.: 5 to 10 mg/kg undiluted. Repeat in 12 hours.	• Severe hypotension; initial transient hypertension; bradycardia; increased frequency of arrhythmias; ventricular irritability; vomiting	• Do not use in patients with digitalis-induced arrhythmia. • Monitor vital signs (especially blood pressure) every 15 minutes until stable. • If patient experiences a *severe, sudden* drop in blood pressure, keep him flat in bed and administer vasopressors.
Cardiogenic shock, hypovolemic shock, hypotension: 5 to 20 mcg/kg/min. by I.V. infusion. Titrate to desired hemodynamic and/or renal response.	• Cardiac arrhythmias; palpitations; widening of QRS intervals; increased heart rate; hypertension; vasoconstriction; pallor; sweating; vomiting; tremors; respiratory difficulty; anginal-type pain; decreased urinary output (when given in large doses)	• Don't use if patient has a pheochromocytoma. • Use cautiously if patient has an uncorrected tachyarrhythmia, or ventricular fibrillation, or an arterial embolism. • Because of deterioration, discard drug after 24 hours or sooner if it becomes discolored. • Administer using an infusion pump. • Monitor vital signs, checking for cardiac conduction abnormalities every 15 minutes. Report changes to doctor. • Measure hourly urinary output. • Mix drug with I.V. solution just before administration. • Don't mix with other drugs in alkaline solution; for example, sodium bicarbonate.
Cardiac and circulatory failure, hypotensive states: 0.5 to 1 mg I.V. bolus or 4 mg in 500 cc of I.V. solution at 1 to 8 mcg/min. 0.1 to 0.2 mg intracardiac. *Severe allergic reactions:* 0.1 to 0.5 ml of 1:1,000 subcutaneously or I.M. Repeat every 10 to 15 minutes, as needed. Or, 0.1 to 0.25 ml of 1:1,000 I.V. *Note:* 1 mg = 1 ml of 1:1,000 or 10 ml of 1:10,000.	• Cerebral hemorrhage; cardiac arrhythmia; widened pulse pressure; precordial pain; tachycardia; hypertension; pulmonary edema; tremor; diaphoresis	• Use with extreme caution in patients with shock (other than anaphylactic), ventricular fibrillation, or degenerative heart disease. • Watch for changes in heart rate if given with propranolol hydrochloride (Inderal*). Never administer with isoproterenol hydrochloride (Isuprel*). • Don't expose to light, heat, or air. • If drug is given I.V., take baseline blood pressure and pulse before beginning therapy. Monitor closely until desired effect is reached; then every 5 minutes until patient stabilizes. • After patient stabilizes, monitor blood pressure every 15 minutes. • If patient experiences sharp increase in blood pressure, reduce flow rate and notify doctor. He may order rapid-acting vasodilators to counteract pressor effects of large doses of epinephrine hydrochloride (Adrenalin Chloride). • Massage site after I.M. or subcutaneous administration to prevent vasoconstriction and necrosis. Phentolamine hydrochloride (Regitine) may be injected locally to neutralize effects. • Discard solution after 24 hours, or if it's discolored or contains precipitate.
Asystole, bradyarrhythmia: 0.02 to 0.06 mg I.V.; then, 0.01 to 0.2 mg I.V. or 5 mcg/min. I.V. *Shock:* 0.5 to 5 mcg I.V.	• Tachycardia; palpitations; bronchial edema; cardiac arrhythmias (especially ventricular tachycardia); chest pain; tremors; vomiting; hypertension, which may be followed by hypotension	• Don't use in patients with preexisting arrhythmia, or tachycardia induced by digitalis toxicity. • Use cautiously in patients with cardiac failure or limited cardiac reserve. • Closely monitor patient's vital signs and urinary output. If heart rate exceeds 110 beats per minute (BPM), slow or discontinue infusion. *Note:* A heart rate over 60 BPM may trigger ventricular arrhythmias in a patient with complete heart block. • Draw blood to obtain arterial blood gas (ABG) measurements. When drug is given for shock, monitor blood pressure, central venous pressure (CVP), electrocardiogram (EKG), and measure hourly urinary output. Adjust infusion rate accordingly. • If precordial distress or anginal pain occurs, stop administering drug immediately. • Propanolol hydrochloride (Inderal*) inhibits beta adrenergic effects of isoproterenol. Give together cautiously. Never administer with epinephrine hydrochloride (Adrenalin Chloride). • Administer using microdrip I.V. tubing or infusion pump. • Discard solution if it becomes discolored or contains precipitate.
Ventricular tachycardia, life-threatening premature ventricular contractions, acute ventricular arrhythmia secondary to myocardial infarction or cardiotonic glycosides: Bolus: 50 to 100 mg (1 to 1.5 mg/kg) I.V. at 25 to 50 mg/min. Maximum dose is 200 mg. Half dosage to elderly or lightweight patients, and to those with congestive heart failure (CHF) or hepatic disease. Repeat bolus every 3 to 5 minutes (two to four times) until arrhythmias subside or side effects develop. Infusion: 2 to 4 g in 500 ml of 5% dextrose in water at 1 to 4 mg/min.	• Convulsions; coma; hypotension; cardiovascular collapse; accelerated ventricular rate; cardiac conduction disorders (particularly atrial fibrillation); bradycardia; cardiac or respiratory depression or arrest; anaphylaxis; vomiting; difficulty swallowing; twitching; tremors; hallucinations	• Don't use in patients with Adams-Stokes syndrome, Wolff-Parkinson-White (WPW) syndrome, heart block, CHF, marked hypoxia, severe respiratory depression, shock, or renal failure. • Don't administer to patients with varying degress of sinoatrial, atrioventricular, or intraventricular heart block. • Draw blood to monitor cardiac enzymes, blood urea nitrogen (BUN), and creatinine. • Monitor heart rate and blood pressure. • Administer using an infusion pump. • Expect additive cardiac depressant effects when administered with phenytoin sodium (Dilantin*).
Cardiac arrest: Bolus: 1 to 3 mEq/kg I.V.; may repeat in 10 minutes. Further dose based on ABG measurement. *Metabolic acidosis:* 2 to 5 mEq I.V. over 4 to 8 hours.	• Alkalosis; hypernatremia	• May be added to I.V. solution, unless solution contains epinephrine hydrochloride (Adrenalin Chloride) or norepinephrine injection (Levophed*), or dopamine hydrochloride (Intropin*). • Don't infuse through I.V. line containing calcium, or drug will precipitate. • During administration, draw blood to obtain ABG and serum electrolyte measurements.

◆ The drugs in this chart are commonly considered first-line cardiac emergency drugs. Your hospital may include others, such as metaraminol bitartrate (Aramine*), norepinephrine injection (Levophed*), calcium chloride, or calcium gluconate. For more information, see the NURSE'S GUIDE TO DRUGS™ or THE NURSE'S DRUG HANDBOOK.

* Available in both the United States and in Canada

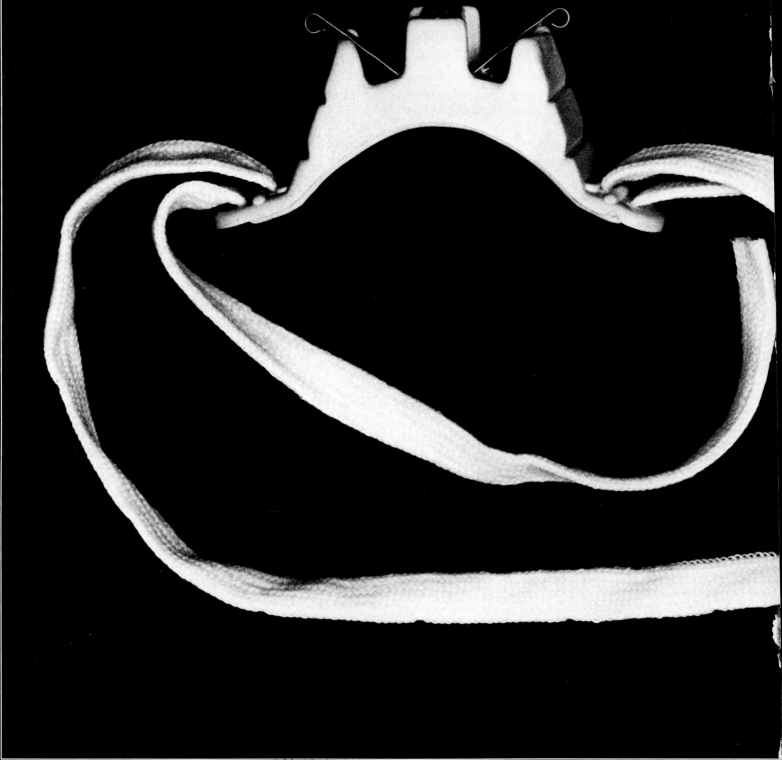

Caring for the Gastrointestinal Patient

Gastrointestinal basics

Tube care

Total parenteral nutrition

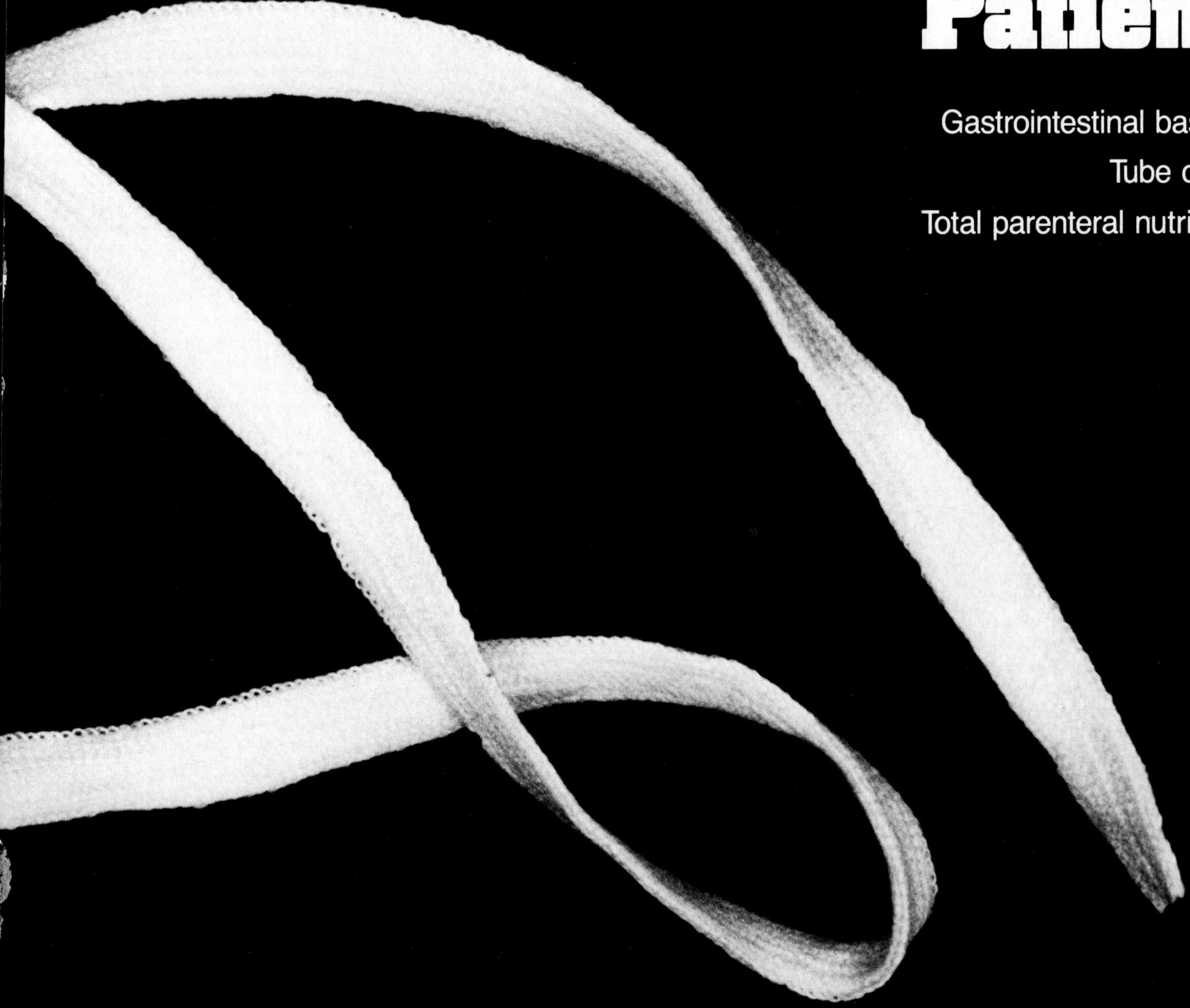

Gastrointestinal basics

As you know, the gastrointestinal tract consists of various organs, all of which perform digestive functions. But, some of these organs perform crucial nondigestive functions also; for example, the liver stores and detoxifies the blood, and the pancreas secretes insulin, which controls carbohydrate metabolism. To help you review all of the digestive tract organs, as well as their specific functions, we've provided you with a detailed chart.

With this foundation in anatomy and physiology, you'll be better equipped to take an accurate patient history and perform a thorough assessment. See the pages following the chart for instructions on assessing your ICU patient.

Learning about GI assessment

To assess your patient's GI tract properly, first obtain a history, as described on page 111. Then, inspect his mouth and throat with a tongue depressor, mirror, and penlight. (For detailed instructions on mouth and throat examination, refer to the NURSING PHOTOBOOK ASSESSING YOUR PATIENTS.) After completing these preliminary steps, inspect, auscultate, percuss, and palpate his abdomen. Then, specifically palpate and percuss his liver, stomach, and spleen. On page 111, we'll give you guidelines for GI inspection and auscultation. (For full instructions on carrying out GI assessment procedures, see the NURSING PHOTOBOOK PERFORMING GI PROCEDURES.)

To complete the assessment, the doctor may order extensive blood studies, X-rays, and invasive or noninvasive diagnostic studies.

Of course, complete GI assessment depends on your understanding of GI structures. The following chart provides a review.

Recognizing GI structures

Mouth and throat

Description
- Consists of lips, cheeks, teeth, tongue, palate, salivary glands, and pharynx.
- Makes up initial portion of digestive tract.

Function
- Teeth break up food, increasing the total surface area of the food, which allows more rapid and efficient digestion.
- Salivary glands produce saliva, which contains mucus and an enzyme, ptyalin. Ptyalin breaks down starches. Mucus helps lubricate and moisten food.
- The tongue moves food into the pharynx by voluntary movement. From there, food is carried into the esophagus by involuntary swallowing.

Esophagus

Description
- Hollow, collapsible, tubelike structure about 10″ (25 cm) long and 1″ (2.5 cm) in diameter. Located behind trachea but in front of the vertebral column.
- Connects mouth to stomach.
- Epiglottis prevents aspiration of liquids and solids.

Function
- Moves food to the stomach by peristaltic contractions, which are stimulated by food and aided by gravity.
- Secretes mucus, which facilitates swallowing and prevents reflux gastric juices from breaking down the esophageal wall.

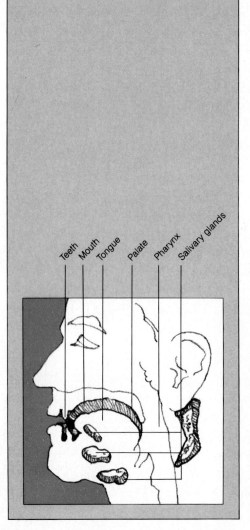

Teeth   Mouth   Tongue   Palate   Pharynx   Salivary glands

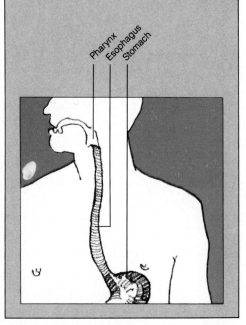

Pharynx   Esophagus   Stomach

Stomach

Description

- Elongated pouchlike structure located in the upper abdomen, below the diaphragm and above the transverse colon.
- Approximately five sixths of stomach lies to left of midline.
- Composed of three parts: the fundus, or food storage area; the body, where gastric juices act on food; and the antrum (pylorus), the site of mechanical breakdown of chyme (partially digested food).
- Cardiac sphincter at proximal end permits food to enter from the esophagus and prevents reflux of gastric contents into the esophagus.
- Pyloric sphincter, at distal end, regulates flow of chyme into duodenum and prevents reflux of duodenal contents.

Function

- Undergoes peristaltic contractions to aid in digestion.
- Secretes gastrin from pylorus, when stimulated by partially digested proteins and distention of stomach (from presence of food). Gastrin is a hormone that causes release of gastric juices, and influences the sphincter contractions that control chyme transport.
- Secretes 2 to 3 l of gastric juices per day from gastric mucosa. Gastric juices contain a high proportion of hydrochloric acid, pepsin, and mucus. The juices mix with food to form chyme. Hydrochloric acid and pepsin help break down the food. Mucus helps prevent self-digestion of the stomach lining.
- Absorbs water, alcohol, and glucose from chyme into the circulatory and lymphatic systems.
- Stores chyme before it enters the small intestine.
- Slowly empties chyme into small intestine by peristalsis and contraction of pylorus and duodenal bulb. Rate of emptying varies with volume and chemical composition of food ingested.

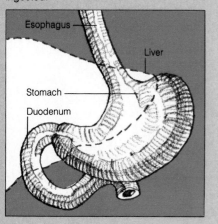

Small intestine

Description

- Tubelike structure about 20' (6 m) long and 1" (2.5 cm) in diameter.
- Extends from the distal end of the pyloric sphincter to the ileocecal valve, filling most of the lower abdominal cavity.
- Divided into three parts: duodenum, jejunum, and ileum. The duodenum, about 10" (25 cm) long, begins at the pylorus and forms a C-shape that curves around the pancreas. The jejunum, which measures about 8' (2.4 m) long, lies coiled in the umbilical region. The ileum, about 12' (3.6 m) long, extends from the jejunum to the ileocecal valve (the junction of the small intestine and the large intestine).
- To facilitate food absorption, 4 to 5 million finger-like projections (or villi) line the interior wall, increasing the surface area available for absorption.
- Releases the hormones secretin and cholecystokinin (pancreozymin) when stimulated by presence of chyme in the duodenum. These hormones activate enzymes from the liver, gallbladder, pancreas, and duodenal mucosa, which break down fats, proteins, and carbohydrates.

Function

- Releases the hormone enterogastrone when stimulated by presence of fats, sugar, and acids in intestine. Enterogastrone inhibits gastric secretion.
- Releases the hormone villikinin when stimulated by presence of chyme in intestine. Villikinin stimulates villi movements.
- Absorbs water and nutrients from chyme into circulatory and lymphatic systems.
- Alternately contracts different segments, to help break up chyme, combine it with intestinal secretions and expose it to the villi for maximum absorption.
- Propels chyme through the small intestine into the large intestine by peristaltic contractions.

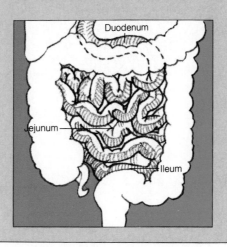

Large intestine

Description

- Tubelike structure about 5' (1.6 m) long and 2½" (6.3 cm) in diameter. Located in the lower abdomen, it extends from the ileocecal valve to the anus.
- Consists of four parts: cecum, a blind pouch about 2" to 3" (5 to 7.5 cm) long located in the lower right abdomen; vermiform appendix, a narrow blind tube about 4" (10 cm) long attached to the distal end of the cecum; colon, a tube about 4' (1.2 m) long, which outlines the abdominal tract and is divided into ascending, transverse, descending, and sigmoid portions; and the rectum, about 7" (17.5 cm) long, located on the anterior surface of the sacrum and the coccyx. Its distal end is called the anal canal.

Function

- Absorbs water and salts from chyme into circulatory and lymphatic systems.
- Secretes mucus, which lubricates and protects intestinal lining.
- Allows slow passage of chyme to colon through the ileocecal valve, which also prevents backflow to small intestine.
- Completes digestion through bacterial action on chyme.
- Facilitates absorption by alternately contracting different segments.
- Propels chyme through intestine by colonic peristalsis. Initiates urge to defecate by mass peristalsis, which occurs several times each day.
- Eliminates digestive wastes.

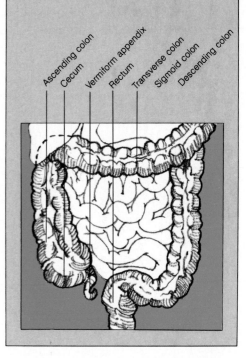

Gastrointestinal basics

Recognizing GI structures continued

Pancreas

Description
- Lobulated structure 5″ to 7″ (12.5 cm to 17.5 cm) long, located behind the stomach. Its wide end connects with the duodenum and its narrow end contacts the spleen.
- Connected with duodenum by pancreatic duct.

Function
- Secretes about 300 to 500 ml pancreatic juice from acinar cells into the duodenum each day. Intestinal hormones secretin and cholecystokinin (pancreozymin) stimulate secretion of juice, which consists of water, bicarbonate, sodium, potassium, zinc, calcium, magnesium, protein, and the enzymes trypsin, amylase, and lipase. The juice breaks down carbohydrates, fats, and proteins.
- Secretes insulin from beta cells and glucagon from alpha cells of the islets of Langerhans, the pancreatic endocrine tissue. Insulin and glucagon move from the pancreas directly into the circulatory system.

Liver

Description
- Large, brownish-red organ located under the right diaphragm in upper portion of the abdomen.
- Largest organ in body, weighing about 3 pounds (1.4 kg) in an adult.
- Right lobe is divided into three segments; left lobe is divided into two segments.
- Glisson's capsule, a thick sheath of connective tissue, surrounds entire organ.
- Supplied with oxygenated blood by hepatic artery and with blood for detoxification and storage (from the stomach, spleen, pancreas, intestines, and mesentery) by portal vein.
- Hepatic vein drains all blood from the liver.
- Connected to common bile duct by hepatic duct.

Function
- Secretes about 700 to 800 ml bile per day. Bile contains bile salts, bile pigments, cholesterol, bilirubin, phospholipids, potassium, sodium, and chloride. Aids in digestion and absorption of fats and fat-soluble vitamins.
- Metabolizes carbohydrates, protein, fat, steroids, minerals, and water.
- Stores glycogen, fat-soluble vitamins, and some water-soluble vitamins.
- Stores large amounts of blood. Regulates blood volume by increasing or decreasing amount of blood flowing through hepatic vein.
- Cleanses blood of any toxic substances.
- Produces prothrombin, fibrinogen, and heparin, which function in the coagulation of blood.

Gallbladder

Description
- Pear-shaped structure about 4″ (10 cm) long located on the liver's undersurface.
- Connected to duodenum's upper portion by biliary duct system.

Function
- Concentrates and stores up to 50 ml bile between periods of digestion.
- With its related ducts (hepatic, cystic, and common bile ducts), forms biliary system. Biliary system provides pathway for flow of bile from liver to duodenum.
- Undergoes muscular contractions with accompanying relaxation of sphincter of Oddi to push bile into duodenum, when stimulated by cholecystokinin (pancreozymin).

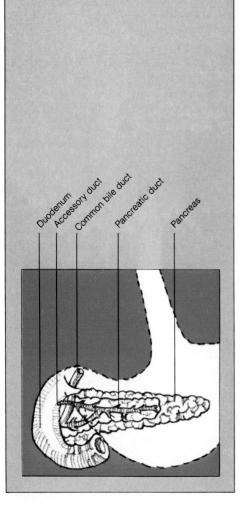

Duodenum   Accessory duct   Common bile duct   Pancreatic duct   Pancreas

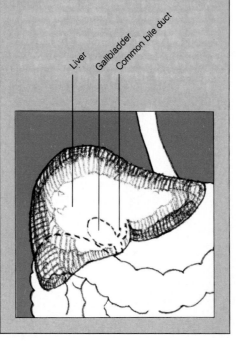

Liver   Gallbladder   Common bile duct

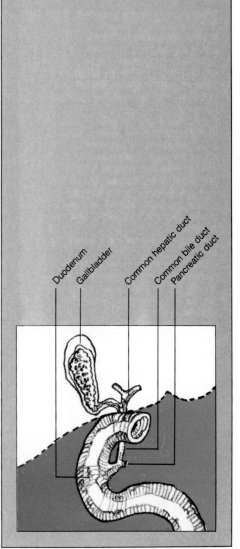

Duodenum   Gallbladder   Common hepatic duct   Common bile duct   Pancreatic duct

DOCUMENTING

Obtaining a GI history

When obtaining your patient's GI history, cover the following topics, using the listed questions as guidelines. If your patient can't respond for any reason, question a family member instead.

Abdominal pain
Do you have pain? If so, where? How long does it last? Is it colicky, constant, or sharp? Does anything relieve it? Do you feel it more when you're in a particular position? Do you have—or have you ever had—an ulcer? When? How were you treated for it? Do you still have pain from it?

Appetite and eating habits
How's your appetite? Have you had a sudden weight loss recently? Do you have excessive gas? Does food stick in your throat? Do you have indigestion or heartburn? Regurgitation? Nausea? Vomiting? If so, what color is the vomitus? Does it contain blood or undigested food? Do you take medicine to stop vomiting?

Bowel symptoms
Do you experience excessive flatulence? How many times a day do you have a bowel movement? Have you noticed a change in your bowel habits recently? Do you have diarrhea or constipation? What color is your stool? What size and shape is it? Does it contain blood or mucus? Is it frothy? Do you use laxatives or enemas? How often? Do you strain to have a bowel movement, without success? Does your abdomen feel distended or rigid? Can you feel a mass in your abdomen? If you have a colostomy or ileostomy, do you have any problems with it?

Liver symptoms
Has your skin color changed? Does your skin itch? What color is your urine? Do you bleed easily? Do you have spider-like discolorations on your skin? Is your abdomen swollen? Do the palms of your hands appear redder than usual? Do you have swelling in your hands, feet, or legs?

In questioning your patient, determine if his signs and symptoms are related to meals or specific foods, positions, or activities. Ask him what aggravates, causes, or relieves his symptoms. Invite him to describe any problems you haven't already covered in your questions.

After you've established your patient's current signs and symptoms, ask him if he's experienced any of them in the past. Also, find out about any diseases he's had, his immunizations, and his past hospitalizations (if any).

In addition, be sure to ask him:
• Have you had any abdominal surgery that we haven't discussed?
• Have you ever had your bowel X-rayed or had a proctoscopy or sigmoidoscopy? If so, when and what for?

Document all findings in your nurses' notes.

Inspecting your patient's abdomen

Before you begin inspection, prepare your patient by having him empty his bladder. Thoroughly explain the assessment procedure to him.

Then, position him flat on his back. Place a pillow under his head and another under his knees. Let him place his hands either at his sides or on his upper chest, whichever he prefers. Proceed, following these steps:
• Expose his abdomen from his xiphoid process to his symphysis pubis, but leave his lower body covered. Now, check his abdomen for its overall form. Is it flat, round, protuberant, or scaphoid? If his abdomen looks distended, you'll auscultate it and check him for ascites. (See the NURSING PHOTOBOOK PERFORMING GI PROCEDURES.)
• Examine his skin for unusual pigmentations, rashes, lesions, hair distribution, or dilated veins. Note any striae or abdominal scars from past trauma or surgery.
• Inspect his abdomen for lumps and masses. Check thoroughly for asymmetry, which may indicate an intra-abdominal mass.
• Examine your patient's umbilicus. Is it red or swollen? If you detect a protrusion that yields to moderate fingertip pressure, suspect an umbilical hernia. Also, check for bluish umbilicus (Cullen's sign), which may indicate intra-abdominal hemorrhage.
• Check his epigastrium for aortic pulsations. To do this, look across his abdomen at eye level. Note the rate, intensity, and location of the pulsation.
• Check his abdomen for peristaltic movement. In a normal patient, you'll see either no motion, or a slight wavelike motion across his abdomen. However, if you see undulating waves (especially accompanied by a distended abdomen and cramps), your patient may have an intestinal obstruction.

Document all of your observations in your nurses' notes.

Auscultating your patient's abdomen

When performing a GI assessment, always auscultate your patient's abdomen before you palpate it. Why? Because palpation may change the frequency of your patient's peristaltic sounds. To auscultate, picture his abdomen divided into quadrants, as shown in the photo. Warm the stethoscope diaphragm in your hands, and place it on your patient's upper right quadrant, above his umbilicus. You should hear intermittent rumbling and gurgling, which are normal bowel sounds. Count these bowel sounds for 1 minute. If all's well, you'll hear 5 to 34 sounds per minute.

Suppose you hear loud bowel sounds occurring more frequently than 34 per minute. Your patient may have a hyperperistaltic, nonobstructed bowel.

If you hear frequent high-pitched, tinkling bowel sounds, or gurgling rushes and loud splashes, your patient may have a bowel obstruction.

What if you don't hear any bowel sounds? Then, auscultate each quadrant—in clockwise order—for 2 to 5 minutes, or until you hear something. If you still don't hear anything in any of the quadrants, your patient may have a paralytic ileus.

Finally, auscultate your patient for friction rub, bruit, or venous hum, as instructed in the NURSING PHOTOBOOK ASSESSING YOUR PATIENTS. A friction rub over your patient's liver or spleen may indicate a hepatic tumor or splenic infarct. Bruits may indicate aortic aneurysm or partial arterial obstruction. Venous hum may indicate hepatic cirrhosis.

Document your findings in your nurses' notes.

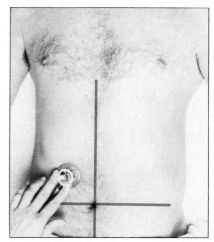

Gastrointestinal basics

How to percuss and palpate your patient's abdomen

1 *Now that you've auscultated your patient's abdomen, get ready to percuss and palpate it. Here's how:*

First, ask your patient if he has any abdominal pain. If he doesn't, start the percussion procedure on his upper right abdominal quadrant, as shown in the photo. However, if your patient does have pain in any quadrant, percuss the affected quadrant last, to prevent muscle guarding. (See page 22 for detailed instructions on positioning your hands for percussion.)

Using uniform finger strikes, percuss each of your patient's quadrants, moving clockwise. As you do so, mentally note where the percussion sounds change from tympanic to dull. This helps you identify abdominal organs and detect possible masses.

Note: A dull sound in your patient's suprapubic area may indicate a distended bladder.

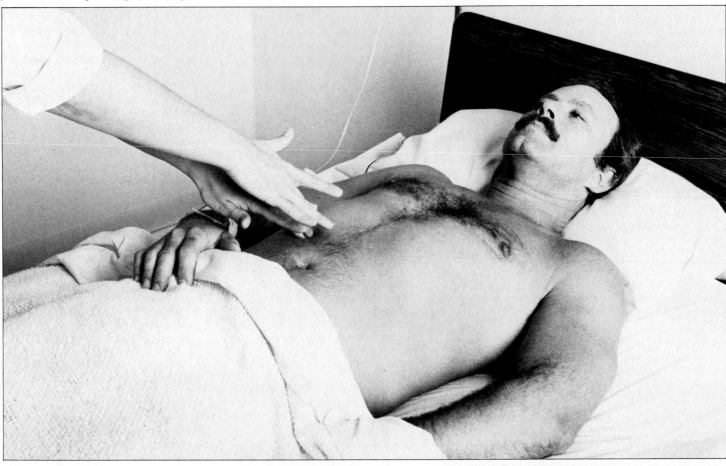

2 After percussing, lightly palpate your patient's abdomen, following the same clockwise order. To palpate, indent your patient's skin about ½″ (1.3 cm) as shown in the photo. Note his skin temperature and moistness. Check for tenderness and possible masses.

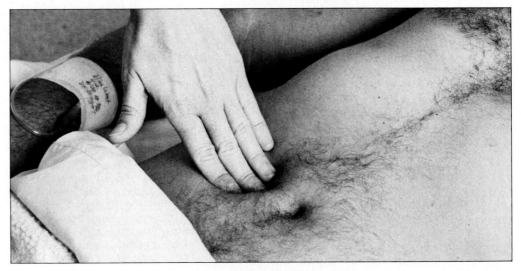

3 Next, deeply palpate his abdomen, following the same clockwise order. To do so, use both your hands to indent your patient's skin more than ½" (1.3 cm), as shown below. Check for organ enlargement, masses, bulges, or swellings. If you detect a mass in your patient's abdomen, note its location, size, shape, consistency, tenderness, and mobility. Also note any pulsations you feel.

If you detect a tender or painful area in your patient's abdomen, check for rebound tenderness or pain, which may indicate peritoneal inflammation or appendicitis. To do this, deeply palpate the tender area. Then, quickly withdraw your fingers. If your patient feels a sharp pain when you do so, he has rebound tenderness.

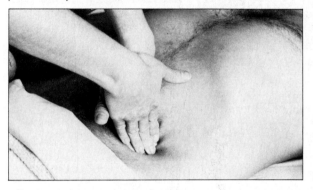

4 To assess your patient's liver, percuss along his right midclavicular line. Percuss upward from his umbilicus and downward from his midsternal level until you hear the percussion sounds change from tympanic to dull. Dullness indicates the liver's borders. Mark the borders and measure the distance between them, which should be 2⅜" to 4¾" (6 cm to 12 cm). If it's greater than 4¾", repeat the percussion procedure at your patient's midline. Here the distance between the upper and lower liver borders should be 1¾" to 3¼" (4.4 cm to 8.3 cm). A measurement greater than 3¼" will confirm an enlarged liver.

Then, deeply palpate the lower edge of his liver, using the bimanual technique shown below. To do so, stand at his right side. Place your left palm under his back, directly under his 11th and 12th ribs. Place your right hand on his abdomen, parallel to his midline. Ask your patient to breathe deeply through his mouth as you press with both hands. You should feel a sharp, firm, regular ridge, which is the liver's lower edge.

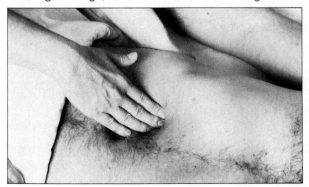

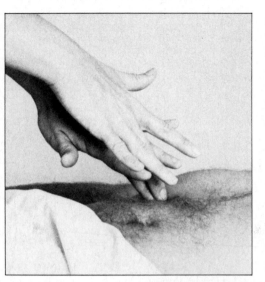

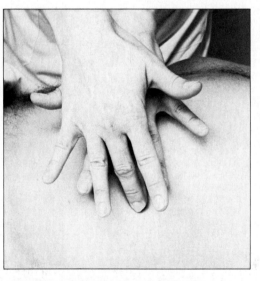

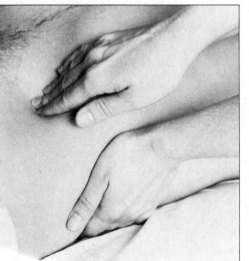

5 Now, percuss his stomach, beginning above and to the right of his umbilicus. Continue across his abdomen to his left anterior axillary line. When the sound changes from dull to tympanic, you're percussing over his stomach. Repeat the percussion in a line 2" (5 cm) above the area just percussed. Continue this process, always percussing 2" above the line you just percussed, until you've determined the size and location of his stomach. No more than five sixths of his stomach should be located left of the median line.

6 To percuss his spleen, begin just under the patient's left midaxillary line, as shown in the photo. Start above the 12th rib (at the 11th intercostal space), and percuss each interspace up to the 8th rib (the 7th intercostal space). If his spleen's normal, you'll hear a tympanic sound as you percuss. If his spleen's enlarged, you'll hear a dull sound. Also percuss his 9th intercostal space at the left anterior axillary line. Then, instruct your patient to breathe deeply and percuss this space a second time.

7 Palpate his spleen by positioning your left hand under his lower left rib cage and your right hand against his lower left costal margin. Tell him to breathe deeply. As he does so, push up with your left hand, and press down with your right fingers. If you feel the spleen's edge, assume the spleen's enlarged about three times its normal size.

Document all findings in your nurses' notes, recording location and size of stomach, liver, and spleen. Record organ enlargement as slight, moderate, or great.

Tube care

Many of your intensive care patients with gastrointestinal problems will require intubation with either a nasogastric (NG) tube or an intestinal tube. You'll use an NG tube for gastric feeding, lavage, or aspiration. You'll use an intestinal tube for intestinal feeding or aspiration. You can also use an intestinal tube to dilate the patient's bowel, if he has a bowel obstruction.

In the following pages, we'll give you descriptions and nursing care information for several different types of tubes. And we'll tell you how to insert an NG tube, in case your hospital's policy permits you to do so.

Have you ever had to treat a patient with a GI hemorrhage? We'll show you how, and cover all the procedures necessary to control his bleeding. We'll also introduce you to the Minnesota tube, a piece of equipment specifically intended to stop bleeding from esophageal varices.

Nurses' guide to gastrointestinal tubes

Do you know when and how to use each of the following gastrointestinal tubes? The chart which follows gives you specific instructions, and outlines your nursing responsibilities. Study it carefully.

In addition, remember these general guidelines when caring for a patient with any type of gastrointestinal tube:
• Before inserting the tube, run water through it to check its patency.
• Immediately after insertion, check tube placement by following the guidelines on page 119.
• Provide good mouth care.
• Keep the skin around the patient's nostrils well lubricated.
• Use proper taping techniques to prevent irritation of skin and nasal passages. Or, use the Deknatel Naso-Gard™ tube holder, as instructed on page 120.
• Observe the patient for signs of tube obstruction, such as nausea, vomiting, distention, discomfort, or lack of drainage. If your patient displays these signs, check the tube for correct placement. If the tube's positioned correctly, irrigate it with normal saline solution, as ordered.
• If you're administering a tube feeding through a gastrointestinal tube, stay alert for these signs of intolerance to the solution: nausea, vomiting, or diarrhea. If you observe any of these signs, stop the feeding and notify the doctor. You may be administering the feeding solution too rapidly.
• To perform gastric lavage when ordered, inject 50 to 100 ml saline solution into the tube. Then, aspirate the fluid or drain it by gravity. Continue to inject and aspirate fluid until the gastric contents are clear of blood or foreign substances. If the tube becomes obstructed, you may need to insert a tube with a larger lumen, or a double-lumen tube.

Note: If you perform gastric lavage to treat a suspected drug overdose, save all lavage specimens and send them to the lab for analysis.

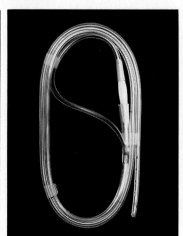

Argyle® Salem Sump®
(nasogastric)

Description
• Double-lumen, 48″ (122 cm) long clear-plastic tube with a blue sump port (pigtail), openings at sides and tip, and markings at 18″, 22″, 26″, and 30″
• Radiopaque Sentinel Line® for X-ray confirmation of placement
• Sump port to help keep gastric mucosa from being drawn into tube during suctioning

Use
• Aspiration of gastric contents
• Administration of tube feedings

Nursing action
• Keep blue pigtail above the level of the patient's stomach to prevent reflux of gastric contents into vent lumen.
• Connect clear port to straight bag drainage, or intermittent or continuous low suction, or clamp it, as ordered. Place any drainage receptacle below the level of the patient's stomach to prevent reflux into the vent lumen.
• If gastric contents reflux into vent lumen, you may irrigate blue pigtail with 30 ml normal saline solution, followed by 10 to 20 cc air.
• Keep tube patent by instilling 30 ml saline solution through clear port or blue pigtail every 2 hours.
• Inject air through blue pigtail after each irrigation.
• For initial feeding, administer water for 2 to 4 hours, or until you're sure of patient's tolerance to tube and infusion.
• Start half-strength tube feedings at a rate of 25 ml/hour, or as ordered. Increase solution to full strength within 24 hours.

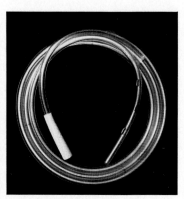

Bard-Parker™ stomach tube
(Levin-type nasogastric)

Description
• Single-lumen, 50″ (127 cm) long clear-plastic tube with openings at tip and along side

Use
• Aspiration of gastric contents
• Administration of tube feedings

Nursing action
• If tube's too limp to insert easily, chill it in a basin of ice. If tube's too stiff, make it more pliant by heating it in a basin of warm water.
• To keep tube patent, irrigate it once every 2 hours with 30 ml normal saline solution, or as ordered.
• Attach tube to intermittent low suction or a drainage bag or bottle, or clamp it, as ordered.
• Before beginning tube feeding, always verify tube placement, using the tests described on page 119.
• Start half-strength tube feedings at a rate of 25 ml/hour, or as ordered. Increase to full-strength solution within 24 hours.

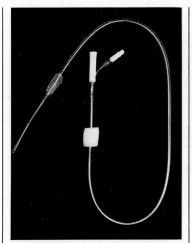

G. Moss™ decompression tube (nasogastric)

Description
● Double-lumen, 35″ (90 cm) long clear-plastic tube with X-ray (radiopaque) tip and foam rubber cushion at nasal opening

Use
● Aspiration of gastric contents

Nursing action
● Before insertion, make sure balloon's intact.
● Insert tube completely and verify its placement in patient's stomach before inflating the balloon.
● Inflate balloon with 30 cc air.
● To position the catheter, pull on it gently until you feel resistance. (In doing so, you'll probably withdraw several inches of catheter from the patient's nostril.) When you feel resistance, the balloon's correctly positioned at the cardia.
● Apply intermittent or continuous low suction, as ordered.
● To ensure tube patency, irrigate tube with 30 ml normal saline solution every 2 hours.

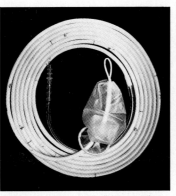

Kaslow® radiopaque (intestinal)

Description
● Single-lumen, 10' (3 m) long rubber tube with centimeter markings
● Available in size 16 French

Use
● For bowel obstruction. When attached to intermittent low suction, allows aspiration of intestinal contents.

Nursing action
● Assist doctor with insertion procedure. Before insertion, test tube for patency and balloon for leaks. Place patient in high Fowler's position with his neck hyperextended.
● After insertion, attach tube to intermittent low suction, as ordered.
● Once every 8 hours (or as ordered), document type and amount of drainage.

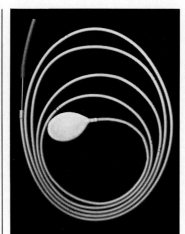

Cantor (intestinal)

Description
● Single-lumen, 10' (3 m) long rubber tube with balloon at distal tip for mercury insertion
● Available in size 16 French

Use
● For bowel obstruction. When attached to suction, allows aspiration of intestinal contents.

Nursing action
● Assist doctor with insertion procedure. Before insertion, test tube for patency and balloon for leaks. For insertion, place patient in high Fowler's position with his neck hyperextended.
● Use a 5 cc syringe with a 21G needle to draw up mercury. Then, inject it directly into the balloon bag's upper portion. Aspirate all the air from the bag.
● To advance the tube into the patient's intestine, position him on his right side (after confirming placement of the tube in his stomach).
● Slowly advance the tube about 1″ every 5 minutes for the next 30 to 60 minutes until it reaches the desired mark.
● Allow gravity to drain tube during insertion. If the tube stops draining at any point, inject 10 cc air.
● Confirm tube's placement in duodenum by aspirating a small amount of fluid. Test aspirate with litmus paper to determine pH. Blue paper indicates alkaline fluid.
● Confirm tube placement by X-ray.
● Attach suction lumen to intermittent low suction, as ordered.
● Once every 8 hours, document type and amount of drainage.

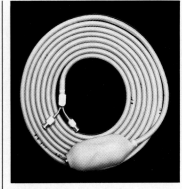

Miller-Abbott (intestinal)

Description
● Double-lumen, 10' (3 m) long rubber tube with centimeter markings
● Available in sizes 12, 14, 16, or 18 French

Use
● For bowel obstruction. When attached to suction, allows aspiration of intestinal contents. Also dilates bowel.

Nursing action
● Assist doctor with insertion procedure. Before insertion, test tube for patency and balloon for leaks. For insertion, place patient in high Fowler's position with his head erect.
● After the tube reaches the stomach, use a 5 cc syringe to insert mercury into balloon lumen.
● Clamp the balloon lumen to prevent accidental mercury withdrawal while suctioning.
● To advance the tube into the patient's intestine, position him on his right side (after confirming placement of the tube in his stomach).
● Slowly advance the tube about 1″ every 5 minutes for the next 30 to 60 minutes until it reaches the desired mark.
● Allow gravity to drain tube during insertion. If the tube stops draining at any point, inject 10 cc air.
● Confirm placement in duodenum by aspirating a small amount of fluid. Test aspirate with litmus paper to determine pH. Blue paper indicates alkaline fluid.
● Confirm tube placement by X-ray.
● Attach suction lumen to intermittent low suction, as ordered.
● Once every 8 hours (or as ordered), document type and amount of drainage.
● Before tube removal, withdraw mercury with a 5 cc syringe.

Tube care

Caring for a patient with a GI hemorrhage

Gerald Crusi, a 48-year-old salesman, is admitted to your intensive care unit with Mallory-Weiss syndrome. After repeated vomiting, he suddenly begins to vomit large amounts of bright red blood, the sign of massive GI hemorrhage. He also displays diaphoresis, chills, tachypnea, weak and thready pulse, pallor, and thirst.

To prevent hemorrhagic shock, you must stop Mr. Crusi's bleeding quickly and replace his lost blood. To do so successfully, you'll need to work with other health care professionals as a team, performing several procedures simultaneously.

In treating Mr. Crusi, your main concerns are: combating hypovolemia; preventing and treating fluid and electrolyte imbalance; controlling bleeding and replacing lost blood; locating the bleeding site; and stopping the bleeding completely. To accomplish these objectives, perform the following procedures as instructed on these pages.

As you do so, keep in mind that your patient's mental status is as important as his physical condition. Reassure him as much as possible. Explain each procedure to him as it's performed, even if he's unconscious. In addition, reassure your patient's family members, and report to them frequently about his condition. Document all procedures in your nurses' notes.

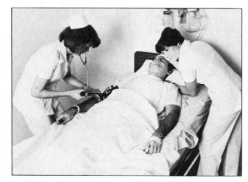

Until the bleeding's controlled, monitor Mr. Crusi's vital signs every 15 minutes. Make sure his airway remains patent. Also, watch him closely for signs of hypovolemic shock, which include: low blood pressure; cold, clammy skin; decreased urinary output; increased respiratory rate; restlessness; and diaphoresis. If you see any of these signs, or if your patient complains of dizziness or nausea, notify the doctor.

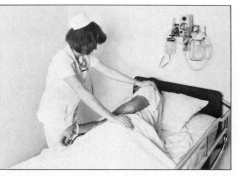

Position Mr. Crusi so he's lying on his side, with his head slightly elevated. This position helps prevent aspiration of vomitus. Cover him with a blanket.

Important: Never place your patient in Trendelenburg position, because his abdominal organs will interfere with respiration and venous return.

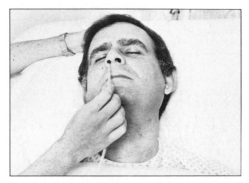

Prepare for nasogastric (NG) tube insertion by placing your patient in high Fowler's position, or as ordered.

Insert the tube as explained on pages 118 to 120. Then, attach the NG tube to intermittent low suction, as ordered. Note the color, amount, and consistency of the aspirated gastric contents.

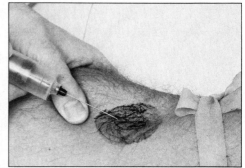

Draw a blood sample for determining type and crossmatch, complete blood cell count (CBC), hemoglobin and hematocrit, and serum electrolyte levels. Also, obtain an arterial sample to determine arterial blood gas (ABG) measurements. Label the samples with your patient's name, his hospital identification number, the date, and time. Send the samples to the laboratory for immediate analysis.

Remember: Keep the arterial blood sample on ice to ensure accurate test results.

Until properly typed and crossmatched blood is available, the doctor may order plasma or albumin administered I.V.

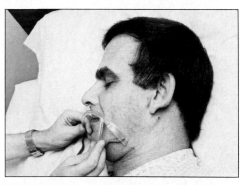

Administer oxygen at a flow rate of 2 to 4 liters via nasal cannula, as ordered. After the doctor gets the results from the ABG measurement, he'll order the oxygen flow rate adjusted accordingly.

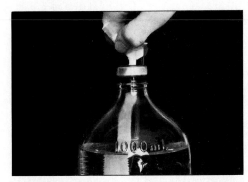

To correct hypovolemia, immediately start an I.V. infusion of normal saline solution, as ordered (unless the doctor specifies plasma or albumin). Don't give your patient any food or fluids by mouth.

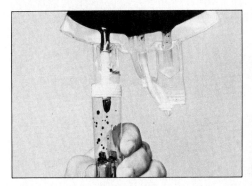

Begin a blood transfusion (as ordered), after Mr. Crusi's blood is typed and crossmatched. If he's already receiving plasma, complete that transfusion first. Then administer fresh blood or packed cells of his own type.

Watch Mr. Crusi closely for any adverse reactions to the blood transfusion, such as diaphoresis, urticaria, chills, or respiratory distress. If any problems develop, stop the transfusion and substitute normal saline solution for the blood. Administer it into the vein at the keep-vein-open (KVO) rate. Then, notify the doctor and return the unused blood and tubing to the lab. If the doctor orders, attempt another transfusion with a fresh bag of blood.

Suppose the doctor doesn't order another transfusion. If after 15 minutes the patient's still having symptoms of blood transfusion reaction, notify the doctor immediately. If the patient's no longer having symptoms, increase the saline solution infusion rate, as ordered.

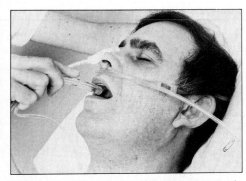

If the hemorrhage isn't self-limiting, get ready to perform iced gastric lavage. Insert a large gauge (36 to 40 French) gastric tube and begin the procedure, as ordered.

During the lavage, have a co-worker closely monitor the patient's blood pressure and pulse for signs of hypothermia. Because of his GI hemorrhage and its resulting hypovolemia, Mr. Crusi's already at risk of hypothermia. Iced gastric lavage greatly increases his risk. (For more information, see the NURSING PHOTOBOOK PERFORMING GI PROCEDURES.)

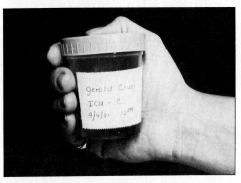

Insert an indwelling (Foley) catheter, as ordered. (For insertion guidelines, see the NURSING PHOTOBOOK IMPLEMENTING UROLOGIC PROCEDURES.) Then, collect and label a sterile urine specimen to send to the lab for analysis.

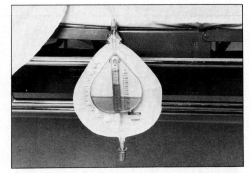

Attach the Foley catheter to a urine meter. Every hour, measure the amount of urine that's collected in the drainage chamber. In your notes, accurately record the amount, color, and consistency of the urine. Also, be sure to keep an accurate fluid intake record. If Mr. Crusi's urine output is less than 30 ml/hour, notify the doctor immediately.

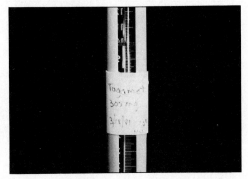

When the patient's condition has stabilized, administer cimetidine (Tagamet*) I.V., as ordered, to keep the bleeding from recurring. Then, prepare the patient for upper GI endoscopy, to locate the bleeding site. The doctor may use the endoscope to apply pressure to stop bleeding in the esophagus, stomach, or duodenum. If the bleeding is from esophageal varices, the doctor may try injecting sclerosing agents through the endoscope directly into the varices to stop the bleeding. A Minnesota or Sengstaken-Blakemore tube may also be used to stop bleeding from varices (see pages 121 to 123).

Alternatively, the doctor may employ angiography to pinpoint the bleeding site and to administer vasopressin (Pitressin Synthetic*) locally. Be prepared to assist the doctor with these procedures, as needed.

If Mr. Crusi's GI bleeding remains uncontrolled, prepare him for surgery (gastric resection), as ordered by the doctor.

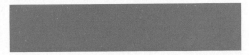

Tube care

How to insert a nasogastric (NG) tube

1 Randy Morrison, a 33-year-old computer programmer with a history of myocardial infarction (MI), has developed paralytic ileus following a cholecystectomy. Because of his cardiac history, you're caring for Mr. Morrison in the ICU. The doctor orders insertion of an NG tube for suctioning Mr. Morrison's gastric contents. If your hospital policy permits, you'll perform the procedure.

Before you begin, wash your hands thoroughly to help prevent contamination. Then, gather this equipment: size 12 to 18 French NG tube or Salem Sump tube (shown here), penlight, Hoffman clamp, cup of water with a straw, irrigation set (including bulb syringe, container, and basin), paper towel, water-soluble lubricant, nonallergenic tape, two bed-saver pads, Skin-Prep, emesis basin, stethoscope, tissues, a safety pin, and normal saline solution (in case tube needs to be irrigated after insertion).

Now, test the tube's patency by running water through it. Also, check it for rough spots and ragged edges. If you're using a vinyl plastic tube, chill or warm it as necessary.

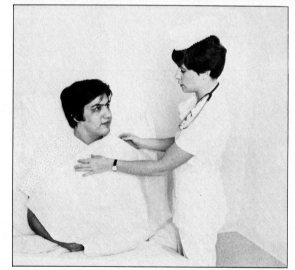

2 Now, explain the procedure to your patient and reassure him. Encourage him to ask questions. Tell him that he may feel some discomfort during the procedure, and agree on a signal he can use to stop the procedure momentarily.

Next, place your patient in a sitting or high Fowler's position. If he's wearing dentures, remove them. Cover his gown and bed linen with bed-saver pads to protect them from spills. Hand him several tissues, as the procedure may stimulate tearing. Also, give him the emesis basin, if he's able to hold it.

Using a penlight, examine his nostrils for possible obstructions or deformities. Then, alternately press each of his nostrils closed and instruct him to inhale through the open nostril. If both nostrils are mechanically obstructed, stop immediately and notify the doctor. He may want you to pass the tube orally. Otherwise, begin the procedure.

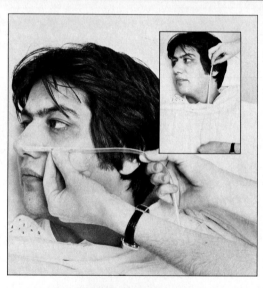

3 Follow this two-step method to determine how much tube to insert. First, use the tube to measure the distance from your patient's earlobe to the tip of his nose, as shown here.

[Inset] Then, measure the distance from his earlobe to the base of his xiphoid process. Total these measurements, and use adhesive tape to mark this length on the tube.

Loosely holding a length of tube between your hands, determine its natural curve. If no curve is evident, shape a curve yourself by coiling the first 5″ (12.7 cm) of tubing tightly around your fingers.

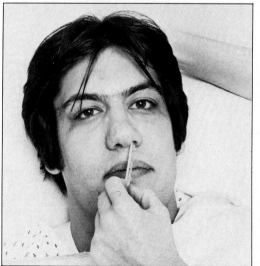

4 Lubricate the first 6″ (15.2 cm) of the tube with water-soluble lubricant.

Now, have your patient hold his head still as you insert the NG tube into an unobstructed nostril, as shown here. Gently advance it along the nasal passage toward the posterior nasopharynx, directing the tube toward your patient's ear on that side.

5 When you feel the tube approaching your patient's nasopharynx, rotate it 180° inward, toward his other nostril. Then, continue to advance the tube gently, until it's in the nasopharynx, pointing toward the esophagus.

Important: If you meet resistance at any point, immediately stop advancing the tube. Instead, use it to probe very gently for the opening to the nasopharynx. Then, try advancing it again. If you're still unable to do so, withdraw the tube completely. Then, relubricate the tube and try inserting it in the other nostril, provided that nostril is unobstructed.

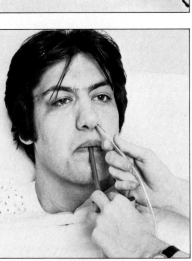

6 What if your patient starts to gag as the tube enters his nasopharynx? Stop advancing the tube immediately, and tell him to take several deep breaths. Or, if he's allowed to drink water, ask him to take a few sips of water through a straw. Either method will relax his pharynx and calm his gag reflex. If your patient can't drink water, have him dry swallow. *Important:* Never give liquids to a patient who is unconscious.

Suppose your patient continues gagging, begins to cough, or becomes dyspneic. Check his mouth with the penlight to see if the tube is coiled in his mouth or throat. If so, withdraw the tube until it's straight. Then, let him rest for a few moments before you continue the procedure.

7 Now, instruct your patient to move his head forward so his chin touches his chest, as shown here. This helps to close his trachea and open his esophagus. Tell your patient to swallow, and continue to advance the tube into his esophagus.

Ask him to sip water or chew ice chips as you advance the tube into his stomach. Or, have him dry swallow. Advance the tubing 3″ to 5″ (7.6 to 12.7 cm) each time he swallows.

Continue inserting the tube until you've reached the premeasured mark. If the tube won't advance that far, you may have inserted it into your patient's trachea. Or, the tube may have curled in the back of his throat. Withdraw the tubing until it's straight, and try again to insert it correctly.

If the tube meets resistance at the 18″ (46 cm) level, it may be blocked by the stomach wall opposite the gastroesophageal junction. Pull the tube back about 4″ (10 cm), rotate it 180°, and reinsert it.

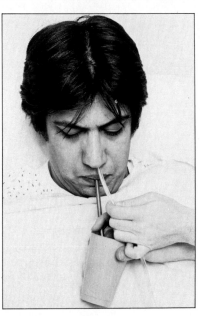

8 At this point in the procedure, you'll want to make sure the tube's in your patient's stomach, not his bronchus. To do this, try at least two of the following tests for proper tube placement.

Here's the first test: Attach a bulb or piston syringe to the end of the tube and try to gently aspirate gastric fluid, as shown here. If you can't withdraw any fluid, the tube may be pressed against the stomach wall, curled in the stomach, or not inserted far enough. In this case, reposition the tube slightly and try again. If you still can't aspirate gastric fluid, the tube may be in your patient's bronchus.

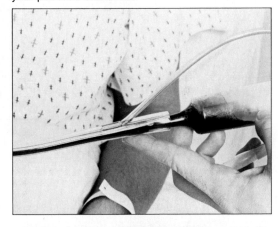

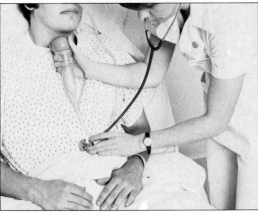

9 Then, try this second test. Place a stethoscope over your patient's stomach. Attach a bulb syringe to the tube and inject some air (about 30 cc) into the tube. Then, listen for air entering the stomach (a swooshing or gurgling sound). Silence indicates that you probably haven't injected air into the stomach, but into your patient's bronchus or esophagus.

For a third test, hold the end of the tube to your ear. You won't hear anything if the tube's in your patient's stomach. But, if it's in his bronchus, you'll hear crackling noises and feel air coming from the tube.

Important: If any test result raises doubts about the tube's position, confirm correct tube placement with an X-ray ordered by the doctor.

Tube care

How to insert a nasogastric (NG) tube continued

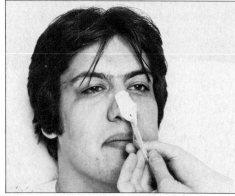

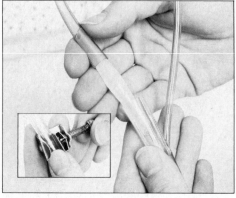

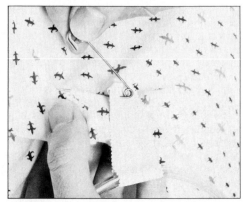

10 When you're sure the tube's properly positioned in his stomach, cut a 3″ (7.6 cm) strip of 1″ (2.5 cm) wide non-allergenic tape. Split the tape lengthwise, leaving a small tab intact at one end. Now, apply Skin-Prep to the top of your patient's nose. When the Skin-Prep feels tacky, place the tab end of the tape over it. Then, spiral one end of the tape around the tube. Bring the other end under the tube and tape it to the top of your patient's nose. Or, instead of taping, you may use the NG tube holder shown below.

Important: Never tape the tube to your patient's forehead. The resulting tension may cause a pressure sore in his nasal passage.

11 Now, if the doctor's ordered suction, as he has for Mr. Morrison, connect the NG tube to the suction tubing, using the tube's adapter. However, if he orders gravity or straight drainage rather than suction, attach the tube to a drainage bag or bottle.

[Inset] Suppose the doctor orders tube feeding. Clamp the tube, using a Hoffman clamp. To keep the tube's end clean, cover it with gauze secured with a rubber band. Or, use a plastic plug to occlude the tube's lumen instead.

Unclamp the tube when you're ready to administer the feeding (according to the prescribed schedule).

Note: If your patient complains of nausea while the tube's clamped, unclamp it and attach it to a drainage receptacle.

12 To prevent the tube from dangling, wrap a piece of adhesive tape around the tube, just above the tube's junction with the suction tubing or just above the end of the unconnected tube. Leave a tab on the tape's ends. Then, using a safety pin, attach the tape tab to your patient's gown, just below his shoulder.

Make your patient as comfortable as possible. To minimize nasal irritation, place a small amount of water-soluble lubricant on the skin around each nostril. Document the procedure in your nurses' notes.

Prevent pressure sores by checking regularly to make sure the tubing's positioned comfortably. Also, provide good mouth care. Irrigate the tube, as ordered. For instructions, see the NURSING PHOTOBOOK PERFORMING GI PROCEDURES.

Using a Deknatel Naso-Gard™ nasogastric tube holder

As an alternative to taping, you may secure your patient's nasogastric tube with a Naso-Gard tube holder. Here's how:
• First, make sure the holder is right side up, as indicated on the front of the guard.
• Place the harness over the patient's ears. Adjust the straps for proper tension by pulling them through the holder's slots until taut (but not tight).
• Now, place the tube securely into the niche behind the nearest nose clip.
• Each day, check the patient's skin under the nosepiece for signs of irritation.
• Check her ears daily for pressure necrosis. Tape folded gauze pads under the straps over her ears to protect her ears.

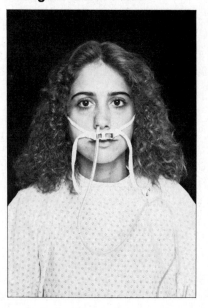

Removing a nasogastric (NG) tube

If the doctor asks you to remove your patient's NG tube, follow these guidelines:
• First, prepare your patient. Explain the procedure to him. Then, place him in high Fowler's position. Use a towel or bed-saver pad to protect his gown and bed linens.
• Unpin the tube from his gown. Remove the tape from his nose.
• Gently rotate the tube to make sure it moves freely. If it doesn't, irrigate the tube with 30 ml normal saline solution.
• When the tube moves freely, inject 30 cc air to clear it of any remaining fluid. Then, clamp the tube, plug its lumen with a plastic plug, or fold the tube in your hand. Occluding the tube will keep gastric fluid from entering your patient's lungs or esophagus during removal.
• Ask your patient to take a deep breath as you quickly, but gently, withdraw the tube. Then, place the tube on a towel, out of the patient's sight.
• As soon as you've removed the tube, tell him to resume breathing. Give him mouth care to make him more comfortable. Also, clean and dry the skin around his nostrils, and lubricate it with water-soluble jelly.
• Document the procedure in your nurses' notes.

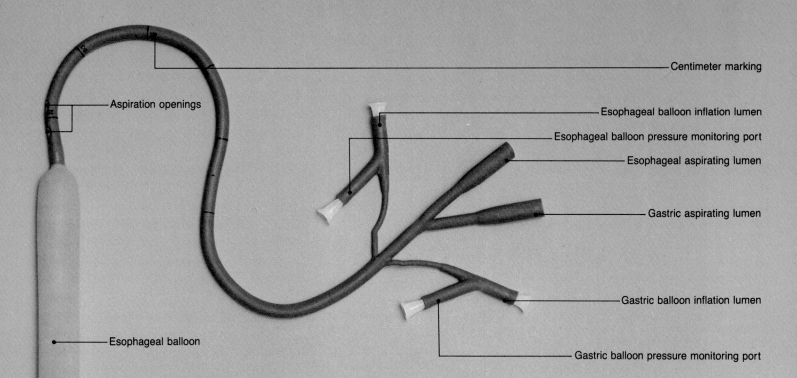

Centimeter marking

Aspiration openings

Esophageal balloon inflation lumen

Esophageal balloon pressure monitoring port

Esophageal aspirating lumen

Gastric aspirating lumen

Gastric balloon inflation lumen

Esophageal balloon

Gastric balloon pressure monitoring port

Gastric balloon

Aspiration openings

Learning about the Davol® Minnesota Four-Lumen Esophagogastric Tamponade Tube

Suppose esophageal varices are causing your patient's GI hemorrhage. The doctor will probably insert a Sengstaken-Blakemore or a Minnesota esophagogastric tube to control the bleeding. These tubes have balloons that, when inflated, press directly against esophageal and gastric varices. This pressure is called tamponade.

In the following photostory, we show you how to use the Minnesota tube. Consider its advantage. Because it has four lumens, you can aspirate esophageal and gastric contents through the same tube that you use to apply tamponade to the varices. The Sengstaken-Blakemore tube has only two lumens, requiring insertion of a separate nasogastric (NG) tube into the esophagus for aspirating. The NG tube must be kept in place for the duration of tamponade.

To understand how the Minnesota tube functions, see the illustration at right. It shows the correct placement of the tube's inflated balloons within the GI tract. The gastric balloon holds the tube in position, as well as applying tamponade to gastric varices. The esophageal balloon provides tamponade to esophageal varices for most of the length of the esophagus. Openings in the tube below the gastric balloon and above the esophageal balloon permit aspiration of esophageal and gastric contents.

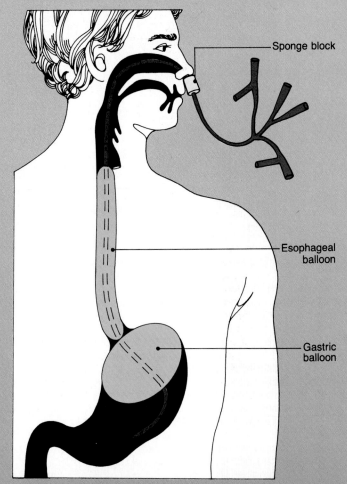

Sponge block

Esophageal balloon

Gastric balloon

Tube care

Assisting with Minnesota tube insertion

1 *The doctor plays the major role in inserting the Minnesota tube. But you'll assist her by preparing the patient, assembling and testing equipment, performing iced gastric lavage, and aspirating gastric and esophageal contents.*

First, obtain the following equipment: Minnesota tube, size 18 French Levin-type nasogastric (NG) tube or size 36 French double-lumen gastric lavage tube (for iced gastric lavage prior to tube insertion), mercury sphygmomanometer, bed-saver pad, water-soluble lubricating jelly, cup of water or ice chips with straw, rubber-shod clamps, 50 cc piston syringe, bottled normal saline solution, large basin with ice (for chilling bottled solution), irrigation set (including bulb syringe, solution container, and small basin), emesis basin, penlight, sponge block or football helmet, two tubing adapters, two suction machines, and scissors (to tape to the bed for use in an emergency).

Wash your hands. Explain the procedure to your patient and reassure him. Place him in semi-Fowler's position, with the head of the bed elevated at least 45°. Place a bed-saver pad across his chest. *Note:* If the patient's unconscious, place him on his left side with the head of the bed elevated at least 45°.

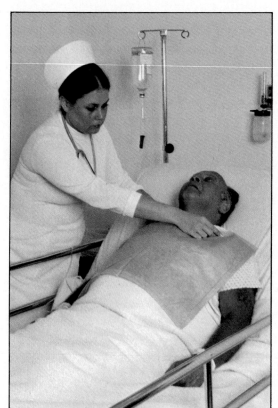

4 Now the doctor's ready to insert the Minnesota tube. To do so, she'll suction the air from the gastric and esophageal balloons. Then, she'll clamp rubber-shod clamps on the balloons' two pressure monitoring ports and insert plastic plugs into the balloons' inflation lumens. Next, she'll advance the first balloon into the patient's nostril. Reassure the patient and tell him to begin swallowing. To keep him from gagging, have him sip water through a straw, chew ice, or dry swallow. Check his vital signs frequently and make sure his airway remains patent.

5 When the 50 cm mark reaches the patient's nostril, the tube's tip should be in his stomach. Using a bulb syringe, immediately aspirate through first the gastric, then the esophageal aspiration lumen. Aspirating through the gastric lumen first will keep the patient from regurgitating gastric juice, blood, and saliva. Gastric aspiration also helps confirm that the tube's properly located.

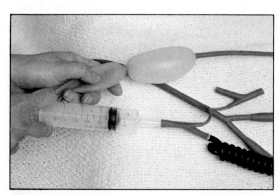

2 Now, test the esophageal and gastric balloons for leaks by inflating each of them with an air-filled 50 cc piston syringe. Submerge the balloons in a basin of water. Watch for any escaping air bubbles. Then, run water through the tubes to check them for patency.

Now you're ready to determine the pressure in the gastric balloon at different inflation levels. To do so, first deflate the balloon. Then, attach a mercury manometer to the pressure monitoring port on the gastric balloon. Inject air into the inflation lumen, as the nurse is doing here.

Note the pressure in the balloon at inflation levels of 100, 200, 300, 400, and 500 cc of air. Record these pressures in your nurses' notes.

Then, deflate both balloons, and coat them with water-soluble jelly.

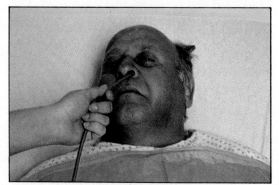

3 Now, use a penlight to inspect the patient for any nasal deformities. If all's well (and if this is a nursing responsibility in your hospital), insert the NG tube into his stomach.

You'll use the NG tube to remove blood clots by performing iced gastric lavage. This reduces the risk of the patient's aspirating blood. First, fill the bulb syringe with 50 ml chilled normal saline solution. Then, attach the syringe to the NG tube, and inject the saline solution into the tube. Withdraw the fluid into the syringe. Repeat the lavage until the return fluid is clear. During lavage, have a co-worker closely monitor the patient's blood pressure and pulse for any signs of hypothermia. After lavage, remove the NG tube.

Note: If large clots obstruct the size 18 French tube, use the double-lumen gastric lavage tube.

6 Now, the doctor will inflate and position the balloons. As she does this, she'll use a mercury manometer to monitor the inflation pressure of the gastric balloon. She'll compare these pressures with the test volume pressures you recorded. After the doctor has correctly positioned the balloons and inflated the gastric balloon with 450 to 500 cc air, she'll clamp the gastric balloon ports, as shown here. Document the amount and inflation pressure of the air injected into the balloons.

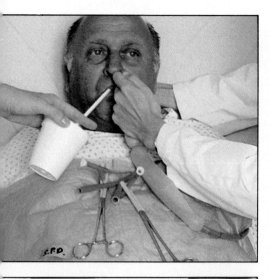

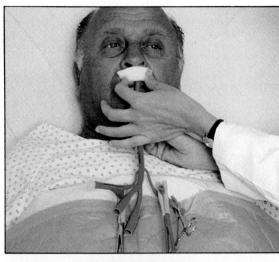

7 Next, the doctor will secure the tube. To do this, she'll gently eliminate slack in the tube by positioning a small sponge block around the tube, just under the patient's nose. Then, she'll tape the tube to the sponge block.

Alternatively, she'll slide a football helmet over the patient's head, and tape the tube to the helmet's mouth guard. This method may hold the tube more firmly in place.

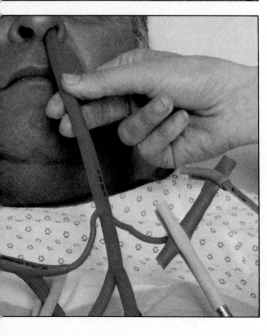

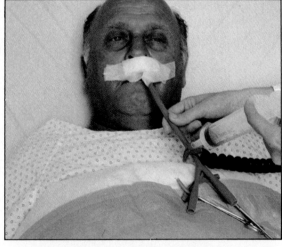

8 Now, you'll administer a second iced gastric lavage through the gastric aspiration lumen, until the aspirate is clear of blood. But, if the bleeding continues, the doctor may inflate the esophageal balloon, as shown here. If the bleeding still won't stop, a gastric varix may be present. To control the bleeding, the doctor will apply external traction on the tube, by increasing the tension on the tube at the point where it's taped.

Important: External traction should be applied for only short periods of time. Within a few hours, it can cause ulceration of the esophageal mucosa.

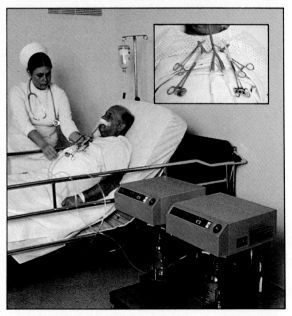

9 After the tube has been inserted and the patient's bleeding brought under control, connect the gastric aspiration lumen to intermittent, low (90 mm Hg) suction, and the esophageal aspiration lumen to continuous high (120 mm Hg) suction (see inset).

Document the procedure, and your patient's reaction to it. Confirm tube placement by obtaining an X-ray. Every 4 hours while the tube's in place, record the amount of drainage and the presence of blood. Give the patient frequent mouth care and keep his nostrils lubricated.

Watch for signs of respiratory distress, such as dyspnea, which may be caused by balloon rupture or release of tension on the tube. At the first sign of distress, cut across the lumens and pull out the tube, using the scissors taped to the bed.

Total parenteral nutrition

A patient with a serious GI disorder probably needs nutrition administered intravenously. This treatment, called total parenteral nutrition (TPN) or hyper-alimentation, provides all the nutrients necessary to sustain the patient and promote his recovery.

In the next few pages, we'll explain:
* the major ingredients of TPN.
* specific TPN additives the doctor might prescribe.
* how TPN's administered, including guidelines for patient care.
* how to prevent complications in a patient with a central I.V. line.

For information about special formulas, such as protein-sparing solution or fat emulsion, see the NURSING PHOTOBOOK MANAGING I.V. THERAPY.

INDICATIONS/CONTRAINDICATIONS

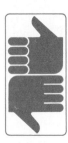

When to administer total parenteral nutrition (TPN)

You'll give TPN when the patient:
* can't tolerate oral or nasogastric tube feeding or when tube feeding is contra-indicated.
* has severe malnutrition.
* has a disorder that renders his GI tract nonfunctional; for example, inflammatory bowel disease, ulcerative colitis, GI fistula, major bowel resection, short bowel syndrome, prolonged paralytic ileus, pancreatitis, or anorexia nervosa.
* has extensive surgical trauma.
* has extensive burns.
* has metastatic cancer with anorexia.
Note: You'll give special TPN preparations to hepatic or renal failure patients.
Never give TPN when a patient has:
* hypercoagulation or bleeding abnor-malities.
* an obstructed or partially thrombosed superior vena cava.
* terminal illness, with all therapy dis-continued.

Learning about TPN components

Wondering how the doctor decides which additives to include in your patient's total parenteral nutrition (TPN) solution? First, the doctor determines your patient's metabolic needs by assessing his physical condition and performing blood studies. Then, he prescribes the appropriate combination of additives in the specific amounts that will help meet your patient's needs.

To understand the functions of TPN additives, study this chart:

TPN additive	Purpose
50% dextrose in water	Provides calories needed for metabolism
Amino acids	Supply protein needed for tissue repair
Potassium	Functions in cellular activity and tissue synthesis
Folic acid	Functions in DNA formation
Vitamin D	Maintains serum calcium levels and functions in bone metabolism
Vitamin B complex	Aids in final absorption of carbohydrates and protein
Vitamin K	Helps prevent bleeding disorders
Vitamin C	Promotes wound healing
Sodium	Helps control water distribution to maintain fluid balance
Chloride	Helps to regulate the acid-base equilibrium and to maintain osmotic pressure
Calcium	Promotes blood clotting; aids teeth and bone development
Phosphate	Minimizes the threat of peripheral paresthesia
Magnesium	Helps absorb carbohydrates and protein
Acetate	Prevents metabolic acidosis
Trace elements (zinc, cobalt, manganese)	Promote wound healing and red blood cell synthesis

---

Learning about total parenteral nutrition (TPN)

Total parenteral nutrition (TPN) is a mixture of 50% dextrose in water, amino acids, and special additives (see the chart at left). In TPN solutions, dextrose and amino acids serve as the major sources of calories. They usually provide about 1,000 calories per liter.

Most TPN solutions have similar amounts of amino acids. And, the dextrose concentration usually approximates 25% of the total TPN solution after 50% dextrose in water is combined with other ingredients. However, dextrose concentrations may vary between 10% and 50%, depending on the quantities of special additives the doctor's ordered. These additives differ from patient to patient, because they're specifically prescribed to meet each patient's particular needs.

Keep in mind that protein-sparing solutions (with one half the usual amount of amino acids) are also available. Also, to supplement the calories provided by a TPN solution, you may give your patient a fat emulsion.

The TPN mixture must be prepared under a laminar flow hood in your hospital's pharmacy. After the correct solution has been delivered to your unit, refrigerate it until the therapy begins.

Important: Before administering any TPN solution, check its expiration date. In most cases, TPN solution must be used within 24 hours of preparation.

Administering TPN
You'll administer TPN through a central I.V. line

resting in the patient's superior vena cava. The doctor may insert the line through the subclavian vein (direct line), or feed it through the jugular vein or a large peripheral vein.

TPN is administered into the superior vena cava to allow adequate dilution of the solution with blood. Otherwise, the high osmolarity of the solution could cause thrombosis at the I.V. catheter tip. Using an infusion pump also helps maintain adequate dilution, by keeping the infusion rate constant.

As you probably know, your patient's body will need time to adjust to the high osmolarity of the TPN solution. So, as ordered, administer 10% dextrose in water before you begin administering TPN. Then, after the adjustment period of 1 to 2 days, begin administering TPN at a slow rate, 1 to 2 l/day for the first 2 days. Doing so will allow the pancreas to secrete enough insulin to handle increased carbohydrate loads. Gradually increase the infusion rate as ordered until you achieve the desired rate, which is usually 3 l/ day.

Remember, always monitor your patient closely when he's receiving TPN therapy. (For guidelines, see the text at right.)

At the end of TPN therapy, reduce the TPN flow rate gradually to allow insulin production to taper off. Otherwise, the patient may experience rebound insulin shock.

For more details on TPN administration, see the NURSING PHOTOBOOK MANAGING I.V. THERAPY.

Caring for a patient receiving total parenteral nutrition (TPN)

To properly care for a patient receiving TPN, observe the following guidelines:
• Closely monitor the flow rate to avoid metabolic complications, such as hyperglycemia or electrolyte imbalance.
• If TPN administration is interrupted for any reason, substitute 10% dextrose in water.
• Monitor your patient's vital signs at least once every 4 hours.
• Test your patient's urine sugar, acetone, and specific gravity every 4 hours. To determine his urine sugar and acetone levels, perform a dipstick test. If test results show a urine sugar level of 2 + or greater—or if you discover a high acetone concentration—notify the doctor. He may increase the TPN solution's insulin level, or order sliding-scale insulin coverage administered subcutaneously.

If, following testing, the specific gravity of your patient's urine is not at the normal level (1.020), the doctor may change the infusion rate or the TPN solution's contents.
• Obtain blood studies for osmolarity and electrolyte, blood sugar, creatinine, blood urea nitrogen (BUN), and trace element levels.
• Weigh your patient at the same time each day to check his fluid balance. Always use the same scale and make sure he's wearing the same clothing.
• Document your patient's daily fluid intake and output and his caloric intake.
• Provide good mouth care, using mouthwash. Brush your patient's teeth twice each day.
• Closely follow the guidelines on central I.V. line care described below.

SPECIAL CONSIDERATIONS

Caring for the patient with a central I.V. line

Unless your patient's receiving a protein-sparing solution, you'll administer total parenteral nutrition (TPN) through a central I.V. line. Keep in mind that certain complications such as infection, air embolism, or thrombophlebitis may be associated with a central I.V. line. Your patient's weakened condition and the TPN solution's high sugar content make him particularly susceptible to infection by such organisms as *Candida, Staphylococcus aureus* or *S. epidermidis*, and *Klebsiella*. However, you can reduce his chance of developing infection or any other complications by following these guidelines:
• Use an infusion pump to keep the infusion rate constant. Never infuse solution too rapidly or attempt to catch up if the infusion is behind schedule.
• Always follow strict aseptic technique when caring for your patient's central I.V. line.
• Check the dressing every 4 hours for cleanliness, good placement, extravasation, or bleeding. Change the dressing at least once every 24 to 48 hours (depending on hospital policy).
• Change the entire I.V. setup (except the catheter) every 24 to 48 hours, (depending on hospital policy). But, if the I.V. tubing disconnects from the catheter (indicated by a wet dressing), or if any part of the equipment is otherwise contaminated, change the I.V. setup immediately.
• To prevent air embolism, have your patient perform the Valsalva maneuver (if the doctor permits) each time you change the I.V. tubing at the catheter site. To do so, he'll lie flat on his back, take a breath, hold it, and bear down. This will help keep air from being sucked into his vein.
• Observe your patient for signs of air embolism, which include dyspnea; blood pressure drop; rise in central venous pressure (CVP); weak, rapid pulse; cyanosis; and loss of consciousness. If you suspect an air embolism, position your patient so he's lying on his left side in Trendelenburg position. This will send air into his heart's right side. From there, it can travel to the lungs, where it can be safely absorbed. Notify the doctor.
• If your patient has pain, soreness, redness, warmth, or swelling at the catheter site, or shows a sudden temperature rise, he may have either an infection or thrombophlebitis. If purulent drainage is also present, he probably has an infection. Notify the doctor of these symptoms.
• If your patient does develop an infection, remove the catheter (if your hospital policy permits you to). Use strict aseptic technique in doing so. After removal, cut off 1" to 2" (2.5 to 5 cm) of the catheter tip with sterile scissors. Then, put the catheter tip in a sterile test tube or container, and send it to the lab for analysis.
• Never use the central TPN line to do a CVP reading, to piggyback any solution, or to take a blood sample.
    Note: When using a peripheral I.V. line to administer nutrition solutions other than TPN (or supplementing TPN), be sure to observe aseptic technique. Use an infusion pump to administer the solution. Also, monitor your patient for signs of infection, thrombophlebitis, and extravasation. For more information, see the NURSING PHOTOBOOK MANAGING I.V. THERAPY.

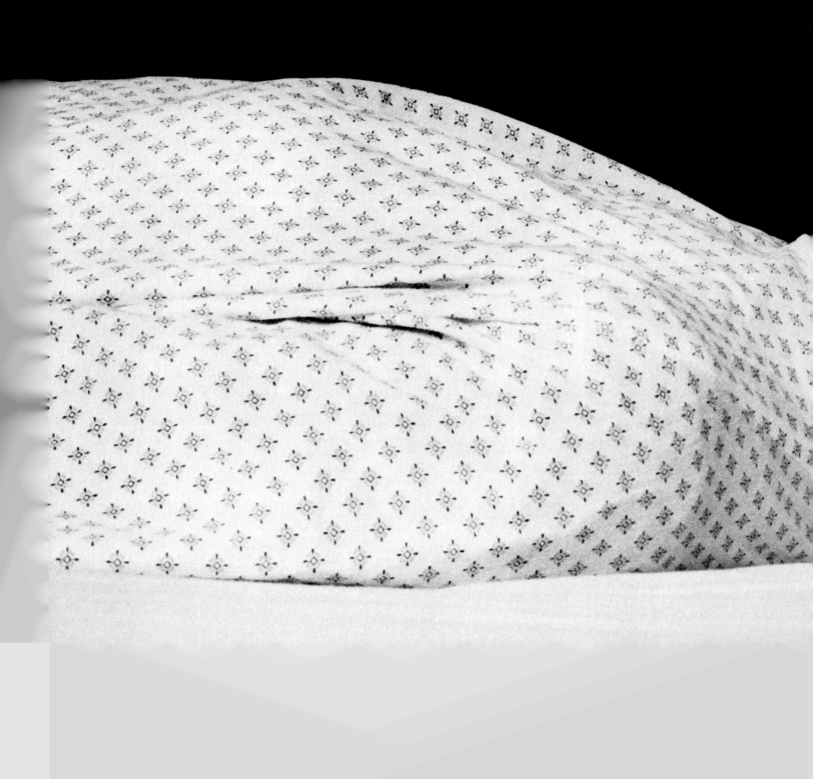

Caring for the Neurologic Patient

Neurologic basics
Special procedures

Neurologic basics

Caring for a patient with a neurologic condition? He'll need special nursing care. To help you provide it, we'll begin with a review of neurologic anatomy and physiology. Then, we'll show you how to conduct a thorough neuro-check, and how to interpret your findings. We'll also tell you what precautions to take if your patient experiences seizures, and how to care for a patient with increased intracranial pressure (ICP).

Understanding the nervous system

The nervous system is the body's telephone system: It receives and regulates internal and external messages and coordinates the body's responses. As you probably know, the nervous system can be separated into these divisions: the central nervous system (CNS), which includes the brain, cranial nerves, and spinal cord; and the peripheral nervous system (PNS), which includes the spinal nerves. The PNS provides a communications network between the CNS and the rest of the body.

Clearly, the CNS and PNS work in concert. But to help you understand how, we'll discuss them separately. Then, we'll consider how the autonomic nervous system (ANS) works. Let's start with the CNS.

The central nervous system (CNS)

The CNS is the body's control center, regulating all body activities. It receives and organizes messages from sensors (eyes, ears, nose, mouth, and skin), and transmits impulses to the muscles' motor nerves.

Take a look at the illustration on the left side of the following page. As you see, we can divide the brain into the regions of the cerebrum, cerebellum, and brain stem (containing the midbrain, pons, and medulla). The cerebrum is the largest part of the brain, and is divided into the right and left hemispheres. The cerebellum lies beneath the cerebrum, in the back of the skull. The pons and medulla—the main sections of the brain stem—lie beneath the cerebrum. The pons is a thick bundle of fibers that bridges the hemispheres and the gap between the medulla and the cerebrum.

The brain is enveloped by three membranes (meninges) that help protect it from shock and infection: the pia mater, the arachnoid, and the dura mater. The narrow subarachnoid space between the arachnoid and the pia mater contains cerebrospinal fluid (CSF). Portions of the dura mater—the falx cerebri and the tentorium—extend into the brain's fissures. The falx cerebri lies in the longitudinal fissure that separates the right and left hemispheres; the tentorium lies in the transverse fissure that separates the cerebrum and cerebellum.

Now, examine the illustration on the right side of the following page. You'll see that the brain's four ventricles contain clusters of capillaries (choroid plexus). These capillaries, as well as the ependymal layer of the spinal cord, produce approximately 21 ml of CSF each hour. From the ventricles, CSF circulates around the brain and spinal cord (see arrows), cushioning them from injury and transporting nutrients and wastes. Eventually, the CSF is absorbed in the brain's venous sinuses through the arachnoid villi (vascular protrusions of the arachnoid). For a healthy adult, the circulating volume of CSF is 100 to 150 ml.

The skull's structure aids in circulation. Numerous tiny openings (foramina) permit nerves and blood vessels to reach the brain and enable the circulation of CSF around the brain and spinal cord.

The spinal column is the second component of the CNS. Encased in the vertebral column, it extends from the coccyx to the base of the skull, where it joins the brain. As with the brain, the meninges and the CSF help protect the spinal cord from injury and infection.

Functionally, the spinal cord is divided into 31 segments.

Each segment gives rise to a pair of nerve roots, one containing motor (efferent) fibers; the other containing sensory (afferent) fibers. The spinal cord conducts afferent impulses in ascending (sensory) tracts to the brain, and efferent impulses in descending (motor) tracts from the brain to organs and muscles. It also acts as a center for reflex action.

The 12 pairs of cranial nerves originate in the brain and innervate internal organs, muscles, and glands. For details on the cranial nerves, refer to page 130.

The peripheral nervous system (PNS)

The paired spinal nerves that connect the CNS with every other receptor and effector in the body constitute the PNS. The spinal nerves are comprised of the 31 pairs of nerve roots that emerge from the spinal cord and innervate the sensory areas (receptors) and motor areas (effectors) of the body.

Another view of the nervous system

The nervous system controls both somatic (voluntary) and autonomic (involuntary) function. For this reason, the nervous system may also be divided in this way: the somatic nervous system, and the autonomic nervous system (ANS). These divisions are based on function, rather than on the location of the nerve pathways.

The somatic nervous system includes skeletal muscle and the CNS itself. The ANS, on the other hand, consists of certain peripheral nerves that innervate the heart, lungs, and other viscera.

Functionally, the ANS is split into *sympathetic* and *parasympathetic* divisions. The sympathetic division accommodates emergency reactions; the parasympathetic division ac-commodates functions of growth, digestion, and reproduction.

Certain characerictics of the ANS distinguish it from the rest of the nervous system. For one thing, we have little control over the actions of these nerves: we cannot willfully control peristalsis, for instance. For another thing, each internal organ receives one set of fibers from the sympathetic nerves and one set from the parasympathetic nerves. Accordingly, impulses from these nerves have an antagonistic action. For example, a sympathetic impulse speeds up the heartbeat; a parasympathetic impulse slows it. This antagonism provides an equilibrium (homeostasis), except when the body requires the dominance of one action over another.

Lateral view of human brain

Cerebrum ——————

Tentorial notch (area) ——————

Pons ——————
Cerebellum ——————
Medulla oblongata ——————

Foramen magnum (area) ——————
Spinal cord ——————

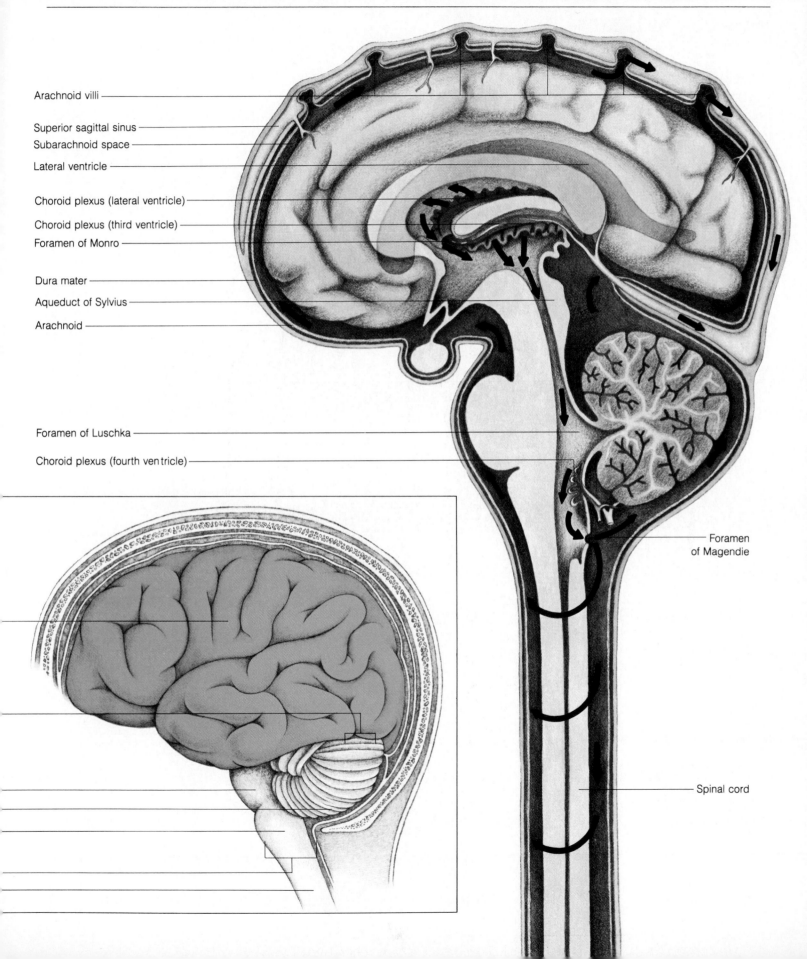

Arachnoid villi

Superior sagittal sinus

Subarachnoid space

Lateral ventricle

Choroid plexus (lateral ventricle)

Choroid plexus (third ventricle)

Foramen of Monro

Dura mater

Aqueduct of Sylvius

Arachnoid

Foramen of Luschka

Choroid plexus (fourth ventricle)

Foramen of Magendie

Spinal cord

Neurologic basics

Learning about the cranial nerves

Nerve	Type	Functions	Evidence of abnormality
I Olfactory	Sensory	• Smell	• Anosmia (inability to detect a specific odor)
II Optic	Sensory	• Sight	• Gross defect in visual field; for example, loss of half the visual field
III Oculomotor	Motor	• Eye movement (up, down, and medial) • Regulation of pupil size • Accommodation • Elevation of upper eyelid	• Lack of consensual pupillary response; improper movement of the eye and eyelid, including ptosis (drooping) of eyelid
IV Trochlear	Motor	• Eye movement (down and lateral)	• Nystagmus (rapid, involuntary eye movements); wandering eye; unparallel gaze
V Trigeminal	Motor	• Chewing movement	• Inability to clench teeth
	Sensory	• Sensations of face, teeth, scalp	• Inability to distinguish sensations on cheeks; absence of blinking and tearing
VI Abducens	Motor	• Lateral eye movement	• Diplopia on lateral gaze
VII Facial	Motor	• Facial expressions	• Asymmetric facial movements: for example, tics or drooping smile; inability to hold eyes shut against resistance or to frown
	Sensory	• Taste; salivary and lacrimal gland secretion	• Inability to taste salty, sour, sweet; increased salivation
VIII Acoustic	Sensory	• Hearing; equilibrium	• Loss of hearing, balance
IX Glossopharyngeal	Motor	• Secretion of saliva; swallowing; gag reflex; reflex control of blood pressure and respirations	• Increased mucus in mouth; impaired gag reflex; nasal speech
	Sensory	• Taste; sensations of tongue	• Inability to determine bitter taste
X Vagus	Motor and sensory	• Swallowing; voice production; slowed heartbeat; accelerated peristalsis; sensations of the larynx and pharynx.	• Difficulty swallowing; loss of voice; hunger sensation; orthostatic hypotension
XI Spinal accessory	Motor	• Shoulder movements; neck rotation; movements of head and viscera; voice production	• Trapezius or sternocleidomastoid muscle weakness
XII Hypoglossal	Motor	• Tongue movement	• Wrinkling of tongue surface; twitching of tongue; dysarthria; dysphagia • Inability of patient to protrude tongue and maintain it in a midline position

What's a neurocheck?

If you've ever cared for a neurologic patient, you're familiar with the assessment procedure called neurocheck (or neurowatch). This procedure's performed periodically to permit an ongoing evaluation of your patient's condition.

Because it's designed to provide fast, frequent assessment information, a neurocheck isn't as thorough as a complete neurologic assessment. But by comparing the results of each neurocheck with preceding ones, you can readily identify subtle changes in your patient's condition. And for a neurologic patient, even subtle changes are significant.

How often do you perform neurochecks? That depends on your patient's condition. Most likely, you'll do them at least every 2 hours. But if your patient's condition is unstable, you may do them as often as every 15 minutes.

In the following photostory, you'll see how to perform a neurocheck. (Keep in mind that your hospital's neurocheck procedure may differ in some ways.) Throughout the procedure, remember to check for bilateral responses, whenever appropriate. Unilateral responses may indicate hemiplegia or some other motor impairment.

Complete each neurocheck with accurate, specific, and complete documentation. Notify the doctor of any changes in your patient's condition. (To learn how to do a complete neurologic assessment, see the NURSING PHOTOBOOK COPING WITH NEUROLOGIC DISORDERS.)

Performing a neurocheck

1 *Julia Martin, a 26-year-old teacher, is recovering from severe head injuries from a car accident. The doctor has ordered a thorough neurocheck every hour. Here's what you'll do:*

If your patient isn't awake, try to awaken her by shaking her gently and calling her name.

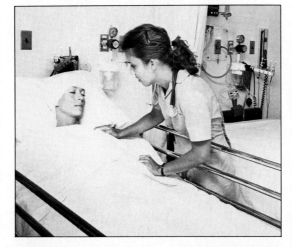

2 What if she doesn't awaken? Try a pain stimulus. Pinch her sternocleidomastoid muscle, as the nurse is doing here. If she responds, observe her pupils for the normal ciliospinal reflex (pupils should dilate).

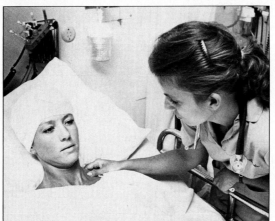

3 Explain the neurocheck procedure to her. If she opens her eyes voluntarily, check her gaze. If both eyes work in unison, consider her gaze conjugate.

Next, look closely at her pupils. Are they equal in size and shape? Are they round? Document their size, using a standard pupil gauge chart like the one shown in the inset.

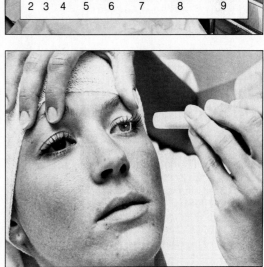

Pupil Gauge (mm)
2 3 4 5 6 7 8 9

4 Now, check to see if her pupils' reaction to light is consensual. To do this, darken the room slightly, if possible. Instruct her not to focus on the light, or her pupils may adjust to the moving light source. Instead, suggest that she focus on an object on the wall. Then, shine your penlight into first one eye, then the other.

Each pupil should constrict in response to light. Her pupil constriction should be consensual: when one pupil constricts in response to light, the other should constrict too.

Be alert for any unexpected reactions. For example, if your patient's oculomotor nerve is compromised, the pupils may dilate, instead of constrict, in response to light. Or, you may see a rhythmic dilation and constriction.

Document the speed of pupillary response: normal, sluggish, or nonreactive. However, keep in mind that nonneurologic factors, such as medication, can affect pupillary response.

Neurologic basics

Performing a neurocheck continued

5 Now, check your patient's extraocular movements (EOMs). Hold your fingers in front of her face, and ask her to keep her eyes on them. Slowly, move your fingers up and down and from side to side, as shown here, and note whether your patient's eyes follow them. Her gaze should be conjugate. This test determines ocular nerve and muscle coordination. (You can also check EOMs by testing for the doll's eye reflex. For details, see page 135.)

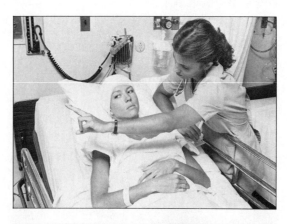

6 Next, check your patient's peripheral visual field. With one hand, hold your penlight directly in front of her eyes, as shown here. Ask your patient to focus on it. Starting at a point beyond her peripheral vision, slowly bring your other hand forward until she can see it.

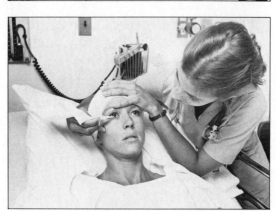

7 Then, check your patient's blink reflex or corneal response. If your patient's awake and alert, you can test her blink reflex by gently rubbing your finger across her eyelashes, or by moving your hand toward her eye. If your patient's drowsy, or you suspect injury to the brain stem or to the fifth or seventh cranial nerves, gently touch a corner of a tissue to the outer aspect of each iris. Her eye should blink and tear.

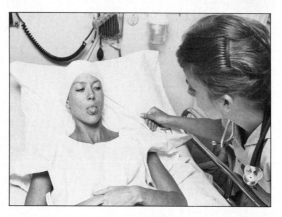

8 To check for hypoglossal nerve response, ask the patient to stick out her tongue. Normally, her tongue will be in a midline position. If it falls to one side, there may be neurologic damage, such as a posterior cranial fossa tumor. Atrophied tongue muscles could also cause the tongue to be pulled toward the stronger, unaffected side.

9 You can check for damage to the facial nerves by asking your patient to show her teeth, smile, or puff out her cheeks. Look for symmetry of her facial movements. If you see drooping of one side of her face or mouth (hemiparesis); asymmetric creases from nose to mouth when she smiles; or other abnormal movements, such as tics; suspect a lesion of the seventh cranial nerve.

10 Does your patient have facial paralysis? A further check can identify central facial palsy, which may affect eye muscles as well as face muscles. Have the patient close her eyes; then, hold her eyebrows up, as shown here. She should be able to keep her eyelids closed while you attempt to open them.

11 Test the trigeminal nerve's sensory function by lightly touching a tissue or cotton wisp to the patient's cheeks. She should be able to identify the sensation and location. Remember to check sensation bilaterally.
Note: Patients who have had a rhizotomy for tic douloureux may not feel this sensation.

12 Test for pain sensation with a pinprick to the forehead, cheeks, and jaw, as shown here. Then, repeat the test using the dull end of the pin. The patient should be able to distinguish between sharp and dull sensations.

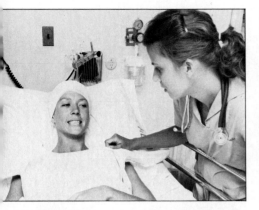

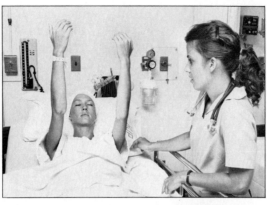

13 Ask the patient to hold her hands above her head with the palms facing the back of the bed, and her eyes shut, as shown. Can she maintain this position and keep her arms steady? If one arm drifts to the side, that side may be weakened or partially paralyzed.

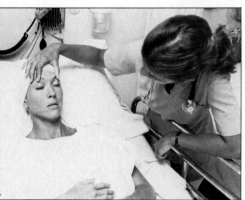

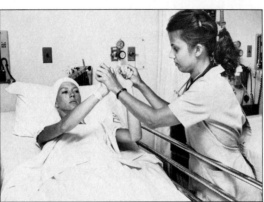

14 Check arm resistance by pushing against the patient's hands, as shown here. Note whether the resistance is equal in each arm (bilateral).

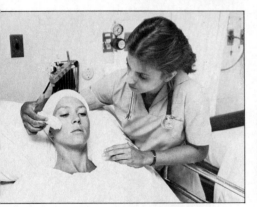

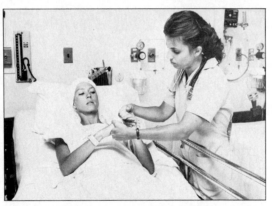

15 Test the patient's grip by asking her to squeeze your hands. Unequal pressure could indicate motor nerve damage to the affected side.

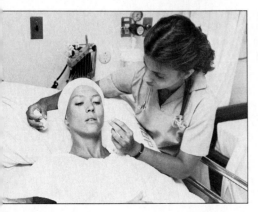

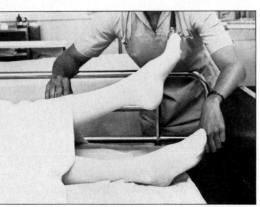

16 Now, ask the patient to hold up her legs, one at a time. She should be able to briefly hold each leg in a raised position. If she can't, suspect motor nerve damage.

Neurologic basics

Performing a neurocheck continued

17 If your patient can lift her legs, test their strength by pressing down on each leg as she attempts to lift it. Note whether the response to your resistance is bilateral.

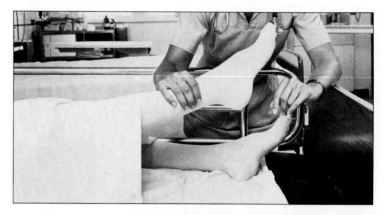

18 Next, check plantarflexion and dorsiflexion by pushing against the bottoms of your patient's feet, as shown here. Note the strength of resistance in both feet and legs.

To check your patient's Babinski response, remove her antiembolism stocking and hold her ankle with one hand. With the other hand, scratch or stroke the sole of her foot near its lateral edge, from her heel upward toward her toes. Use a painless stimulus and stroke with moderate force. The toes should curl. If the toes fan and the big toe dorsiflexes toward the patient's head (positive Babinski), suspect an upper motor neuron lesion.

Repeat the test on her other foot.

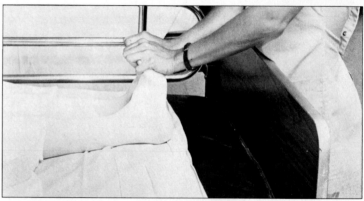

19 To check for ankle clonus, flex the patient's knee and hold her foot. Dorsiflex her foot quickly, toward her head. Rhythmic contractions of the calf muscle and foot indicate damage to upper motor neurons.

Note: Knee and wrist clonus can be tested similarly.

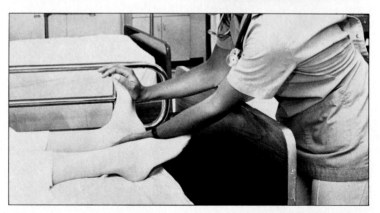

20 Observe the patient's level of consciousness. Is she awake and alert? Is she drowsy or confused? Stuporous? Comatose? Is she aware of her surroundings? Does she know where and who she is? Is she oriented with respect to time? When you record your findings, remember to *describe* your patient's behavior—don't merely label it.

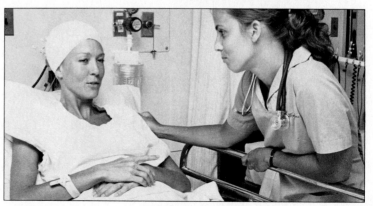

Recognizing brain stem involvement

If her brain stem's damaged, your patient may not exhibit the doll's eye reflex; or she may display decorticate or decerebrate posturing. Here's what to look for:
• *Doll's eye reflex:* Hold your patient's eyelids open. If her eyes appear fixed straight ahead, quickly—but gently— turn her head to one side. If the doll's eye reflex is absent, her eyes will remain fixed in the center of her eye sockets. Normally, the eyes appear to move conjugately in the opposite direction.
• *Decorticate posturing:* Touch your patient, or give her a pain stimulus, such as a pinch. If she exhibits decorticate posturing, her arms will draw up in full flexion on her chest, as shown below, and her legs will extend stiffly.
• *Decerebrate posturing:* Touch your patient or give her a pain stimulus. If she responds with decerebrate posturing, her arms and legs will extend stiffly, and her palms will turn outward, as shown at bottom. Consider decerebrate posturing a sign that's even more ominous than decorticate posturing.

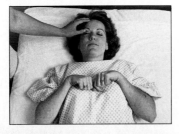

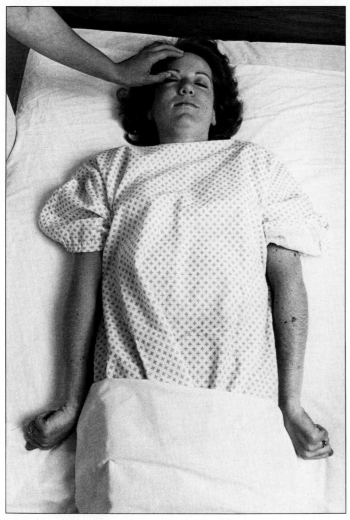

Taking seizure precautions

Is your patient likely to suffer a seizure? To find out, review his patient history, along with the results of skull X-rays, computerized axial tomography (CAT) scans, and contrast studies performed to locate possible brain lesions. Evidence of lesions or brain trauma suggests that your patient's seizure-prone.

In addition, stay alert for possible seizures if your patient has any of these problems:
• history of seizure disorders; for example, epilepsy
• toxic conditions; for example, alcohol or drug withdrawal, or heavy metal poisoning
• neurocirculatory disorders; for example, subarachnoid hemorrhage or cerebrovascular accident (CVA)
• metabolic disorders; for example, uremia, hypocalcemia, or eclampsia
• infections; for example, meningitis, brain abscess, or encephalitis
• hyperpyrexia.

If you've determined that your patient's at risk of seizure, protect him with padded bedrails—raised, of course, at all times. If the patient wears dentures, remove them. During a seizure, they may become dislodged, obstructing breathing.

Helping your patient during a seizure

If your patient has a seizure, do your best to keep him from injuring himself. Here's how:
• If the patient's in bed, keep the padded side rails up. If he's out of bed, help him to the floor to prevent injury.
• If possible, remove his glasses, if he's wearing them. Loosen tight clothing.
• Place a soft cloth between his teeth to prevent him from biting his tongue, if possible. However, never force his jaws open.
• Turn the patient's head to one side to allow saliva drainage. Suction drainage, if possible.
• Place a small pillow beneath his head, but take care not to flex his neck and obstruct his airway.
• Don't restrain him. Doing so won't stop the seizure and it can make it more severe. Instead, hold his hands gently to keep them from hitting the bed or floor.
• Stay with the patient until the seizure has passed.
• As the seizure subsides, reassure and reorient him. Don't offer him food or drink until he's fully alert. Administer oxygen if ordered by the doctor.

After the patient's regained consciousness, ask him if he experienced an aura immediately before the seizure. An aura may include a pungent smell, nausea or indigestion, a rising or sinking feeling in the stomach, a dreamy feeling, an unusual taste, or visual disturbances.

Document the patient's recollections, as well as your observations, in your nurses' notes. Describe the patient's behavior during the seizure, including whether he was incontinent or cyanotic. Did his eyes deviate to one side? Did signs of the seizure start in one extremity, or on one side of the body? A careful description can help the doctor determine the seizure's cause. In addition, note how long the seizure lasted, and how quickly the patient regained complete consciousness. Notify the doctor of the patient's seizure.

Note: Another seizure before the patient fully regains consciousness could indicate status epilepticus. Maintain a patent airway, and ask someone to notify the doctor at once. Anticipate immediate administration of diazepam (Valium*) I.V. Suction patient, if possible.

*Available in both the United States and in Canada

Neurologic basics

Caring for the patient with elevated intracranial pressure (ICP)

Does your patient have increased intracranial pressure (ICP)? Use special consideration when planning his nursing care. Many nursing procedures—even routine ones, like repositioning—tend to raise a patient's ICP. A cluster of nursing procedures done all at once may dangerously spike his ICP. That's why you should do your best to schedule stressful procedures at different times. This chart will show you how to minimize or avoid other stresses that endanger your patient.

Note: The doctor may decide to monitor your patient's ICP with an invasive intracranial monitoring system. For details on the ventricular catheter, subarachnoid screw, and epidural sensor, see the NURSING PHOTOBOOK USING MONITORS.

Nursing order	Rationale	Additional considerations
Maintain oxygenation; avoid hypoxia and/or hypercapnia	• A CO_2 excess and/or O_2 deficit in arterial blood stimulates cerebral vasodilation, increasing cerebral blood flow (CBF). • Increasing CBF raises ICP.	• Maintain a patent airway. • Monitor arterial blood gas (ABG) measurements closely. • Hyperventilate the patient before suctioning, to minimize CO_2 accumulation during the procedure. • Limit suctioning to 10 to 15 seconds.
Maintain venous outflow from the brain	• Obstructions to venous outflow increase capillary pressure and diminish absorption of cerebrospinal fluid (CSF). • Decreased outflow permits CO_2 and lactic acid to accumulate in the brain. Both stimulate cerebral vasodilation. • ICP rises when venous outflow slows. • As a response to rising ICP, blood pressure may drop, causing cerebral ischemia.	• Do not place patient flat or in Trendelenburg position, unless the doctor orders. Instead, elevate the patient's head 30°, or as the doctor orders. • Position the patient's head and neck directly above his midline to avoid compressing a jugular vein. • If the patient has an endotracheal tube in place, make sure the tape securing it doesn't compress the jugular veins.
Avoid increasing intrathoracic or intra-abdominal pressure	• Added thoracic or abdominal pressure can spike ICP by increasing pressure on central veins.	• Do not place patient in Trendelenburg position, even for insertion of jugular or subclavian vein catheter, unless the doctor orders. • Do not ask the patient to execute a Valsalva maneuver, even during insertion of jugular or subclavian vein catheter. Instead, expect the doctor to minimize the danger of air embolism by using a syringe to apply suction to the catheter. • Do your best to prevent the patient from using the Valsalva maneuver during bowel movements. Keep his stools soft with an appropriate diet and/or stool softeners. However, do not administer an enema. • Prevent isometric muscular contractions. Assist your patient when he sits up, and instruct him not to push against the bed's footboard. But if the doctor orders, you may perform passive range-of-motion (ROM) exercises for the patient. • Ask the patient to exhale when you turn him. • Avoid hip flexion. When catheterizing a female patient, for example, flex her legs as little as possible.
Prevent wide or sudden variations in systemic blood pressure	• Normally, autoregulation maintains cerebral perfusion pressure (CPP) at a level equal to mean systemic arterial pressure (MSAP) minus ICP. But autoregulation may fail when ICP is high. If so, CPP fluctuates with systemic blood pressure. Thus, an increase in systemic arterial pressure (SAP) increases cerebral blood flow (CBF), elevates ICP, and worsens cerebral edema. • Conversely, decreases in SAP may produce cerebral ischemia, allowing CO_2 and lactic acid to accumulate.	• Use blood pressure and ICP monitors to evaluate the effect of stressful nursing procedures; for example, endotracheal tube insertion, suctioning, chest physiotherapy, and repositioning. Document your findings carefully. • Minimize pain with a sedative or topical anesthetic, as ordered by the doctor. • If ordered, use muscle relaxants to calm a combative patient during procedures like endotracheal tube insertion. However, avoid using restraints, unless ordered by the doctor. • Rapid-eye-movement (REM) stages of sleep may cause a rise in ICP. Never perform stress-producing procedures during REM sleep.
Prevent systemic infection (sepsis)	• Systemic infection may produce increased cardiac output and vasodilation, increasing CBF.	• Notify doctor promptly if the patient's temperature increases. • If the patient's undergoing ICP monitoring, change the tubing and the dressing on the insertion site daily. • Maintain scrupulous aseptic technique when changing any equipment or dressing. • If the patient has a ventricular catheter in place, obtain a CSF sample daily, and send it to the lab for culturing. *Note:* Before obtaining a CSF sample from the drainage bag, remove the bag and tubing and replace them with sterile ones. Never open the CSF drainage bag while it's attached to the patient, or you risk infecting him.

Special procedures

Your neurologic patient may experience difficulty maintaining correct body temperature. For example, if a lesion presses on his hypothalamus (the temperature control center in the diencephalon), his body temperature may rise or drop sharply. To maintain his body temperature within the normal range, you may use a special temperature control (hyper- or hypothermia) blanket system.

Or, if your patient's experiencing a rise in intracranial pressure (ICP), you may use this blanket system to induce hypothermia. By doing so, you reduce the brain's oxygen needs, and decrease cerebral edema.

The lumbar puncture (spinal tap) is another special procedure your neurologic patient may undergo. The doctor may perform this procedure to obtain cerebrospinal fluid samples, or—under unusual circumstances—to relieve increased ICP. In the following pages, you'll learn your role during a lumbar puncture.

Using the Blanketrol® Hyper-Hypothermia System

1 *To maintain your patient's body temperature in the normal range, you may use a temperature-control system like the Blanketrol Hyper-Hypothermia System made by Cincinnati Sub-Zero Products, Inc. In this photostory, you'll learn how to set up this equipment.*

To begin, gather the equipment shown in these photos. Make sure the blanket is pre-filled with water. Then, check the blanket for signs of leakage. If you see any damp spots, replace the blanket before proceeding. In addition to the equipment shown here, you'll need nonallergenic tape, scissors, Skin-Prep, and a disposable blanket cover supplied by the manufacturer.

Note: If your patient requires a rapid temperature adjustment, you may need an additional blanket, which you'll place on top of the patient. (For details, check the manufacturer's instructions.)

Lift the water reservoir cover and check the water level. The reservoir should be filled with distilled water ½" to 1" above the copper tubing visible at the reservoir opening. If necessary, add more distilled water. (The reservoir holds about 2½ gallons of water.)

Note: To prevent bacterial growth, an antibacterial agent may be added to the water. Check the manufacturer's instructions for recommendations.

Now, make sure the master control toggle switch is in OFF position; then, plug the Servo controller panel into the Blanketrol machine. Insert the machine's three-prong plug into a properly-grounded outlet.

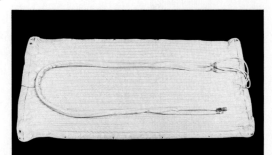

Hyper-hypothermia blanket

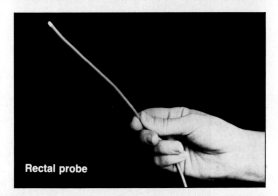

Rectal probe

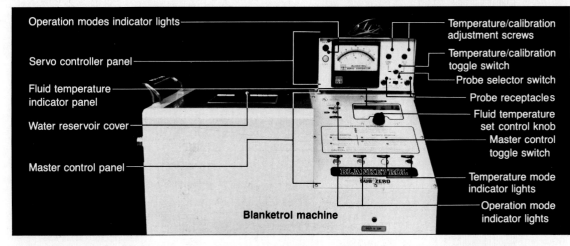

Operation modes indicator lights

Servo controller panel

Fluid temperature indicator panel

Water reservoir cover

Master control panel

Temperature/calibration adjustment screws

Temperature/calibration toggle switch

Probe selector switch

Probe receptacles

Fluid temperature set control knob

Master control toggle switch

Temperature mode indicator lights

Operation mode indicator lights

Blanketrol machine

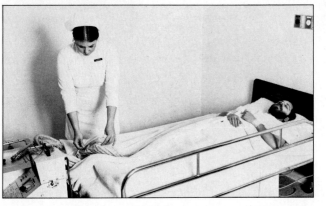

2 Explain the equipment to the patient, and answer his questions. Record his vital signs, and perform a thorough neurocheck. This provides a baseline for assessing the patient's response to therapy.

Then, cover the blanket with the disposable blanket cover, as the nurse is doing here.

Special procedures

Using the Blanketrol® Hyper-Hypothermia System continued

3 Turn the patient on his side, and position the blanket under him.

Nursing tip: If your patient's skin is in poor condition, consider protecting him from possible burns by placing a bath blanket between him and the Blanketrol blanket.

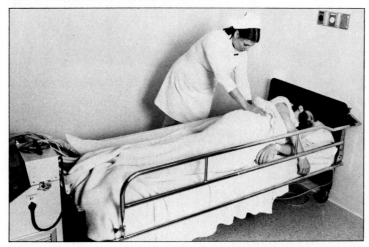

5 Turn the patient on his side and insert the rectal probe. Advance it about 6″ into his rectum. Apply Skin-Prep and tape the probe to his leg or buttocks. *Note:* You may use a skin or esophageal probe instead of a rectal probe, depending on the patient's condition.

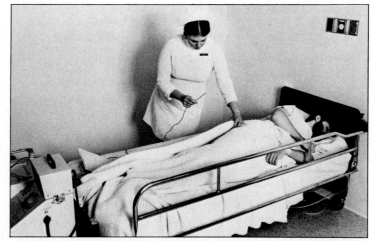

4 Now you're ready to connect the blanket cables to the side of the Blanketrol machine. To do so, grasp the female adapter on the blanket cable and slide the collar backward. Then, push the female coupling over one of the male couplings on the lower left side of the Blanketrol machine. Let the collar snap into place; then, gently pull the cable to assure a secure connection. As this photo shows, the nurse has already secured the female adapter to the male coupling.

Next, slide the collar back on one of the machine's female couplings, as the nurse is doing here, and insert the cable's male adapter into it. Push in the cable's male adapter until you hear a click.

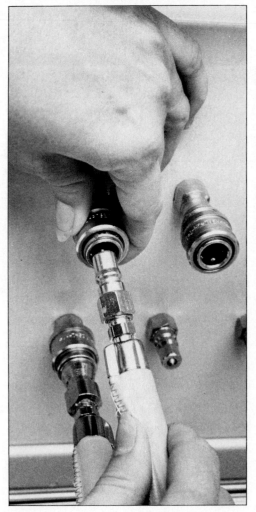

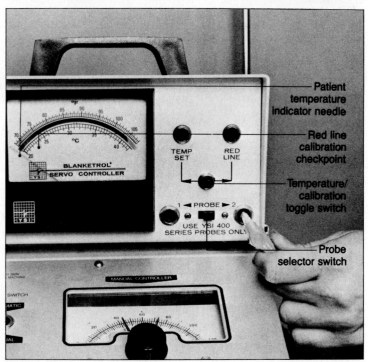

6 Insert the probe's plug into one of the probe receptacles, as shown here. Choose whichever is more convenient. Then, push the probe selector switch toward the probe receptacle that you're using.

To calibrate the Blanketrol unit, push the temperature/calibration toggle switch toward the right, and watch the patient temperature indicator needle. The needle should come to rest directly over the red line calibration checkpoint. If it doesn't, continue to hold the toggle switch and use your scissors to turn the screw labeled RED LINE, until the needle rests over the red line. Then, release the toggle switch. (You may also use a dime to turn the screw.)

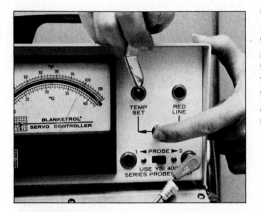

7 When the machine's calibrated, you're ready to set the temperature ordered for your patient. To do so, press the temperature/calibration toggle switch to the left, toward TEMP SET. If the needle reading isn't the same as the doctor ordered, adjust it by turning the TEMP SET screw until it is. Release the toggle switch.

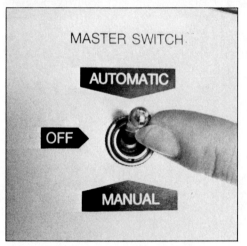

8 Now, push the master control switch to the AUTOMATIC position. The automatic cycle indicator will light, and water will begin to circulate through the system. The automatic setting maintains the patient's temperature at the preset level. (Use the MANUAL setting to treat two patients at once. See the manufacturer's instructions for details.)

Check the patient's vital signs every half hour, until they're stable. At least once an hour, check the patient for signs of edema, inflammation, skin color changes, and other signs of burns or frostbite. Monitor the patient's heart rate and conduct neurochecks throughout treatment.

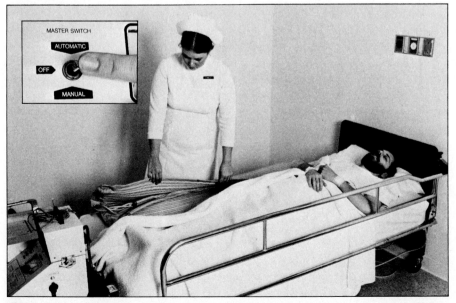

9 To discontinue blanket use, first turn off the master control toggle switch (see inset photo) and remove the rectal probe. Disconnect the machine's plug from the wall outlet. Then, take the blanket out from under the patient, and remove the disposable blanket cover. Disconnect the blanket cables from the side of the machine, and fold the cables inside the blanket, as the nurse is doing here.

Assisting with a lumbar puncture

The doctor may perform a lumbar puncture (spinal tap) for these reasons: to obtain cerebrospinal fluid (CSF) samples; to measure CSF pressure; to introduce a contrast medium or air into the subarachnoid space for a myelogram or pneumoencephalogram; or to remove CSF to reduce intracranial pressure caused by a subcutaneous subarachnoid hemorrhage.

Suppose the doctor wants to measure CSF pressure and obtain CSF samples. What's your role? Follow these guidelines:
• Gather the equipment he'll need: sterile disposable lumbar puncture tray (which includes a manometer), two pairs of sterile gloves, grease or wax pencil, paper cup, and a face mask for the doctor.
• Explain the procedure to the patient and answer his questions. Assure him that the doctor will anesthetize the puncture site, but inform him that he will feel some pressure. Tell him to remain still throughout the procedure. Finally, ask him to empty his bowel and bladder.
• Unless the doctor prefers an alternate position, place the patient on his side, with his spine curved and his back at the bed's edge. Ask him to draw his knees up to his chin. (If the patient can't maintain a knee/chest position, ask another nurse to support him by placing one hand behind his neck and the other hand behind his knees.)
• As the doctor performs the procedure, reassure the patient. Using the manometer, the doctor will measure CSF pressure; then, he'll fill the test tubes with CSF samples and cap them. Use the grease pencil to mark the test tubes (as directed), and place them in the paper cup.
• After the procedure, ask your patient to lie flat. Explain that he must remain in that position for 4 to 6 hours (as ordered), to reduce the chance of developing a spinal headache. Encourage him to drink plenty of liquids, to help his body replace lost CSF.
• Fill out the necessary lab slips, and send the CSF samples to the lab at once. *Important:* Never refrigerate CSF samples.
• Document the procedure, including CSF pressure readings and the amount of CSF withdrawn. Note the color and clarity of the CSF samples, including the presence of blood or purulence.
• Check the puncture site at least every 2 hours for edema or CSF leakage.
• Continue to conduct neurochecks, as ordered.

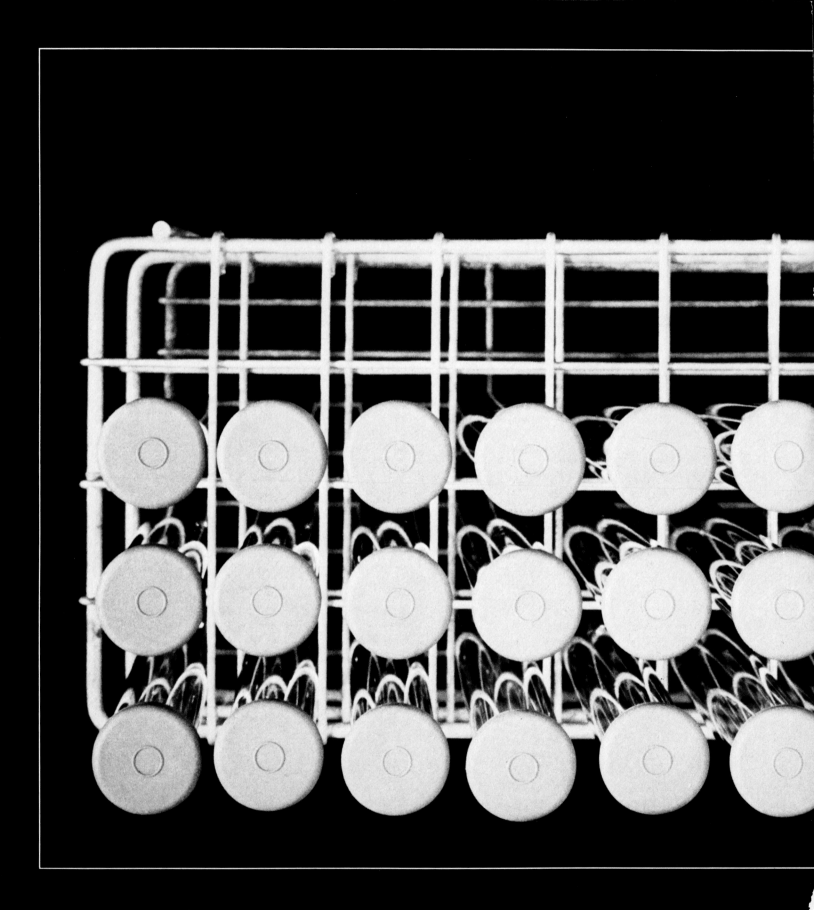

Managing Special ICU Challenges

Fluids and electrolytes
Common problems
Stress management

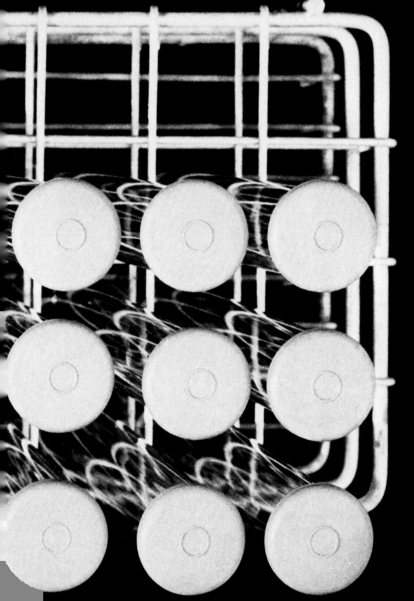

Fluids and electrolytes

As you know, critically ill patients need continuous monitoring for fluid and electrolyte imbalances. The signs and symptoms of these imbalances may be subtle, particularly in their early stages. So, each patient requires close observation for symptoms, and careful daily weighing. In addition, an accurate record of his daily intake and output must be kept.

Do you know which patients are likely to develop an imbalance, so you can be alert for their earliest signs and symptoms? If not, we'll spell this out for you on the following pages. We'll also explain how to determine your patient's fluid balance, by correlating his weight with his intake and output record. To help you in detecting and effectively treating specific imbalances, we've provided a detailed chart listing signs and symptoms and nursing considerations.

To treat your patient's fluid imbalance (and some electrolyte imbalances), you may use an infusion pump. So, on these next few pages, we'll also tell you how to use the Cutter infusion pump.

Learning about the Cutter Dependaflo™ Volumetric Infusion Pump

Status alarms (lights and sound):

OCCLUSION: Activates with pressure build up of about 14 pounds per square inch, which may be caused by kinking, clogging, a closed roller clamp, or infiltration at the venipuncture site. Pump stops automatically.

INFUSION COMPLETE: Activates when preset volume to be infused has been delivered. At this point, pump switches to 1 ml/hr (1 microdrip/min.) keep-vein-open (KVO) rate.

HIGH/LOW FLOW RATE: Activates when an electronic malfunction occurs. Pump stops automatically.

BATTERY LOW: Activates when battery requires recharging.

DOOR OPEN: Activates when pump door isn't completely latched. Pump stops automatically.

AIR IN LINE: Activates when sensor detects air bubbles larger than ⅜" (1 cm). Pump stops automatically.

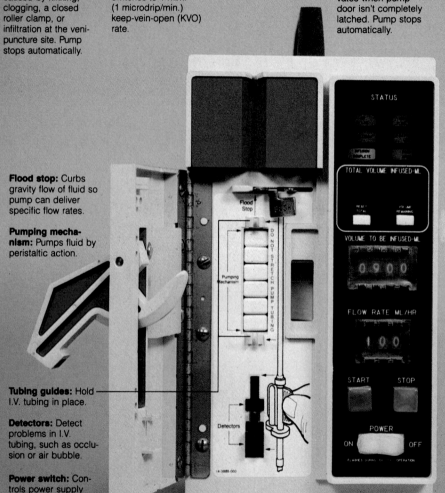

Flood stop: Curbs gravity flow of fluid so pump can deliver specific flow rates.

Pumping mechanism: Pumps fluid by peristaltic action.

Tubing guides: Hold I.V. tubing in place.

Detectors: Detect problems in I.V. tubing, such as occlusion or air bubble.

Power switch: Controls power supply to machine.

Total volume infused: At any time during infusion, provides readout of amount already infused, ranging from 1 to 9999 ml.

Volume remaining button: When pressed, displays amount remaining to be infused.

Reset button: Clears total volume infused display.

Volume to be infused: Indicates amounts ranging from 1 to 9999 ml. Set by pressing upper keys (to decrease numbers) or lower keys (to increase numbers).

Flow rate: Ranges from 1 to 499 ml/hr (1 to 499 microdrip/min.). Set by pressing upper keys (to decrease numbers) or lower keys (to increase numbers).

Start button: Starts pump operation.

Stop button: Stops pump operation.

When administering fluids to correct your critically ill patient's fluid imbalance, you may use an infusion pump. With an infusion pump, you can infuse solutions at a specific rate far more accurately than with the gravity-and-clamp system.

On the following pages, we'll show you how to use the Cutter infusion pump (shown above).

You'll need a special administration (pump) set, which includes volume-calibrated tubing designed to measure the volume to be delivered. The pump also uses a peristaltic pumping mechanism, which exerts pressure on the I.V. tubing, rather than directly on the fluid. (To learn about other types of pumps, see the NURSING PHOTOBOOK MANAGING I.V. THERAPY.)

Using the Cutter infusion pump

1 *Jeanne Stokes, a 35-year-old telephone operator with a history of acute renal failure, is admitted to your ICU. She's dehydrated from severe vomiting. She also has a urinary tract infection. The doctor orders 5% dextrose in water to replace her lost fluids. Because you want to carefully monitor her fluid intake, you'll use an infusion pump to administer the solution. Here's how to use a Cutter pump:*

Assemble a Cutter pump set (I.V. tubing set), an I.V. bag or bottle, an I.V. pole, and an infusion pump. Explain the procedure to your patient, and wash your hands.

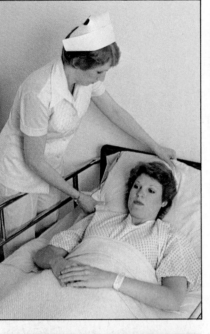

2 Next, attach the pump to an I.V. pole. Plug the power cord into an outlet. Open the pump chamber door.

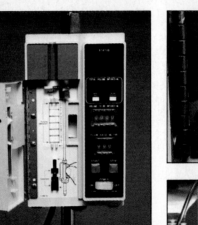

3 Then, spike the I.V. bottle with the Cutter I.V. tubing set. Make sure the tubing's roller clamp is closed. Hang the bottle on the I.V. pole.

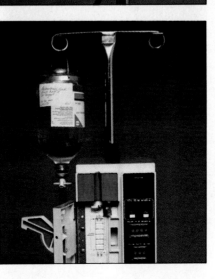

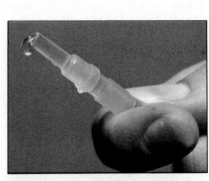

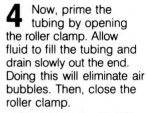

4 Now, prime the tubing by opening the roller clamp. Allow fluid to fill the tubing and drain slowly out the end. Doing this will eliminate air bubbles. Then, close the roller clamp.

Be sure to cap the I.V. tubing with a plastic tip.

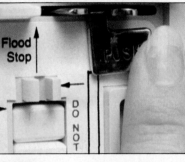

5 Now you're ready to insert the I.V. tubing set into the pump chamber. First, open the FLOOD STOP (the metal tab marked PUSH).

6 Then, locate the I.V. tubing set's occlusion chamber (a rigid, clear-plastic piece). Insert the occlusion chamber into the pump's detectors so that its ridged part faces outward.

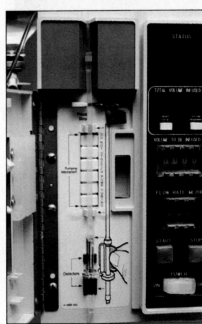

7 Without stretching the tubing, push it first into the guides above and below the pumping mechanism, and then through the open FLOOD STOP.

Fluids and electrolytes

Using the Cutter infusion pump continued

8 Close and latch the pump chamber door, as shown here. Open the roller clamp.

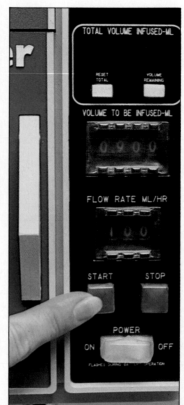

9 Next, set the volume to be infused by pressing the keys above or below the VOLUME TO BE INFUSED display. Be sure the volume you set does not exceed the amount in the I.V. bottle. If the bottle drains completely, air might enter the patient's vein.

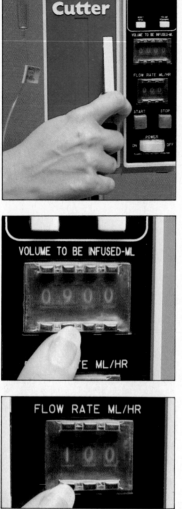

10 Set the FLOW RATE at the desired level by pressing the keys above and below the FLOW RATE display.
   Perform venipuncture. Then, remove the cap from the I.V. tubing and attach the tubing to the patient's I.V. catheter.

11 To check pump functions, turn the POWER switch on. Then, make sure the red STOP button lights, indicating that power's being supplied to the pump. Check to see that four 8's appear for a few seconds in the TOTAL VOLUME INFUSED display. Make sure that all alarm windows light up, and that the audio alarm sounds.

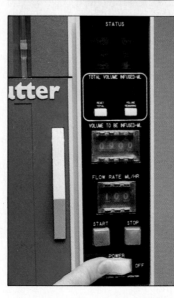

12 Finally, to begin infusion, press the green START button. When you do this, all alarm lights and sounds should cease. The TOTAL VOLUME IN-FUSED display will begin showing a counting.
   In your nurses' notes, document the solution infused, the flow rate, and the volume to be infused.
   Note: If you decide to change the flow rate during infusion, press the STOP button first. Make the change, and then press the START button.
   Suppose the AIR IN LINE alarm rings suddenly. Immediately press the STOP button. Then open the FLOOD STOP. When air reaches the tubing's Y connector, quickly close the roller clamp. Draw air out of the Y port with a syringe. Then, secure the tubing in the FLOOD STOP and close the FLOOD STOP. To resume infusion, press the START button.

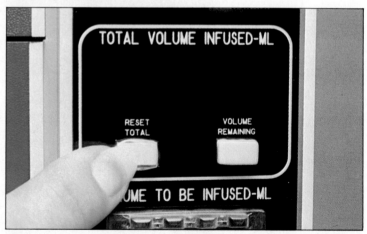

13 After the preset volume has been infused, the INFUSION COMPLETE alarm sounds. The pump automatically switches to the 1 ml/hr keep-vein-open (KVO) rate.
   When the INFUSION COMPLETE alarm sounds, replace the used I.V. bottle with a new one. To do so, first press the STOP button. Set the desired VOLUME TO BE INFUSED and FLOW RATE. Spike and hang the new bottle. Then, you may press the RESET button, to return the TOTAL VOLUME INFUSED display to zero. Or, you may choose not to reset the TOTAL VOLUME INFUSED. If so, the new volume infused will be included in a running total. Finally, press the START button.
   Document the I.V. bottle change in your nurses' notes. Record solution infused, flow rate, volume already infused, and volume to be infused.

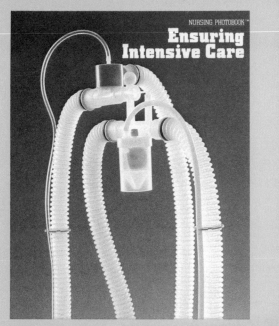

NURSING PHOTOBOOK™
Ensuring Intensive Care

Grow in confidence and expertise with this new NURSING PHOTOBOOK, *Ensuring Intensive Care*. Step-by-step photographs and clear, concise captions show you how to effectively manage:

- respiratory support systems
- cardiac and hemodynamic monitors
- nasogastric tube care
- intracranial pressure monitors
- seizures
- and much more.

You'll learn new nursing procedures...emergency techniques...and special intensive care skills to help you meet the challenge of intensive care nursing. Examine this important PHOTOBOOK for 10 days absolutely free. Send in the order card today!

10-DAY FREE TRIAL

USE THE CARD ABOVE TO:

1. Subscribe to the NURSING PHOTOBOOK™ series (and pay only $15.95 per book).

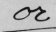

2. Buy *Ensuring Intensive Care* without joining the series (and pay only $17.95 for each copy).

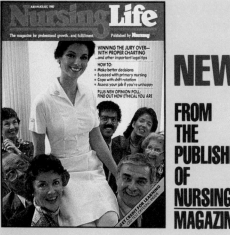

NEW!

FROM THE PUBLISHER OF NURSING84® MAGAZINE.

Mail the postage-paid card at right. ▶

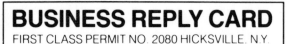
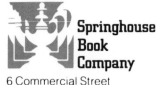
Introduce yourself to the NURSING PHOTOBOOK™ series

…the remarkable breakthrough in nursing education that can change your career. Each book in this unique series contains detailed *Photostories*…and tables, charts, and graphs to help you learn important new procedures. And each handsome PHOTOBOOK offers you • 160 illustrated, fact-filled pages • brilliant, high-contrast, photographs • convenient 9″ × 10½″ size • durable, hardcover binding • carefully chosen bibliography • complete index. Watch the experts at work showing you how to… administer drugs…teach your patient about his illness and its treatment…minimize trauma… understand doctors' diagnoses…increase patient comfort…and much more. Discover how you can become a better nurse by joining this exciting new series. You can examine each PHOTOBOOK at your liesure…for 10 days *absolutely free!*

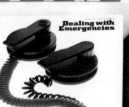

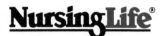
At last! A magazine that helps you with "the other side" of nursing. The things they didn't (and couldn't) teach you in nursing school.

NursingLife tells you how to be a better nurse…how to find greater fulfillment in your career…how to grow on the job.

It's all about the skills today's nurses need to round out their professional lives.

Become a subscriber to this exciting new magazine. Just tear off and mail this card today. There's no need to send money now. This is a no-obligation, free trial offer!

If order card is missing, send your order to:

Nursing Life®

P.O. Box 1961
One Health Care Circle
Marion, Ohio 43305

Monitoring your patient for fluid and electrolyte imbalance

Any patient who loses large amounts of body fluid from vomiting, wound drainage, or excessive diuresis will experience fluid and electrolyte imbalance. So will a patient who is receiving treatment such as hormonal therapy, electrolyte replacement, or vitamin administration.

In addition, be prepared for fluid and electrolyte imbalances in a patient who:
• has experienced severe trauma; for example, in an automobile accident.
• has severe burns.
• has a high fever.
• has liver, heart, or kidney malfunction.
• has just undergone major surgery.
• is severely malnourished.
• has a restricted diet, such as a low-sodium diet.

To find out specific symptoms and treatments for fluid and electrolyte imbalances, see the chart on the following pages.

In addition to being overhydrated or dehydrated, or having an excess or deficiency of a particular electrolyte, your patient could experience the *shift to the third space*. Many patients with severe burns, trauma, or infection, as well as postsurgical patients, experience this movement of fluids and protein from the blood vessels to the interstitial spaces. The shift may be local or widespread. Patients with this condition may exhibit pallor, tachycardia, low blood pressure, weak pulse, cold extremities, disorientation, and coma. Of course, they require treatment for their primary condition. They also need I.V. replacement of the shifted fluids and protein.

Once inflammation and trauma subside, the shift naturally reverses itself. But, until it does, these patients need careful monitoring for *hypo*volemia. When the fluids and protein begin to shift back into the blood vessels, reduce fluid and protein replacement, and carefully monitor the patient for *hyper*volemia.

How to determine your patient's fluid balance

To correctly determine your patient's fluid balance, you must maintain an accurate intake and output record. Study the sample below to learn how to make your record as complete as possible. Don't forget to include in your record any fluid added or removed by special procedures, such as peritoneal dialysis (if this information isn't recorded on a special dialysis record).

How do you use the information in the intake and output record to determine your patient's fluid balance? Every 24 hours, add all items on the record's intake portion. Then, add all items on the output portion. The intake sum has a positive value and the output sum has a negative value.

To find the 24-hour body fluid balance, combine the negative output sum and the positive intake sum. If intake is greater than output, the balance will be positive. If output is greater than intake, the balance will be negative.

Check the balance against the patient's daily weight, because his fluid loss or retention will be rapidly reflected in a weight change. A positive intake and output balance of 1 liter accounts for 2.2 pounds (1 kg) of weight gain. A negative balance of the same amount accounts for 2.2 pounds (1 kg) of weight loss.

Weighing your patient accurately

When obtaining your patient's daily weight, observe the following guidelines:
• Use the same scale each day.
• Weigh the patient at the same time each day (preferably before he eats breakfast).
• Make sure the patient's wearing the same (or similar) clothing each time you weigh him.
• Remove all items that would add to the patient's own weight. If you can't remove an item, weigh its equivalent separately. Then, subtract its weight from the patient's total weight.
• Correlate the patient's weight with a 24-hour tally of his intake and output record.

Coping with fluid and electrolyte imbalance

Use the chart on the following pages to help you determine whether your patient's experiencing fluid and electrolyte imbalance. If he is, observe these general guidelines:
• Weigh the patient daily.
• Maintain an accurate intake and output record.
• Observe the patient for signs and symptoms. Immediately report any changes to the doctor.
• Closely monitor all laboratory test results. Immediately report any changes to the doctor.
• To treat your patient's particular problem, apply the nursing considerations specified in the chart.

24-HOUR INTAKE AND OUTPUT RECORD (IN ML)			
ORAL INTAKE (Include tube feedings)	11 to 7	7 to 3	3 to 11
None (NG tube in place)	—	—	—
8-Hour **oral intake** totals	0	0	0
PARENTERAL FLUID INTAKE (Blood, plasma, TPN, fat emulsions, I.V. solutions. Document time started.)			
1000 ml D₅W with 0.45% NaCl at 11PM	600	400	
1000 ml D₅W at 10AM		800	200
1000 ml D₅W at 4PM			900
8-Hour **parenteral fluid intake** totals	600	1200	1100
ALL OTHER INTAKE (For example, irrigation fluid)			
NG tube irrigation	120	120	120
8-Hour **all other intake** totals	120	120	120
8-Hour total intake	720 + 1320 + 1220		
Total 24-Hour Intake	= 3260		
URINE OUTPUT (Urethral catheter - C; Ureteral - U. Describe urine, if significant.)			
C; Dark yellow, concentrated	600	1000	800
8-Hour **urine output** totals	600	1000	800
ALL OTHER OUTPUT (Emesis, gastric drainage, wound drainage, blood, bile, liquid stool)			
NG tube drainage	200	150	120
Diaphoresis (Moderate-M; Profuse-P)	P	M	M
8-Hour **all other output** totals	200	150	120
8-Hour total output	800 + 1150 + 920		
Total 24-Hour output	= 2870		

Fluids and electrolytes

Nurses' guide to fluid and electrolyte imbalances

Problem
Dehydration

Causes
• Decreased water intake from dysfunctional thirst mechanism
• Antidiuretic hormone (ADH) insufficiency
• Diuretic phase of renal disease
• Excessive use of diuretics
• Administration of osmotic agents (such as mannitol or dextrans) which may increase diuresis
• Hyperglycemia (in uncontrolled diabetes) leading to osmotic diuresis
• Fever with excessive diaphoresis
• Excessive gastrointestinal fluid losses from nasogastric drainage, diarrhea, or vomiting

Signs and symptoms
• Low-grade fever
• Flushed skin, dry mucous membranes, poor skin turgor
• Hypotension
• Rapid pulse
• Thirst
• Muscle weakness
• Alteration in urine output (usually oliguria)
• Elevated hematocrit and serum sodium level
• Weight loss
• Lethargy, disorientation, coma (in severe dehydration)

Nursing considerations
• For prevention, administer any hypertonic solutions cautiously, staying alert for signs of dehydration.
• Observe patient closely for insensible water loss from hyperventilation and excessive diaphoresis.
• Administer fluids, as ordered.

Problem
Overhydration

Causes
• Increased water ingestion, including psychogenic water ingestion
• Excessive ADH secretion
• Oliguric phase of renal disease
• Excessive administration of I.V. fluids

Signs and symptoms
• Weight gain
• Muscle weakness
• Moist rales; dyspnea
• Increased blood pressure
• Lethargy, apathy, disorientation
• Possible reduced hematocrit
• Possible reduced serum sodium level (from dilution)
• Abdominal cramping

Nursing considerations
• For prevention, exercise caution when administering hypotonic solutions such as 0.45% NaCl.
• For prevention, administer fluids cautiously (at specified rates), especially to cardiopulmonary disease patients.

Problem
Hypokalemia (serum potassium level below 3.5 mEq/l)

Causes
• Thiazide and osmotic diuretic therapy
• Potassium-free I.V. therapy (for a patient receiving nothing by mouth)
• Renal disease such as tubular acidosis and Fanconi's syndrome
• Excessive aldosterone secretion
• Acid-base imbalance
• Excessive gastrointestinal fluid losses from nasogastric suctioning, vomiting, diarrhea, or intestinal fistula
• Malnutrition or malabsorption syndrome
• Laxative abuse
• Trauma with associated loss of potassium in urine

Signs and symptoms
• Arrhythmias, enhanced effectiveness of digitalis (to the point of toxicosis), presence of U wave and depressed S-T segment on EKG waveform.
• Muscle weakness, fatigue, leg cramps
• Drowsiness, irritability, coma
• Anorexia, vomiting, paralytic ileus
• Polydipsia

Nursing considerations
• Place patient on cardiac monitor, as ordered. Observe him for changes in heart rate, rhythm, and EKG pattern.
• Treat arrhythmias by correcting potassium imbalance, as ordered; method depends on serum level and severity of symptoms. Doctor may order: increased potassium intake in diet, or oral potassium supplements (diluted to prevent irritation and to facilitate absorption); or, in emergency, slow administration of diluted potassium chloride I.V. (with patient on cardiac monitor). Monitor patient for signs and symptoms of sudden hyperkalemia onset.
• Monitor serum potassium level to determine effects of replacement therapy.
• Determine source of potassium loss; for example, wound or fistula drainage. Analysis of drainage sample electrolyte content will help indicate amount of daily loss.
• Observe patient for digitalis toxicosis.
• Observe patient for signs of alkalosis, such as irritability, confusion, diarrhea, and nausea.
• Never give potassium when patient's urine output is below 600 ml/day.

Problem
Hyperkalemia (serum potassium level above 5.5 mEq/l)

Causes
• Excessive administration of potassium chloride
• Renal disease
• Use of potassium-sparing diuretics by renal disease patients
• Destruction of cells by burns or trauma, with subsequent potassium release
• Aldosterone insufficiency
• Acidosis, for example, diabetic ketoacidosis

Signs and symptoms
• Cardiac symptoms, including bradycardia, lethal arrhythmias, and cardiac arrest; EKG waveform shows peaked T wave and narrow QRS complex, progressing to widened QRS complex, then flat to absent P wave and asystole
• Apathy, confusion, tingling
• Areflexia, numbness, muscle weakness
• Abdominal cramping, nausea, diarrhea
• Oliguria
• Acetone breath and acetone in urine (indicating metabolic acidosis)

Nursing considerations
• Place patient on cardiac monitor, as ordered. Observe him for changes in heart rate, rhythm, and EKG pattern.
• Restrict ingestion of potassium in diet.
• In an emergency (when potassium excess causes EKG changes or the serum potassium level exceeds 6 mEq/l), administer I.V. glucose, insulin, and sodium bicarbonate, as ordered. This treatment will help shift potassium into the cell. *Note:* Treatment's effects last about 4 hours.
• Check serum potassium levels to monitor shift of potassium in and out of cells. With I.V. treatment, potassium shifts rapidly into cells. When I.V. treatment is discontinued, potassium shifts back into blood.
• Follow I.V. treatment with one or both of the following, as ordered: sodium polystyrene sulfonate (Kayexalete*), an exchange resin, administered orally, through a nasogastric tube, or as an enema; or dialysis. If these treatments are prolonged, monitor patient for resulting hypokalemia.

*Available in both the United States and in Canada

EKG lead II waveforms

Hypokalemia   Hyperkalemia

Problem

Hypocalcemia (serum calcium below 8.5 mg/dl)

Causes

- Hypoparathyroidism
- Chronic renal failure
- Inadequate vitamin D and calcium intake
- Chronic malabsorption syndrome
- Cancer
- Hyperphosphatemia
- Hypomagnesemia
- Cushing's syndrome
- Acute pancreatitis

Signs and symptoms

- Muscle tremors, muscle cramps, tetany, tonic/clonic seizures, paresthesia
- Paralytic ileus
- Alteration in normal blood clotting mechanisms, causing bleeding
- Arrhythmias, hypotension, lengthened Q-T interval with normal T wave on EKG waveform
- Anxiety, irritability, twitching, convulsions, Chvostek's sign, Trousseau's sign

Nursing considerations

- Place patient on cardiac monitor, as ordered. Observe him for changes in heart rate, rhythm, and EKG pattern.
- Administer calcium gluconate or calcium chloride 10% I.V., as ordered.
- Provide calcium in diet, as ordered.
- Administer vitamin D if deficiency is present, as ordered.
- Monitor serum calcium levels every 12 to 24 hours. Report a calcium deficit less than 8 mEq/l.
- Monitor blood's prothrombin time and platelet levels.
- Administer any ordered antacids with caution; some contain calcium.

Problem

Hypercalcemia (serum calcium above 10.5 mg/dl)

Causes

- Long-term immobilization (causes calcium displacement from bone to blood)
- Hyperparathyroidism
- Hypophosphatemia
- Metastatic carcinoma
- Alkalosis
- Thyrotoxicosis
- Vitamin D toxicosis
- Prolonged thiazide diuretic therapy
- Addison's disease

Signs and symptoms

- Drowsiness, lethargy, headaches, depression, apathy, irritability, confusion, personality change
- Increased incidence of kidney stones, with associated flank pain
- Muscular flaccidity
- Nausea, vomiting, anorexia, or constipation
- Polydipsia
- Polyuria
- Hypertension; enhanced effectiveness of digitalis, to the point of toxicosis (administration of digitalis may cause arrhythmias); shortening of Q-T interval of EKG waveform; decreased effectiveness of cardiac contractions, leading to cardiac arrest
- Pathologic fractures

Nursing considerations

- Place patient on cardiac monitor. Observe him for changes in heart rate, rhythm, and EKG pattern.
- Monitor serum calcium level frequently. Watch for cardiac arrhythmias if serum calcium level exceeds 5.7 mEq/l.
- If patient's on digitalis, check his digitalis serum level before administering each daily dose. Assess him for signs of digitalis toxicosis, such as vomiting, headache, fatigue, and arrhythmias.
- Administer the following medication, as ordered: loop diuretics (never thiazide diuretics) and fluid therapy, to enhance renal calcium excretion; mithramycin (Mithracin); corticosteroids; phosphate binders.
- Administer any ordered antacids with caution; some contain calcium.
- Check urine for renal calculi and acidity.

Problem

Hyponatremia (serum sodium below 135 mEq/L)

Causes

Hyponatremia associated with excess fluid
- Inappropriate ADH syndrome
- Excessive intake of hypotonic fluids

Hyponatremia associated with dehydration
- Administration of salt-removing diuretics
- Salt-wasting nephritis
- Excessive gastrointestinal fluid losses from nasogastric suctioning, vomiting, or diarrhea
- Severe diaphoresis
- Potassium depletion
- Trauma, such as surgery or burns
- Aldosterone insufficiency
- Severe malnutrition

Signs and symptoms

Hyponatremia associated with excess fluid
- Headache, anxiety, lassitude, apathy, confusion
- Anorexia, nausea, vomiting, diarrhea, cramping
- Hyperreflexia, muscle spasms, muscle weakness

Hyponatremia associated with dehydration
- Irritability, tremors, seizure, coma
- Dry mucous membranes
- Low-grade fever
- Hypotension, tachycardia
- Decreased urine output ranging from oliguria to anuria

Nursing considerations

- Correct sodium and water imbalance through diet and administration of I.V. solutions, as ordered.
- During administration of normal saline solution, observe patient closely for signs of hypervolemia (such as dyspnea, rales, and engorged neck or hand veins).
- During treatments, monitor neurologic and gastrointestinal symptoms, to detect improvement or deterioration.
- Monitor sodium and potassium levels closely.

Problem

Hypernatremia (serum sodium above 145 mEq/l)

Causes

Hypernatremia associated with excess fluid
- Excessive administration of large amounts of sodium chloride solution I.V.
- Excessive aldosterone secretion

Hypernatremia associated with dehydration
- Dehydration *without sodium loss,* from decreased water intake, severe vomiting, or diarrhea
- Excessive administration of osmotic diuretics
- Hypercalcemia with polyuria and dehydration
- Neurohypophyseal dysfunction (as in diabetes insipidus)
- Renal tubular disease
- Dysfunctional thirst mechanism

Signs and symptoms

Hypernatremia associated with excess fluid
- Weight gain
- Pitting edema in extremities
- Hypertension
- Shortness of breath (only in severe imbalance)
- Agitation, restlessness, convulsions (only in severe imbalance)

Hypernatremia associated with dehydration
- Lethargy, irritability, tremors, seizures, coma
- Dry mucous membranes; rough, dry tongue; flushed skin
- Low-grade fever
- Oliguria
- Intense thirst

Nursing considerations

- Monitor hourly urine output.
- Replace water volume, as ordered, administering fluids with caution.
- Check serum sodium levels every 6 hours.
- Monitor vital signs closely. Watch for increasing pulse rate and hypertension.
- Observe patient for signs of hypervolemia.

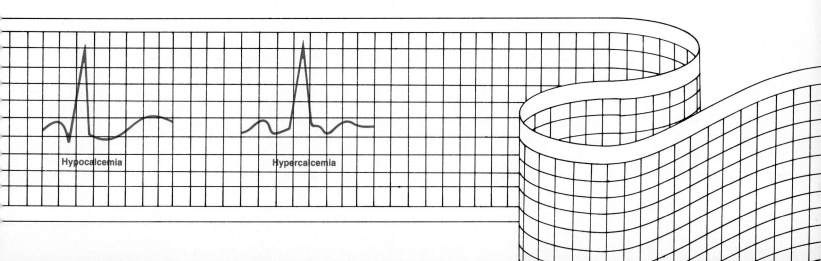

Fluids and electrolytes

Nurses' guide to fluid and electrolyte imbalances continued

Problem
Hypophosphatemia (serum phosphate level below 3.5 mg/dl)

Causes
• Chronic alcoholism (usually entails decreased phosphate intake)
• Prolonged phosphate-free or low-phosphate total parenteral nutrition (TPN) therapy
• Hyperparathyroidism, with resultant hypercalcemia
• Excessive use of phosphate-binding gels such as aluminum hydroxide
• Malabsorption syndrome
• Chronic diarrhea

Signs and symptoms
• Anorexia
• Mental confusion
• Muscle weakness, muscle wasting, tremors, paresthesia
• Hemolytic anemia
• Hypoxia with peripheral cyanosis
• Hypercalcemia

Nursing considerations
• Monitor calcium, magnesium, and phosphorus levels, and report any changes immediately.
• Administer potassium phosphate I.V., as ordered.
• Provide phosphate in diet, or give oral phosphate supplements, as ordered. Monitor patient for signs of hypocalcemia when giving supplements.
• If patient's receiving phosphate-binding gels such as aluminum hydroxide (Amphojel*), discontinue their use.

*Available in both the United States and in Canada

Problem
Hyperphosphatemia (serum phosphate level above 4.5 mg/dl)

Causes
• Excessive use of phosphate-containing laxatives or enemas
• Acute and chronic renal failure
• Excessive I.V. or oral phosphate therapy
• Cytotoxic agents
• Vitamin D toxicosis
• Hypocalcemia
• Hypoparathyroidism

Signs and symptoms
• Usually asymptomatic
• Possible metastatic calcifications
• With hypocalcemia, neuromuscular changes including cramps, tetany, or seizures

Nursing considerations
• Administer phosphate-binding gels such as aluminum hydroxide (Amphojel*), as ordered.
• Monitor serum calcium, magnesium, and phosphorus levels. Report any changes immediately.
• Observe patient for signs of hypocalcemia, such as muscle twitching and tetany.
• Discontinue antacids, such as Maalox* and Mylanta*.

Problem
Hypomagnesemia (serum magnesium level below 1.5 mEq/l)

Causes
• Starvation syndrome
• Malabsorption syndrome
• Postoperative complications after bowel resection
• Prolonged TPN therapy without adequate magnesium
• Excessive administration of mercurial diuretics
• Excessive GI fluid losses from nasogastric suctioning, vomiting, diarrhea, or fistula
• Hyper- and hypoparathyroidism

Signs and symptoms
• Dizziness, confusion, delusions, hallucinations, convulsions
• Tremors, hyperirritability, tetany, leg and foot cramps, Chvostek's sign
• Arrhythmias and vasomotor changes
• Anorexia and nausea

Nursing considerations
• If patient needs antacids, give Maalox* or Mylanta* (as ordered).
• Take seizure precautions, such as keeping side rails up, and initiating neurochecks.
• Replace magnesium losses, as ordered. Infuse magnesium replacement slowly, observing patient for bradycardia and decreased respirations.
• Monitor serum magnesium levels every 6 to 12 hours during replacement therapy. Report abnormal levels immediately.

Problem
Hypermagnesemia (serum magnesium level above 2.5 mEq/l)

Causes
• Renal failure
• Adrenal insufficiency
• Excessive ingestion of magnesium (for example, in the form of antacid gels such as Maalox* and Mylanta*)
• Excessive use of magnesium-containing laxatives such as Milk of Magnesia

Signs and symptoms
• Drowsiness, lethargy, confusion, coma
• Bradycardia, weak pulse, hypotension, prolonged Q-T interval on EKG waveform, heart block, cardiac arrest (with serum levels of 25 mEq/ l)
• Vague neuromuscular changes (may include tremors and hyporeflexia)
• Vague GI symptoms, such as nausea

Nursing considerations
• Discontinue Maalox* and Mylanta*, if patient's receiving them.
• Administer calcium gluconate I.V. as ordered. Note that calcium enhances digitalis action.
• In renal failure, perform dialysis as ordered, to remove excess magnesium.
• Monitor serum magnesium levels to determine effectiveness of treatment. Watch for respiratory distress if serum magnesium levels exceed 10 mEq/l.

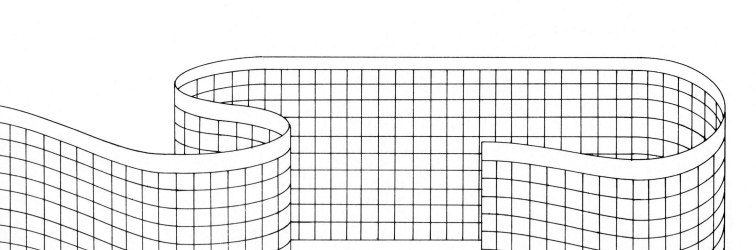

Common problems

When caring for an ICU patient, you'll use every means ordered to intensively treat his primary illness. But that's not your *only* concern—your patient's illness makes him extremely vulnerable to secondary complications arising from nosocomial infection or immobilization. And, because ICU care depends heavily on electrical monitoring and support equipment, he also risks receiving an electrical shock. So, ironically, just when your patient's defenses are the weakest, his therapy multiplies the threats to his health.

From the moment he enters the ICU to the moment he leaves, your patient needs vigilant protection against these threats. To provide it, you'll need to know:
• how to prevent or treat common types of infections.
• what safety measures can reduce the risk of electrical shock.
• how long-term immobilization affects your patient's body systems.

To find out this information, study the charts, text, and illustrations on the following pages.

Preventing infection

Your ICU patient's normal defense mechanisms are gravely compromised by his illness. Under these circumstances, what can you do to prevent infection?

First, you can reduce the pathogens in his environment. In doing so, keep in mind that pathogens may be transmitted in the following ways:
• through the air in the form of contaminated water vapor or dust
• through contact, either direct (transfer of microorganisms from host to patient) or indirect (transfer of microorganisms in contaminated dressings, instruments, foods, or in droplets spread from sneezing and coughing)
• through a common vehicle, such as contaminated blood or I.V. solution
• through an insect vector.

To interrupt these transmission routes and reduce the presence of pathogens, take regular precautions. Change dressings and solutions every 24 hours, and I.V. tubing every 24 to 48 hours, according to hospital policy. Properly dispose of soiled dressings and used syringes. Does your patient have a tracheostomy? Give aseptic tracheostomy care. To reduce the risk of introducing new pathogens into the ICU, restrict all visitors with upper respiratory tract infections; if you have a cold yourself, wear a mask. Finally, report any

inadequate housekeeping you see.

In addition to promoting an aseptic environment, bolster your patient's defense mechanisms by following these general guidelines:
• Perform nursing procedures using aseptic or clean technique, whichever is appropriate.
• Wash your hands between treating two different patients.
• Isolate patients with communicable infections, as necessary.
• Provide adequate nutrition to promote tissue healing and immune system function.
• Remove indwelling (Foley) catheters and I.V. lines, as soon as practical.
• Take measures to relieve patient stress (see pages 10 to 13).

Observing the precautions listed above will greatly reduce cross-contamination in the ICU. Also, whenever possible, collaborate with the nurse epidemiologist. And always comply with your hospital's standardized procedures for wound and instrument care, using criteria established by the Joint Commission on Accreditation of Hospitals (JCAH), or the American Hospital Association (AHA). For more information, consult the NURSING PHOTOBOOK CONTROLLING INFECTION.

For identification and treatment of specific ICU infection problems, see the chart that begins below.

Nurses' guide to common ICU infections

Problem	Causes	Signs and symptoms	Prevention	Nursing management
Bacteremia or septicemia	• Contaminated I.V. system or infected I.V. insertion site • Septic thrombophlebitis • Urinary tract infection	• Chills, fever, lethargy, fatigue • Tenderness, swelling, pus, phlebitis at I.V. insertion site • Blood cultures positive for *Staphylococcus aureus, S. epidermidis, Klebsiella* species, *Enterobacter* species, or *Serratia marcescens* • Cloudy, bloody, or foul-smelling urine; burning on urination; urinary frequency • Hypotension progressing to multisystem failure, from septic shock	• Use strict aseptic technique when inserting any I.V. catheter. Change I.V. dressings, tubing and solution every 24 hours, or according to hospital policy. Always check I.V. solutions for clarity and expiration date. • For guidelines on preventing urinary tract infection, see the following page. • For guidelines on care of central I.V. lines, see page 125.	• Report signs of local infection. • Obtain culture from infection site, if exudate is present. • Administer antibiotics, as ordered. • Continue appropriate preventive measures.

Common problems

Nurses' guide to common ICU infections continued

Problem	Causes	Signs and symptoms	Prevention	Nursing management
Respiratory tract infection	• Aspiration • Contaminated oxygen or ventilating equipment • Reduced respiratory defense mechanisms • Trauma; for example, an endotracheal tube irritating the patient's trachea • Immobilization	• Altered breath sounds, including bronchial and bronchovesicular sounds, and transient fine rales • Change in color, odor, or consistency of sputum • Sputum culture positive for *Escherichia coli, Klebsiella* species, *Streptococcus pneumoniae, Proteus* species, *Serratia marcescens,* or *Pseudomonas aeruginosa* • Sudden productive cough followed by chills, fever • Chest X-ray revealing consolidation	• Assess breath sounds for changes. • Turn patient every 2 hours to mobilize secretions. Ask patient to cough and deep breathe every 2 hours. • Use aseptic technique when suctioning. • Follow hospital policy for cleaning inhalation equipment. • Use sterile water in humidifer; change water every 24 hours or more frequently, as needed. • Obtain sputum cultures, as ordered. • Adhere to respiratory and physical therapy programs.	• Report symptoms of infection immediately. • Confirm infection with sputum culture. • Administer antibiotics, as ordered. • Continue appropriate preventive measures.
Wound infection	• Postoperative complication • Patient self-contamination	• Fever, headache, fatigue • Redness, tenderness, inflammation, pus, pain at wound site, wound dehiscence, wound fails to heal or heals irregularly • Wound culture positive for *Staphylococcus aureus, S. epidermidis, Klebsiella* species, *Enterobacter* species, *Serratia* species, *Actinobacillus* species, or *Aspergillus* species	• Use aseptic technique when changing dressing. Remember to wash your hands carefully. • Change dressing, as ordered, at least every 24 hours; more frequently if drainage is excessive. Apply antimicrobial ointment, as ordered. • Consult nurse epidemiologist, if you perceive a pattern in infection incidence.	• Immediately report any signs of infection or any alteration in the healing process. (However, expect delayed healing in a diabetic patient or a patient receiving steroids.) Culture site, as ordered. • Encourage adequate nutritional support. • Debride wound, as ordered, to assist in new tissue growth. • Continue appropriate preventive measures.
Urinary tract infection	• Improper urinary catheter care • Neurogenic bladder • Urine retention • Urine reflux into bladder or ureters	• Fever, chills, lethargy • Cloudy, bloody, or foul-smelling urine • Bladder spasms • Urinalysis reveals abundance of white blood cells • Culture positive (with 100,000 colonies per ml urine) for *Klebsiella* species, *Streptoccus pneumoniae, Serratia marcescens,* or *Proteus rettgeri*	• Remove indwelling (Foley) catheter as soon as possible. • Perform catheter care according to hospital policy. • Use a closed drainage system. • Do not allow tubing or drainage bag to touch floor. • Do not irrigate catheter, unless ordered. • Encourage patient to increase fluid intake, especially of fluids containing ascorbic acid.	• If you note cloudy, bloody, or foul-smelling urine, send specimen to lab for culture. • If patient's catheterized, use a syringe at catheter resealing site or sampling port to obtain a culture specimen. • Remove Foley catheter as soon as it is practical. • Administer sulfonamides or antibiotics, as ordered. • Continue appropriate preventive measures.

Guarding against electrical hazards

The monitors, ventilators, and other electrical equipment used in an ICU are invaluable aids in patient care. But, as beneficial as they are, they do present the threat of electrical shock and burns. To protect your patient and yourself, follow these guidelines:

• Learn the proper use of electrical equipment.

• Before use, always check equipment for frayed wires, loose connections, damaged plugs, and any other damage or defects. Report defective equipment, and remove it from the unit.

• Check electrical outlets before use. Report any defective outlets.

• Plug all equipment used on a single patient into a cluster of closely associated wall outlets.

• Ground all equipment properly. Never use an adapter for connecting a three-prong plug to a two-prong outlet.

• Avoid using extension cords.

• Never touch both a patient who's connected to electrical equipment, and a conductive surface at the same time. If a piece of electrical equipment (an electric bed, for example) isn't grounded properly, or if it's leaking even small amounts of electrical current, you may unwittingly create a dangerous new circuit. The illustration below shows how this situation endangers both you and your patient.

• Report any tingling sensations you get from a machine as well as any sparking, smoking, or overheating you observe. Disconnect the equipment as quickly as possible, taking measures to protect the patient's well-being if he's dependent on the equipment.

• Do not touch exposed portions of any intravascular or intracardiac catheters (such as direct pacer wires) unless you're wearing rubber gloves.

• Cover pacemaker box terminals with a rubber glove, if they aren't insulated.

• Wipe up spilled liquid quickly. Never use electrical equipment as a place to set wet items or food trays.

Managing defibrillation safely

As you know, an electrical shock delivered during defibrillation (or cardioversion) can be life-saving. But in order to safely perform this procedure, you must follow these specific guidelines:

• If your patient's receiving oxygen, turn it off before beginning defibrillation.

• To prevent electrical arcing, check the paddles to make sure they're smooth and free of cracks and caked gel.

• Apply fresh gel to the paddles just before use. But avoid using too much, or electrical burns may result.

• Before initiating the charge, check to be sure you're not standing on a wet surface. Then, announce that you're defibrillating the patient and make sure your co-workers step back from the bed.

• Always keep the paddles at least 2″ apart when in use.

• Check the machine's watt-seconds or joules reading to confirm that it equals the prescribed amount of electrical current.

• Thoroughly remove all gel from the defibrillator paddles after each use.

Understanding immobility

Not so long ago, a patient who'd suffered a myocardial infarction (MI) was confined to complete bed rest for weeks. These days, a patient recovering from an MI resumes some type of physical activity within several days. Why? In large part, because health care professionals now recognize the debilitating effects of prolonged immobilization. These ill effects can affect every part of the patient's body, and may complicate and prolong his recovery.

No matter what type of condition your ICU patient has, he'll spend most of his time on bed rest. For a moment, consider his plight. In the ICU, one or more of these factors restrict—or eliminate entirely—his opportunity to move normally:

• his condition itself; for example, paralysis, or an injury requiring a body cast

• medical or nursing procedures; for example, peritoneal dialysis

• equipment, such as pressure monitoring equipment; ventilators; I.V. pumps and tubing; and indwelling (Foley) catheters and drainage bags

• hospital policy. In many ICUs, patients aren't permitted to leave their beds without supervision.

• psychological factors, such as social isolation, depression or ICU syndrome (see page 13).

Recognizing immobilization's effects

What does prolonged immobilization mean for your patient? The chart beginning on the next page explains some of the changes you can expect to see—and tells you how to minimize their ill effects.

Keep in mind that changes in one body system inevitably affect others. Consider, for example, the far-reaching effects of nitrogen depletion, a metabolic disturbance caused by severe illness. Within the first few days of critical illness, your patient's likely to excrete large amounts of nitrogen. The resulting negative nitrogen balance contributes to loss of muscle mass, and muscle atrophy—processes that also come from simple muscle disuse.

Consider, too, the effects of immobilization on your patient's hematologic system. During immobilization, his blood volume decreases, as does the number of oxygen-carrying red blood cells. Because his lung capacity is also compromised by immobilization, your patient may not get the oxygen he needs.

In addition, immobilization may lead to

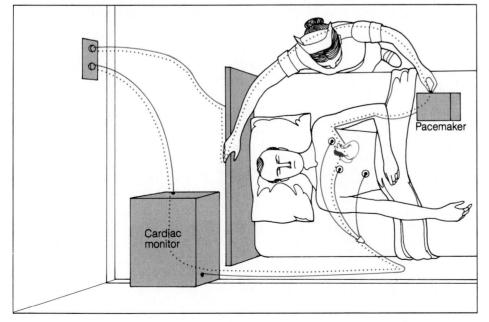

Pacemaker

Cardiac monitor

Common problems

Understanding immobility continued

hypercoagulability. This increases his risk of pulmonary embolism and thrombophlebitis.

What you can do

Not surprisingly, the best way to combat the ill effects of immobilization is by mobilizing the patient, to whatever extent his condition permits. If your patient's confined to his bed, perform passive range-of-motion (ROM) exercises at least three times a day (unless the doctor instructs otherwise). By doing so, you maintain joint function and muscle tone, despite the patient's inactivity. For detailed instructions on performing ROM exercises—as well as information on the difference between active and passive ROM exercises—see the NURSING PHOTOBOOK PROVIDING EARLY MOBILITY.

Look for opportunities to work passive ROMs into your nursing routine; for example, perform them while you give the patient a bed bath. As you work, explain what you're doing and why. Remember, the patient may worry that exercises will hamper his recovery. Take care to assure him that exercising actually *speeds* his recovery. Also, take this opportunity to teach him some exercises he can perform actively. For example, teach him leg and foot exercises to stimulate circulation and help prevent thrombophlebitis.

Keep in mind that when your patient resumes activity, or even changes position from recumbent to sitting, he's likely to experience fatigue, dyspnea, or the dizziness of postural hypotension. To avoid exhausting the patient, plan a steady but *gradual* return to activity. (As an example, see the in-house cardiac rehabilitation program described in the NURSING PHOTOBOOK GIVING CARDIAC CARE.)

Finally, don't overlook the psychological effects of immobilization. Provide support by reassuring the patient about his condition (if you can do so honestly). Encourage him to discuss his fears and frustrations, especially if his immobilization will be prolonged. Help him to resume routine self-care as soon as he's able. And finally, promote his interaction with his family, and encourage them all to participate in planning the patient's care.

Nurses' guide to immobility hazards

This chart tells you how you can minimize immobility's effects. Of course, you'll adjust your nursing care for each patient, depending on his primary condition.

Important: If your patient develops a complication, carefully assess it to determine whether it's caused by immobility, or the patient's primary condition. For example, tachycardia may result from stimulation of the sympathetic nervous system during immobilization—or, it may result from myocardial infarction. Your accurate assessment is essential.

System
INTEGUMENTARY (SKIN)

Complications
• Painful, reddened areas
• Decubitus ulcers

Nursing intervention
• Turn and position your patient regularly.
• Observe *all* skin surfaces, especially bony prominences, for pressure signs, such as blanched or reddened areas.
• Keep your patient's skin clean and dry.
• When necessary, use special equipment to minimize pressure on your patient's body; for example, an egg crate, air, or water mattress; flotation pads; and heel and elbow protectors.
• Gently massage *around* (never on) pressure areas to stimulate circulation.
• From a distance of 18″ (46 cm), apply a heat lamp 15 minutes daily, if ordered. *Caution:* Check the patient's skin frequently to prevent burns.
• Avoid irritating your patient's skin, by using a drawsheet or sheepskin to move him.
• Make sure your patient is on a high-protein, low-calcium diet, with plenty of fluids.
• Explain all procedures to your patient.

System
SKELETAL

Complications
• Backaches
• Osteoporosis from disuse

Nursing intervention
• Turn and position your patient regularly, according to his needs.
• Make sure that his body's well aligned and that his joints and muscles are properly supported.
• Perform complete range-of-motion (ROM) exercises at least three times a day.
• Periodically, try to stand your patient upright, or use a tilt table.
• Make sure your patient has a high-protein, low-calcium diet, with plenty of fluids.
• Check his urine for sediment, which may indicate early formation of renal calculi. If you note any sediment, send a urine specimen to the lab for analysis. Document the results, and notify the doctor, if necessary.
• Explain all procedures to your patient.

System
MUSCULAR

Complications
• Contractures
• Decreased muscle tone
• Muscle atrophy

Nursing intervention
• Turn and position your patient regularly, according to his needs.
• Make sure that his body's well aligned, and that his joints and muscles are properly supported.
• Perform complete ROM exercises at least three times a day.
• Use supportive devices, as needed, such as footdrop stops, splints, trochanter rolls, and hand rolls.
• Whenever possible, reduce edema by elevating extremities.
• Hyperextend your patient's hips at least three times daily, if his condition permits.
• Explain all procedures to your patient.

System
CARDIOVASCULAR

Complications
- Decreased myocardial tone
- Venous stasis, causing decreased cardiac output and edema
- Thrombus formation
- Orthostatic hypotension
- Increased heart rate

Nursing intervention
- Place your patient in high Fowler's or a seated position, if his condition permits. If he's in a seated position, place his feet flat on the floor or on a footstool, to alleviate pressure on the backs of his knees.
- When seating your patient upright in bed, raise the head of the bed gradually.
- When possible, use standing transfers to move your patient from one place to another.
- Apply antiembolism stockings, as ordered.
- Make sure that your patient has a high-protein, low-calcium diet, with plenty of fluids (unless this is contraindicated).
- Gradually increase your patient's activities.
- Instruct your patient to exhale slowly when moving in bed to prevent him from performing a Valsalva maneuver.
- Explain all procedures to your patient.

System
RESPIRATORY

Complications
- Reduction of lung capacity
- Pooling of respiratory secretions
- Respiratory infections
- Hypostatic pneumonia
- Atelectasis
- Respiratory acidosis
- Pulmonary emboli

Nursing intervention
- Turn and position your patient regularly, according to his needs.
- Make sure that your patient's body is well aligned and that his joints and muscles are properly supported.
- Encourage your patient to cough and deep breathe, to fully expand his lungs and clear secretions.
- Observe and assess your patient's respiratory patterns and breath sounds.
- Be prepared to administer intermittent positive pressure breathing (IPPB) treatments, as ordered.
- Encourage the use of incentive spirometry and blow bottles, as needed.
- Perform chest physiotherapy frequently.
- Percuss and vibrate your patient's chest to loosen secretions, as needed.
- Explain all procedures to your patient.

System
GENITOURINARY

Complications
- Urinary retention
- Renal calculi
- Urinary tract infections

Nursing intervention
- Unless your patient has an indwelling (Foley) catheter in place, follow this procedure: When a female patient needs to void, place her in a seated position to allow good urine drainage. If your patient's a male, have him stand, if he's able. Also, provide privacy.
- Observe your patient's pubic symphysis for bladder distention. If you suspect distention, palpate the area to confirm your findings.
- Minimize formation of new calculi by acidifying your patient's urine. Make sure he gets adequate amounts of vitamin C. Encourage him to drink orange or cranberry juice, or administer urine acidifiers, as ordered.
- Don't give your patient foods that leave an alkaline ash residue, such as tomato or grapefruit juice.
- Check his urine for sediment, which may indicate developing renal calculi. If you note any sediment, send a specimen to the lab for analysis. Document the results, and notify the doctor, if necessary.
- Explain all procedures to your patient.

System
GASTROINTESTINAL

Complications
- Anorexia
- Constipation

Nursing intervention
- If your patient can eat, make sure he has a balanced diet, with many of his food preferences and plenty of bulk. Arrange for your patient to have several small meals throughout the day instead of three large ones.
- Provide your patient with 1,000 to 2,000 ml of fluid daily, unless contraindicated.
- Be ready to administer stool softeners and laxatives, as needed.
- Check your patient's bowel movement history. If he's constipated, make sure his medication isn't causing the problem.
- Provide privacy for your patient when he's defecating. When possible, place your patient in a sitting position in a bathroom or commode chair.
- Gradually increase your patient's activities.
- Explain all procedures to your patient.

System
NEUROLOGIC AND PSYCHOLOGICAL

Complications
- Dependency
- Disorientation
- Decreased motivation
- Insomnia

Nursing intervention
- Gradually increase your patient's physical activities. Encourage him to participate in his care and to do as much for himself as possible.
- Hold frequent conversations with your patient to orient him. Keep him involved and informed on all aspects of his care and therapy. (For more guidelines on orienting your patient, review pages 10 to 13.)
- Provide your patient with intellectual stimulation. For example, suggest he receive visitors; read newspapers, books, and magazines; or work crossword puzzles (as permitted by his condition and hospital policy).

Stress management

No one has to tell you that ICU nursing is stressful. And that's not necessarily bad. Stress can be a stimulus that inspires you to do your best. And performing well under pressure can be exhilarating.

But stress has its negative side, too. When it becomes intense—or when it's unrelieved for long periods—it's devitalizing. That's when you're in danger of burnout—lingering feelings of depression, hopelessness, and apathy that don't lift when you go home.

In order to combat burnout, you need to know how to recognize it. On these pages, we'll tell you what danger signs to look for, and what actions to take against them.

Burnout: A special ICU hazard

Joy Lawry's been an ICU nurse for almost a year now, and she's good at her job. She prides herself on going an extra mile for her patients. If another nurse is late for the next shift, she'll willingly stay overtime to pick up the slack. Or, if one of her patients is unstable, she's likely to sit with him and his family all night, long after her shift's over. And if he dies? She's genuinely bereaved, and may mourn for several days.

Joy's patients and colleagues consider her exceptionally dedicated. Her patients, unquestionably, receive top-notch care. But how about Joy? Is she thriving on the pace and emotional

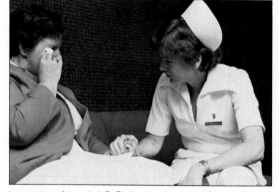

intensity of her job? Or is she headed for professional burnout?

Stress in the ICU

Maybe you've never experienced burnout yourself. But chances are, you've known someone like Joy. Like you, she chose ICU nursing because she enjoys challenges, and gets satisfaction out of helping patients who need expert nursing care. Ironically, a highly-motivated nurse like Joy Lawry is particularly prone to burnout.

When you think about it, it's not surprising. In the ICU, you know that an emergency may occur at any time—or, that several emergencies may occur at once. No matter what happens, you expect yourself to act quickly and skillfully. You never forget that a misjudgment can be life-threatening.

And of course, ICU nursing is *emotionally* stressful. Some of your patients die, despite your efforts, and grieving family members turn to you for support.

Some nurses, like Joy, cope with the inherent stress of ICU nursing by redoubling their efforts. Eventually, physical and emotional exhaustion open the door to burnout.

Another side of burnout

But some nurses find another way to cope with stress. Consider Marian Gelfi, for example. Bright and efficient, she immerses herself in the technical side of nursing. Marian can accurately interpret an unusual EKG strip at a glance, yet she never takes time to sit and talk with an anxious patient. She tends to depersonalize her patients by thinking of them as cases: "We're having a lot of

trouble stabilizing the cardiac case that came in this morning," she may tell you. If you ask her how a patient's feeling today, she's likely to recite his vital signs. And if a patient dies, she takes it in stride, seemingly unmoved.

In short, Marian has distanced herself emotionally from her work. But while effective in the short run, emotional distancing takes its toll. No one can switch off her emotions at the beginning of a shift, and turn them on again 8 hours later. Nurses like Marian, who pride themselves on their detachment, may find that it has a profoundly negative effect on their personal lives.

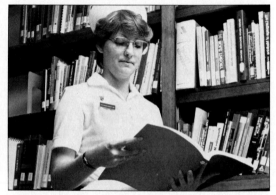

So what's the answer? How can you find the middle ground between overinvolvement and complete emotional detachment? Begin by analyzing *your* coping mechanisms. Many nurses who've experienced burnout say that it took them by surprise; that their lives had been seriously affected before they knew what was happening. Don't let this happen to you. By identifying problems before they become overwhelming, you can take steps to solve them.

Recognizing danger signs

How can you tell if you're headed toward burnout? Consider yourself at risk if you:
• dread going to work and frequently call in sick.
• feel plagued by headaches, insomnia, tooth and gum sensitivity, or minor disorders such as colds and indigestion.
• feel professionally inadequate, as though nothing you do is quite enough.
• feel as though you never get away from the job, even on your days off.
• feel irritable much of the time.
• seem unable to make decisions or long-term plans.
• withdraw from personal contact with your patients and their families, or avoid patients with certain conditions.
• engage in spells of inappropriate laughing or crying.
• label or categorize your patients; for example, "the senile old lady in bed B."
• let off steam with cold, cynical, or sarcastic remarks; for example, "Mrs. Borden's family is so upset, they drive me nuts."

Acknowledgements

- spend significant amounts of time gossiping and complaining about work with co-workers.
- lack initiative and are unable to concentrate on the job, resulting (for example) in more medication errors.
- take less pride in your physical appearance.
- need drugs or alcohol in order to relax.
- notice changes in eating and elimination patterns.

Taking action
Let's say you recognize some of these danger signs in your behavior. The next step is to pin down the cause. Ask yourself these questions:
- *How well do I handle stress?* Are your coping mechanisms effective? If not, even small amounts of stress can become overwhelming. Adopting some or all of the stress-reducing techniques listed on the right may help.
- *Is anything in my personal life contributing to stress on the job?* Make sure your professional problems don't begin at home. If you're dissatisfied with your personal life, changes in your professional life aren't likely to help.
- *Are my goals and expectations realistic?* For example, do you find yourself wishing you could save a dying patient? Or, are you angry with yourself if the nursing care you give is anything less than perfect? If so, you may unwittingly be setting yourself up for disappointment and disillusionment.
- *Is my unit understaffed or poorly run?* If so, everyone's working under additional stress. Knowing that you're not caring for patients as well as you could is demoralizing. Take positive action. Instead of simply griping about conditions with co-workers, schedule a private appointment with your supervisor and offer constructive suggestions for change. For example, if additional staff is out of the question, suggest staggering responsibilities so that nurses alternate stressful duties with less stressful ones. Although your supervisor's probably aware of the unit's problems, she doesn't have your perspective on them. Listen to her views and proposed solutions. Then, support her plan of action, and encourage your co-workers to do likewise.
- *Are you suited, professionally and emotionally, for ICU nursing?* If your training hasn't prepared you adequately, you'll naturally feel overwhelmed. Additional education and training may be the answer, if you're committed to ICU nursing.

But maybe you're really not sure that ICU nursing's for you. Do you find dealing with critically ill patients emotionally draining? Would you be happier with fewer—or less demanding—responsibilities? If so, consider trying another type of nursing. Don't consider such a change to be a defeat. Remember, recognizing what's best for you—and then taking steps to achieve it—is an antidote to burnout. You'll be happier—and you'll be a better nurse for it.

Rx for stress

How you can reduce stress:
- Acknowledge your feelings. Recognizing signs of stress—and then dealing with them—is a sign of strength.
- Don't live and breathe your job. Cultivate a social life that's unrelated to work. Take regular vacations—at least twice a year, if possible.
- Don't make working overtime a regular practice.
- Plan time to relax when you leave the job. Instead of hurrying home, sit in a park for 20 minutes and relax. Or relax in the bathtub as soon as you get home. In other words, break the day's hurried, stressful pattern. But beware of relying on alcohol or drugs to help you relax.
- Find physical outlets for stress, such as swimming, jogging, or walking. But avoid competitive sports unless you're a good loser.
- Avoid boredom on the job by looking for new challenges. For example, try writing articles for a nursing publication, or taking a 6-month sabbatical to continue your education.

Your hospital administration can help reduce your unit's stress by:
- maintaining a high staff-to-patient ratio.
- assigning senior ICU staff members to orient and teach new staff members.
- promoting support groups, led by a psychiatric liaison, to encourage staff members to ventilate feelings in a constructive way.
- using nurse consultants to analyze unit practices and unit morale, and to make recommendations.
- permitting staff members to transfer or rotate without recriminations.
- recognizing the need for regular work breaks and vacations, and encouraging nurses to take them.

We'd like to thank the following people and companies for their help with this Photobook:

ALLIED HEALTHCARE PRODUCTS, INC.
Gomco Division
St. Louis, Mo.

CINCINNATI SUB-ZERO PRODUCTS, INC.
Cincinnati, Ohio

CRITIKON, INC.
Tampa, Fla.

CUTTER MEDICAL
Division of Cutter Laboratories, Inc.
Emeryville, Calif.

DAVOL, INC.
Subsidiary of C.R. Bard, Inc.
Cranston, R.I.

DEKNATEL
Division of Howmedica, Inc.
Floral Park, N.Y.

GOULD, INC.
Medical Products Division
Oxnard, Calif.

HEWLETT-PACKARD
Waltham, Mass.

OHIO MEDICAL PRODUCTS
Division of AIRCO, Inc.
Madison, Wis.

PORTEX, INC.
Wilmington, Mass.

PURITAN-BENNETT CORPORATION
Bellmawr, N.J.

Dr. Arthur Bogert, D.O.
Metropolitan Hospital
Parkview Division
Philadelphia, Pa.

Dr. John Simelaro, D.O.
Chief of Pulmonary Medicine
Osteopathic Medical Center of Philadelphia
Philadelphia, Pa.

Also the staffs of:
ROLLING HILL HOSPITAL AND DIAGNOSTIC CENTER
Intensive Care Unit
Elkins Park, Pa.
Ann Ashton, R.N.
Divisional Coordinator, ICU
Dr. Jeffrey Weisman, D.O.

HOSPITAL OF THE UNIVERSITY OF PENNSYLVANIA
Philadelphia, Pa.

Selected references

Books

Andreoli, Kathleen, et al. COMPREHENSIVE CARDIAC CARE, 4th ed. St. Louis: C.V. Mosby Co., 1979.

ASSESSING YOUR PATIENTS. Nursing Photobook™ Series. Springhouse, Pa.: Springhouse Corporation, 1981.

Burton, George, et al. RESPIRATORY CARE. Philadelphia: J.B. Lippincott Co., 1977.

Castle, Mary. HOSPITAL INFECTION CONTROL: PRINCIPLES AND PRACTICE. New York: John Wiley and Sons Inc., 1980.

Cherniack, Reuben M. PULMONARY FUNCTION TESTING. Philadelphia: W.B. Saunders Co., 1977.

Chusid, Joseph G. CORRELATIVE NEUROANATOMY AND FUNCTIONAL NEUROLOGY, 16th ed. Los Altos, Calif.: Lange Medical Publications, 1976.

Claus, Karen E., and June T. Bailey. LIVING WITH STRESS AND PROMOTING WELL-BEING. St. Louis: C.V. Mosby Co., 1980.

Comroe, Julius H. Jr., et al. THE LUNG—CLINICAL PHYSIOLOGY AND PULMONARY FUNCTION TESTS, 2nd ed. Chicago: Year Book Medical Publishers, Inc., 1962.

Comroe, Julius H. Jr. PHYSIOLOGY OF RESPIRATION—AN INTRODUCTORY TEXT. Chicago: Year Book Medical Publishers, Inc., 1974.

CONTROLLING INFECTION. Nursing Photobook™ Series. Springhouse, Pa.: Springhouse Corporation, 1981.

COPING WITH NEUROLOGIC DISORDERS. Nursing Photobook™ Series. Springhouse, Pa.: Springhouse Corporation, 1981.

Davis, Joan E., and Celestine B. Mason. NEUROLOGIC CRITICAL CARE. New York: Van Nostrand Reinhold Co., 1979.

DEALING WITH EMERGENCIES. Nursing Photobook™ Series. Springhouse, Pa.: Springhouse Corporation, 1981.

Dubay, Elaine C., and Reba D. Grubb. INFECTION: PREVENTION AND CONTROL, 2nd ed. St. Louis: C.V. Mosby Co., 1978.

Gilroy, John, and John S. Meyer. MEDICAL NEUROLOGY. London: The MacMillian Company, 1969.

Given, Barbara A., and Sandra J. Simmons. GASTROENTEROLOGY IN CLINICAL NURSING. St. Louis: C.V. Mosby Co., 1975.

GIVING CARDIAC CARE. Nursing Photobook™ Series. Springhouse, Pa.: Springhouse Corporation, 1981.

Holloway, Nancy M. NURSING THE CRITICALLY ILL ADULT. Reading, Mass.: Addison-Wesley Pub. Co., 1979.

Hurst, J. Willis, et al. THE HEART, 3rd ed. New York: McGraw-Hill Book Co., 1974.

Kintzel, Kay C., ed. ADVANCED CONCEPTS IN CLINICAL NURSING, 2nd ed. Philadelphia: J.B. Lippincott Co., 1977.

Luckmann, Joan, and Karen C. Sorenson. MEDICAL-SURGICAL NURSING: A PSYCHOPHYSIOLOGIC APPROACH. Philadelphia: W.B. Saunders Co., 1980.

McKinney, Brian. PATHOLOGY OF THE CARDIOMYOPATHIES. Woburn, Mass.: Butterworth Publishers, Inc., 1974.

Meltzer, Lawrence E., et al. CONCEPTS AND PRACTICES OF INTENSIVE CARE FOR NURSE SPECIALISTS. Bowie, Md.: Charles Press Publishers, 1969.

Meltzer, Lawrence E., et al. INTENSIVE CORONARY CARE, 3rd ed. Bowie, Md.: Charles Press Publishers, 1977.

Metheny, Norma M. NURSES' HANDBOOK OF FLUID BALANCE, 3rd ed. Philadelphia: J.B. Lippincott Co., 1979.

NURSE'S GUIDE TO DRUGS™. Nursing80 Books. Springhouse, Pa.: Springhouse Corporation, 1980.

NURSING DRUG HANDBOOK™. Nursing81 Books. Springhouse, Pa.: Springhouse Corporation, 1981.

PERFORMING GI PROCEDURES. Nursing Photobook™ Series. Springhouse, Pa.: Springhouse Corporation, 1981.

PROVIDING EARLY MOBILITY. Nursing Photobook™ Series. Springhouse, Pa.: Springhouse Corporation, 1981.

PROVIDING RESPIRATORY CARE. Nursing Photobook™ Series. Springhouse, Pa.: Springhouse Corporation, 1981.

Roberts, Sharon L. BEHAVIORAL CONCEPTS AND THE CRITICALLY ILL PATIENT. Englewood Cliffs, N.J.: Prentice-Hall, Inc., 1976.

Shafer, Kathleen N., et al. MEDICAL-SURGICAL NURSING. St. Louis: C.V. Mosby Co., 1975.

Stroot, Violet R., et al. FLUIDS AND ELECTROLYTES: A PRACTICAL APPROACH, 2nd ed. Philadelphia: F.A. Davis Co., 1977.

USING MONITORS. Nursing Photobook™ Series. Springhouse, Pa.: Springhouse Corporation, 1981.

Watson, Jeanette E. MEDICAL-SURGICAL NURSING AND RELATED PHYSIOLOGY. Philadelphia: W.B. Saunders Co., 1972.

Wenger, Nanette K., et al. CARDIOLOGY FOR NURSES. New York: McGraw-Hill Book Co., 1980.

Periodicals

Bailey, June T., et al. *The Stress Audit: Identifying the Stressors of ICU Nursing,* JOURNAL OF NURSING EDUCATION. 19:15-25, June 1980.

Bruce, Derek, et al. *Resuscitation from Coma Due to Head Injury,* CRITICAL CARE MEDICINE. 6:254-269, July-August 1978.

Colley, Rita, and Jeanne Wilson. *How to Begin Hyperalimentation Therapy: Meeting Patients' Nutritional Needs with Hyperalimentation,* NURSING79. 9:76-83, May 1979.

Colley, Rita, and Jeanne Wilson. *Managing the Patient on Hyperalimentation: Meeting Patients' Nutritional Needs with Hyperalimentation,* NURSING79. 9:57-61, June 1979.

Eyman, Linda N. *Pre-Operative Classes for the Gastric Bypass Patient,* PENNSYLVANIA SOCIETY OF GASTROINTES-TINAL ASSISTANTS NEWS UPDATE. pp. 16-18, August 1980.

Gehrke, Mary. *Identifying Brain Tumors,* JOURNAL OF NEUROSURGICAL NURSING. 12:90-92, June 1980.

Helton, Mary C., et al. *The Correlation Between Sleep Deprivation and the Intensive Care Unit Syndrome,* HEART AND LUNG. 9:464-468, May-June, 1980.

Jones, Cathy. *Monitoring Recovery After Head Injury: Translating Research into Practice,* JOURNAL OF NEUROSURGICAL NURSING. 11:192-198, December 1979.

Levy, Madelyn M., and Judith A. Stubbs. *Nursing Implications in the Care of Patients Treated with Assisted Mechanical Ventilation Modified with Positive End-Expiratory Pressure,* HEART AND LUNG. 7:299-305, March-April 1978.

Mylrea, Kenneth C. and L. Burke O'Neal. *Electricity and Electrical Safety in the Hospital,* NURSING76. 6:52-59, January 1976.

Noble, MaryAnne. *Communication in the ICU: Therapeutic or Disturbing?* NURSING OUTLOOK, 27:195-198, March 1979.

Regestein, Quentin R., and Jane E. Barbiasz. *Sleep Disorders: Recognizing Them in Patients,* JOURNAL OF PRACTICAL NURSING. 30:21-22, November-December 1980.

Seybert, Patricia L., et al. *The LeVeen Shunt: New Hope for Ascites Patients,* NURSING79. 9:24-31, January 1979.

Shubin, S. *Burnout: The Professional Hazard You Face in Nursing,* NURSING78. 8:22-27, July 1978.

Smith, Marcy J.T., and Hans Selye. *Reducing the Negative Effects of Stress,* AMERICAN JOURNAL OF NURSING. 79:1953-1955, November 1979.

Storlie, Frances J. *Burnout: The Elaboration of a Concept,* AMERICAN JOURNAL OF NURSING. 79:2108-2111, December 1979.

Twombley, Marilyn. *The Shift into Third Space,* NURSING76. 8:38-41, June 1978.

Wilson, Jeanne, and Rita Colley. *Administering Peripheral and Enteral Feedings: Meeting Patients' Nutritional Needs with Hyperalimentation,* NURSING79. 9:62-69, September 1979.

Index

A

Abdomen
  auscultation, 111
  inspection, 111
  percussion and palpation, 112-113
    liver assessment, 113
    spleen assessment, 113
    stomach assessment, 113
Acid-base compensation, evaluating, 27
Adapting patient's ICU environment, 11
Adventitious sounds, nurses' guide to, 24
Airways, artificial, nurses' guide to, 28-29
Alveolar-arterial oxygen gradient
    (A-aDO$_2$), 20
Anatomy and physiology
  cardiovascular, 60-61
  gastrointestinal, 108-110
  neurologic, 128-130
  respiratory, 18-19
Angina, assessing pain of, 66
Apnea, 21
Apneusis, 21
Arrhythmias, cardiac, nurses' guide to,
    80-83
Arterial blood gas measurements
  interpreting, 26
  nurses' guide to, 27
Arterial blood pressure
  measuring, 63
  variance among arteries, 84
  See also Hemodynamic monitoring.
Artificial airways, nurses' guide to, 28-29
Assessment
  cardiovascular, 62-63
  chest, 20-26
  gastrointestinal, 108, 111-113
  neurologic, 131-135
Asthma, signs and symptoms, 24, 26
Atelectasis, 23-25, 51
Atrial pressure. See Right atrial
    pressure.
Auscultation
  abdomen, 111
  chest areas, 23-26
  heart, cardiac auscultation areas, 63

B

Balancing and calibrating, pressure
    monitoring equipment, 88-89
Bard-Parker nasogastric tube, 114
Barrel chest, 22
Bennett ventilators
  MA-1 volume-cycled, 45
  PR-2 pressure-cycled, 45
Biot's pattern, 21
Bird Mark 7, pressure-cycled ventilator, 45
Bite block, using an endotracheal
    tube holder as, 36
Blanketrol hyper-hypothermia blanket
    system, how to use, 137-139
Blood gas measurements, arterial. See
    Arterial blood gas measurements.
Bournes Bear 1, volume-cycled ventilator, 45
Bowel
  sounds, assessing, 111
  symptoms, obtaining history of, 111

Bradypnea, 21
Breath sounds
  abnormal, 24
  adventitious, nurses' guide to, 24
  bronchial or tracheal, 23
  bronchovesicular, 23
  vesicular, 23
Bronchitis, 24, 26
Burnout, professional, 154-155

C

Calibrating pressure monitoring equip-
    ment. See Balancing and calibrating.
Cantor intestinal tube, 115
Cardiac
  conduction
    explained, 61
    measuring, 71
    See also Electrocardiogram, and
        Monitors, cardiac.
  cycle, explained, 61
  emergency drug guide, 104-105
  output, measuring, 97
Cardiopulmonary resuscitation during
    code, 101-102
Cardiovascular
  assessment, 62-63
  emergency
    calling a code, 101-103
    cardiopulmonary resuscitation
        during, 101-103
    crash cart contents, 100
    emergency drug guide, 104-105
    nursing role during, 100
    providing emotional support, 104
  history, obtaining a, 62
Central I.V. line, patient care, 125. See
    also Total parenteral nutrition.
Central venous pressure
  evaluating, 63
  setting up PA catheter to measure, 94-95
Chest
  assessment, 20-26
    adventitious sounds, nurses' guide to, 24
    auscultation, 23-26
    breath sounds, nurses' guide to, 23
    common lung conditions, signs and
        symptoms, 25-26
    inspection, 22
    palpation, 23-26
    percussion, 22, 24-26
  drainage system. See Thoracic
      drainage system.
  electrodes. See Electrodes, placement of.
  pain, assessing, 66
Cheyne-Stokes pattern, 21
Circulation
  interaction of respiratory and systemic, 19
  intrapulmonary, 18-19
Compensation, acid-base. See Acid-
    base compensation.
Compliance, 18, 45
Conduction, cardiac. See Cardiac conduction.
Congestive heart failure, without effu-
    sion, 24, 25
Consolidation, 23, 25
Continuous cardiac monitoring. See

Monitors, cardiac.
Continuous positive airway pressure (CPAP), 49
CPR. See Cardiopulmonary resuscitation.
Cranial nerves, 130
Crash cart, contents of, 100
Critikon Dinamap 845 monitor
  checking accuracy, 88
  using, 85-87
Cutter Dependaflo Volumetric Infusion
    Pump. See Infusion pump.

D

Damped waveform, troubleshooting guide, 98
Death, helping the family confront, 15
Decerebrate posturing, 135
Decorticate posturing, 135
Defibrillation, during code, 102
Dehydration, 146
Dinamap monitor. See Critikon Dinamap
    845 monitor.
Doll's eye reflex, 135
Drainage system, thoracic. See Thoracic
    drainage system.
Drugs, cardiac emergency, 104-105

E

Electrical hazards, guarding against, 151
Electrocardiogram (EKG)
  placing chest electrodes, 66-67
  running 12-lead EKG, 67-70
  waveforms
    interpreting, 71
    recognizing, 70
Electrodes, placement of
  EKG chest, 66-67
  five-electrode monitor, 74
  three-electrode monitor, 74
Emergency, cardiovascular. See Car-
    diovascular, emergency.
Emotional
  stress
    of nurse, 154-155
    of patient, 10
  support, how to provide, 10, 13-15, 104
Emphysema, 23-24, 26
Endotracheal tube, problems of, 41-42
Endotracheal tube holder, using as
    bite block, 36
Eupnea, 21
Expiratory reserve volume, 20

F

Finger clubbing, 22
Fluid and electrolyte imbalances
  coping with, 145
  determining fluid balance, 145
  monitoring for, 145
  nurses' guide to, 146-148
Functional residual capacity (FRC), 20
Funnel chest, 22

G

Gastric suction, 119, 122-123
Gastrointestinal (GI)

anatomy and physiology, 108-110
assessment, 111-113
    percussing and palpating abdo-
        men, 112-113
hemorrhage, patient care, 116-117
tubes, nurses' guide to, 114-115

H

Hardwire cardiac monitoring. *See*
    Monitors, cardiac.
Heart
    anatomy, 60
    rate and rhythm, assessing, 71
    sounds, nurses' guide to, 65
    See also Cardiovascular.
Hemodynamic monitoring
    invasive
        assembling equipment for, 89
        balancing and calibrating equipment, 88
        pros and cons, 88
        pulmonary artery (PA) catheter, 94-97
        setting up equipment for arterial line, 90-93
    noninvasive, 85-88
    troubleshooting
        damped waveform, 98
        other common problems, 99
Hemorrhage, GI. *See* Gastrointestinal
    (GI), hemorrhage.
History. *See* Patient, history, obtaining.
Hyperalimentation. *See* Total parenteral
    nutrition.
Hypercalcemia, 147
Hyper-hypothermia blanket system, 137-139
Hyperkalemia, 146
Hypermagnesemia, 148
Hypernatremia, 147
Hyperphosphatemia, 148
Hyperpnea, 21
Hypocalcemia, 147
Hypokalemia, 146
Hypomagnesemia, 148
Hyponatremia, 147
Hypophosphatemia, 148

I

Iced gastric lavage, 117, 122-123
ICU syndrome, coping with, 13
Immobility
    hazards of, nurses' guide to, 152-153
    understanding, 151-152
Infection
    common ICU, nurses' guide to, 149-150
    preventing, 149
Infusion pump, Cutter Dependaflo volumetric
    learning about, 142
    using, 143-144
Inspection and palpation
    interpreting findings, 64
    performing
        abdomen, 112-113
        chest, 22-23
Inspiratory reserve volume, 20
Inspiron venturi mask, 44
Intensive care
    environment, adapting patient's, 11
    nursing, special challenge of, 9

patient,
    adapting environment of, 11
    emotional stress of, 10
    ICU syndrome of, 13
    sensory imbalance of, 10
    sleep deprivation of, 12
    teaching about ICU, 9
Intermittent demand ventilation (IDV), 54
Intermittent mandatory ventilation (IMV), 54
Intestinal tubes, guide to, 115
Intracranial pressure (ICP), elevated,
    patient care, 136
Intrapulmonary circulation, 18-19

K

Kaslow radiopaque intestinal tube, 115
Kussmaul's, respiratory pattern, 21

L

Lazarus complex, 104
Liver, symptoms, documenting, 111
Lumbar puncture, nursing role in, 139
Lung
    anatomy and physiology, 18-19
    breath sounds, 23-24
    common conditions of, signs and
        symptoms, 25-26
    volumes, 20
    See also Respiratory.

M

MA-1 ventilator, positive end-expiratory
    pressure attachment, using, 47-48
Mallory-Weiss syndrome, 116-117
Miller-Abbott intestinal tube, 115
Minnesota four-lumen esophagogastric
    tamponade tube, 117, 121-123
    explained, 121
    insertion, assisting in, 122-123
Monilial infection, oral, treating, 36
Monitoring, hemodynamic. *See* Hemo-
    dynamic monitoring.
Monitors, cardiac
    comparing systems, 74-75
    initiating, 76-78
    troubleshooting, 79
    understanding, 72-73
    See also Electrocardiogram (EKG).
Moss decompression nasogastric
    tube, 115
Mouth care, 36
Myocardial infarction, assessing pain of, 66

N

Nasal endotracheal airway
    coping with problems of, 41
    guide to, 29
Nasogastric tube
    guide to, 114-115
    inserting, 118-120
    removing, 120
    securing with a tube holder, 120
Nasopharyngeal airway, guide to, 28
Negative inspiratory pressure, 20

Nerves, cranial. *See* Cranial nerves.
Neurocheck
    conducting, 131-134
    explained, 131
Neurowatch. *See* Neurocheck.

O

Ohio 560, volume-cycled ventilator, 45
Oral endotracheal airway
    coping with problems of, 41-42
    guide to, 29
    removing, 36-37
    repositioning, 35
    suctioning, 34
    taping, 34
Oral esophageal airway, guide to, 28
Organic brain syndrome, 13
Oropharyngeal airway
    guide to, 28
    inserting, 30
Overhydration, 146
Oxygen dissociation curve, 26

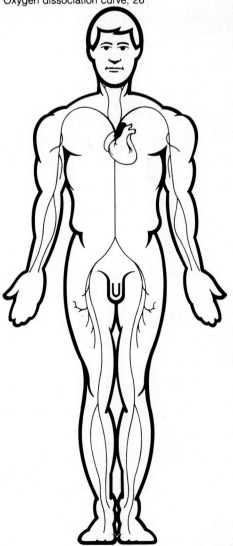

Index

P

Pain, chest. *See* Chest, pain.
Palpation, cardiovascular
  interpreting findings, 64
  palpating arteries, 63
Patient
  family of, helping them cope, 14, 15, 104
  history, obtaining
    cardiovascular, 62
    gastrointestinal, 111
    respiratory, 21
  intensive care, problems of, 9-13
    See also Intensive care, patient.
PEEP. *See* Positive end-expiratory pressure.
Percussing and palpating
  abdomen, 112-113
  chest, 22-23
  heart, percussing, 63
  sounds, percussion, 22
Physiology. *See* Anatomy and physiology.
Pigeon chest, 22
Pleural
  effusion, 25
  friction rub, 24
Pneumothorax, 25, 51
Positive end-expiratory pressure (PEEP)
  indications/contraindications of, 46
  patient care during therapy, 49
  understanding, 46
  using MA-1 ventilator PEEP attach-
    ment, 47-48
  weaning from, 53
Posturing
  decerebrate, 135
  decorticate, 135
Pressure-cycled ventilator. *See* Ventila-
    tors. *See also specific model.*
Pressure monitoring equipment. *See*
    Balancing and calibrating, *and*
    Hemodynamic monitoring.
Pulmonary
  function tests, 52
  resistance, 18
  See also Respiratory.
Pulmonary artery (PA)
  catheter
    explained, 94
    measuring cardiac output, 97
    measuring PA wedge pressure, 96-97

    setting up equipment for, 94-95
    troubleshooting, 98-99
  pressure (PAP)
    setting up equipment to measure, 94-95
    waveform of, 97
  wedge pressure (PAWP), measuring, 96-97
Pulmonary capillary wedge pressure
  (PCWP). *See* Pulmonary artery
    wedge pressure.
Pulse
  amplitude, assessing, 63
  arterial, interpreting, 64
Pump, infusion. *See* Infusion pump,
    Cutter Dependaflo volumetric.

R

Rales, coarse, fine, medium, 24
Residual volume, 20
Respirators. *See* Ventilators.
Respiratory
  anatomy and physiology, 18-19
  gas exchange, 19
  history, obtaining, 21
  patterns, nurses' guide to, 20
  terms, defined, 20
Resting minute ventilation, 20
Rhonchi, sibilant, sonorous, 24
Right atrial pressure, setting up equip-
    ment to measure, 94-95

S

Salem sump tube, Argyle, 114.
Seizure precautions, 135
Sengstaken-Blakemore tube, 121, 122
Spinal tap. *See* Lumbar puncture.
Stress, professional, 154-155
Suctioning, mouth and trachea, 31-33
Swan-Ganz® catheter. *See* Pulmonary
    artery (PA) catheter.

T

Tachypnea, 21
Tactile fremitus, 23
Thermal blanket. *See* Hyper-hypo-
    thermia blanket system.
Thoracic drainage system
  explained, 54
  using, 55-57
Tidal volume, 20
Total lung capacity, 20
Total parenteral nutrition (TPN)
  explained, 124
  indications/contraindications, 124
  patient care, central I.V. line, 125

Tracheostomy
  guide to, 29
  patient care
    daily, 38-39
    for ventilator-dependent patient, 40
  trach tube
    emergency reinsertion of, 40
    problems of, 41-42
    weaning patient with, 53-54
Trach tube. *See* Tracheostomy.

U

Urine sugar, testing for, 125

V

Varices, esophageal and gastric, 117, 121-123
Ventilators
  complications, coping with, 51
  MA-I ventilator PEEP attachment,
    using, 47-48
  pressure- and volume-cycled, compared, 45
  warning signals, responding, 50
  weaning patient from, 52-54
  See also specific model.
Venturi
  device, 43
  effect, 43
  mask
    explained, 43
    using an Inspiron, 44
Vital capacity, 20
Volume-cycled ventilators. *See* Ventila-
    tors. *See also specific model.*

W

Weaning
  conventional weaning, 54
  determining proper time, 52
  from positive end-expiratory pressure, 53
  from ventilator, 52
  intermittent demand ventilation, 54
  intermittent mandatory ventilation, 54

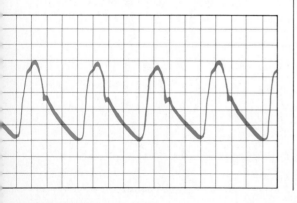